Injectable Fillers in Aesthetic Medicine

Mauricio de Maio • Berthold Rzany

Injectable Fillers in Aesthetic Medicine

Second Edition

Springer

Mauricio de Maio
Clínica Médica Dr Mauricio de Maio
São Paulo
São Paulo
Brazil

Berthold Rzany
RZANY & HUND
Privatpraxis für Dermatologie und
Ästhetische Medizin
Kurfüstendamm
Berlin
Germany

ISBN 978-3-662-49998-6 ISBN 978-3-642-45125-6 (eBook)
DOI 10.1007/978-3-642-45125-6
Springer Heidelberg New York Dordrecht London

Softcover reprint of the hardcover 2nd edition 2014

Printed on acid-free paper

Springer is part of Springer Science+Business Media (www.springer.com)

Foreword II

During my residency in plastic surgery at The John Hopkins Hospital in the mid-1970s, I visited the Stanford University plastic surgery program, where I saw residents, faculty and researchers literally "squeezing" collagen out of cow hides in an attempt to create an injectable material to fill out soft tissue depressions. Fascinated by this concept, I joined the original plastic surgical advisory board of the Collagen Corporation in the early 1980s. The original commercial collagen product was viewed more as a "wrinkle filler", and to a great degree was embraced in the market place more by dermatologists to treat wrinkles non-operatively, than by scalpel-wielding plastic surgeons. While the field of aesthetic dermatology evolved in part triggered by this original collagen product (enhanced of course by lasers, neurolytics, and other topical advances), plastic surgeons, for the most part, stuck with surgery.

Mauricio de Maio was the first plastic surgeon to appreciate the full aesthetic potential of the use of fillers in total facial rejuvenation, not simply in the treatment of wrinkles. I first met Mauricio 15 years ago, when he was a young.

Brazilian plastic surgeon using hyaluronic fillers. I was immediately taken by his artistic brilliance in the assessment of facial anatomy and proportion and his revolutionary approach in correcting disproportion, asymmetry and aging via injectable fillers, rather than surgery. I have watched his career evolve from a little-known Brazilian artistic pioneer, to an internationally, experienced master injector and physician. His techniques, his selection of ever evolving products and his own self-critique and constant striving for safety and improved outcomes have placed him at the highest level amongst his world-peers in aesthetic plastic surgery and dermatology.

The importance of this book is the combined input of facial aesthetic medical pioneer and aesthetic dermatology master, Berthold Rzany, along with that of Mauricio de Maio. For as the world of "fillers" has evolved from the original bovine collagen product to various hyaluronic acids and beyond, and the location of their placement and volume goes deeper than the skin. The combined expertise of aesthetic dermatology and aesthetic surgery now work hand in hand to evaluate patients, consider various treatment options, promote patient safety, and improve predictable aesthetic outcomes.

This book is a "must-read" manual, reference and desk-top text for all practitioners working with "fillers" in the "aesthetic medical space".

I congratulate the authors as well as thank them for creating and updating this much needed body of work.

G. Patrick Maxwell, MD, FACS
Maxwells Aesthetics, Plastic and
Reconstructive Surgery,
South Nashville,
TN, USA

Foreword I

It has been 5 years since the publication of the 1st edition of Drs. De Maio and Rzany's book *Injectable Fillers in Aesthetic Medicine*. During this time a revolution has occurred in our understanding of facial anatomy and its relationship to the aging process as well as the development of new and improved products. We no longer "cookbook" the nasolabial fold or lips in all patients alike, but have evolved our understanding of the development of folds, creases and atrophy related to the aging process. It is the incorporation of these new principles to the practice of aesthetic medicine that makes this new 2nd edition a hallmark in our understanding of injectable correction and an invaluable guide to personalizing the practice in practical terms. Of extreme importance are the chapters that set the stage for injecting, injectable products and their applications, patient evaluation and selection of treatment and development of a treatment plan. Rather than simply separating injection areas, as has previously been done, this guide gives the clinician a broader view of facial aging, then interprets the areas together for a more complete program to reverse facial aging. The attention to "blind spots" for patients and physicians instruct as how to evaluate patient needs in a fresh new manner. This gives the physician a plan to treat the aging face and satisfy the patient. The emphasis on "Do's", "Don'ts", 'Key points" and "FAQ's" summarize the essentials of each chapter in a readable, yet complete guide to injectable facial treatment.

This is the first practical compendium for a new era of injectable filler treatment of the aging face. In this case, the 2nd edition is not just an update, but a new approach to facial treatment. It is the closest experience to a tutorial lesson with two masters of aesthetic facial injection treatment.

Gary D. Monheit, MD
Departments of Dermatology and Ophthalmology
Total Skin & Beauty Dermatology Center, P.C.,
University of Alabama at Birmingham
Birmingham, AL, USA

Preface

The book on injectable fillers was our first book and was like our book on botulinum toxin A very successful. Why did we decide on an update? Of course the 1st edition still stands its ground in many aspects. However, during the last years we have seen many changes in the filler market. Fillers have been withdrawn from the market (some for very good reasons!), and new fillers did appear. Furthermore, we have improved, too. We increased the number of indications we can offer, and we advanced our injection techniques. Furthermore, we made a great step forward in how we analyze our patients and how we set up the most optimal treatment strategy – the treatment plan – that includes the doctors' *and* the patients' perspectives.

The tasks of this book though remain unchanged: first, to give an overview on the most common biodegradable and nonbiodegradable fillers and how to approach them and, second, to lead through the most common indications of the face and other body areas. This book kept the hands-on approach from the 1st edition. However, we included new features. From our last common book on Male Aesthetics, we included the "Do's", "Don'ts", and the "Key Points" to highlight the most important points. Last but not least, we tried to be as specific as possible. However, in case we missed something or something appears to be unclear or even wrong, please do not hesitate to contact us by mail, and we will both try to answer your questions as clearly and quickly as possible.

Berlin, Germany
São Paulo, Brazil

Berthold Rzany
Mauricio de Maio

About the Authors

Berthold Rzany

Berthold Rzany is a dermatologist and clinical epidemiologist in private practice (RZANY & HUND) in Berlin, Germany. Between 2002 and 2011 he held the position of C3-Professor of Evidence Based Medicine in Dermatology at the Department of Dermatology and Venereology at the Charité Universitätsmedizin. He studied medicine in Freiburg, Germany; Vienna, Austria; and Harvard Medical School, Boston, USA. He received his dermatological education at the Department of Dermatology at the University of Freiburg, Germany, and worked as a consultant in dermatology in Mannheim, Fakultät für Klinische Medizin, University of Heidelberg. He has a special interest in aesthetic medicine and tries to incorporate evidence-based medicine in aesthetic medicine. He is the author of several leading publications in the field of Aesthetic Medicine. He likes teaching and frequently gives hands-on workshops on botulinum toxin A and injectable fillers. He is also a consultant for various companies for these substances.

Conflict of interest Berthold Rzany is a speaker and/or advisor for the following filler companies (2013): Merz Pharmaceuticals, Q-Med Galderma, Teoxane Laboratories and Sinclair Pharmaceuticals.

Mauricio de Maio

Dr. de Maio is a board certified plastic surgeon from the Brazilian Society of Plastic Surgery and member of the International Society of Aesthetic Plastic Surgery. Dr. de Maio graduated in Medicine in the Medical School of the University of Sao Paulo in 1990. He specialized in plastic surgery in Brazil in 1996. He obtained his Master's Degree in Medicine in 1997 and Doctorate in Sciences in 2006 at the University of Sao Paulo, Brazil. He was a clinical assistant professor of the Plastic Surgery Department of the University of Sao Paulo from 1996 to 2002. Dr. de Maio has authored scientific publications and articles as well as published several books including the following books he coauthored with B. Rzany: *Fillers in Aesthetic Medicine*, 2006; *Botulinum Toxin in Aesthetic Medicine*, 2007; and *The Male Patient in Aesthetic Medicine*,

2009, by Springer-Verlag – Germany. He is actively involved in research and teaching in international training courses in America, Europe, and Asia-Pacific as well in consulting companies.

Conflict of interest Mauricio de Maio is a speaker and advisor for the following filler company (2013): Pharm-Allergan.

Acknowledgments

The 2nd edition of this book would not have been possible without the help of many others. First, we would like to thank our patients and colleagues with whom during the last years we advanced together discovering new indications and techniques. We would like to thank those who helped us with their skills and support during the completion of this book. Furthermore, we would like to take this opportunity to thank Mrs. Ellen Blasig from Springer Heidelberg for her guidance and her continuous support, which enabled us to keep the project going.

From the German team, we are grateful to Julian Wiora and Twyla Michnevich for proofreading the text. From the Brazilian team, we would like to thank the staff, who are always prompt in providing support with new tasks: Mrs. Liliann Amoroso Ribeiro and Lilian de Toledo Lima.

Abbreviations

BoNT-A	Botulinum toxin A
CE	Conformité Européenne
CaHa	Calcium hydroxylapatite
CIA	Cosmetic investment advisor
FDA	Food and Drug Administration
HA	Hyaluronic acid
HEMA	Hydroxyethylmethacrylate
HIV	Human immunodeficiency virus
KTP laser	Kaliumtitanphosphat (potassium titanyl phosphate) laser
PLLA	Poly-l-lactic acid
PMMA	Polymethylmethacrylate
SMAS	Submuscular aponeurotic system
SOOF	Suborbicularis oculi fat

Contents

1 Overview on Injectable Fillers: Efficacy and Safety 1
1.1 Introduction 1
1.2 Classification of Fillers 1
1.2.1 Classification by Biodegradability 2
1.2.2 Classification by the Quality of Clinical Data 2
1.3 Biodegradable Fillers 2
1.3.1 Collagen 2
1.3.2 Hyaluronic Acid 5
1.3.3 Combination of Hyaluronic Acid with Other Substances 7
1.3.4 Alginates 8
1.3.5 Poly-l-lactic Acid 8
1.3.6 Calcium Hydroxylapatite 10
1.4 Nonbiodegradable Fillers 11
1.4.1 Silicone 11
1.4.2 Polyacrylamide 12
1.4.3 Polyalkylimide 13
1.5 Combination of Nonbiodegradable and Biodegradable Fillers 13
1.5.1 Polymethylmethacrylate and Collagen 14
1.5.2 Hydroxyethylmethacrylate and Hyaluronic Acid 15
1.6 Combining Different Fillers in One Area 15
1.7 General Approach to New Fillers 15
References 16

2 Selection of Patients 21
2.1 Introduction 21
2.2 General Rules 22
2.3 The First Consultation 24
2.4 The Facial Thirds System 25
2.5 The Ideal Patient 25
2.6 The Aging Patient 25
2.7 The Patient with Facial Imperfections 26
2.8 The Patient You Do Not Want to Treat 27
2.9 The Dysmorphic Patient 28
References 28

3 Requirements and Rules . . . 31
3.1 General Requirements . . . 31
3.1.1 Introduction . . . 31
3.1.2 Documentation . . . 31
3.1.3 Charts . . . 31
3.1.4 Photographs . . . 32
3.1.5 Consent . . . 33
3.1.6 Treatment Plan . . . 33
3.1.7 Staff . . . 33
3.2 Technical Requirements . . . 34
3.2.1 Room . . . 34
3.2.2 Chair . . . 34
3.2.3 Mirror . . . 34
3.2.4 Small Things . . . 34
3.2.5 First Aid Kit . . . 34
3.2.6 Tips, Tricks and Key Points . . . 35
3.3 The 13 General Rules . . . 35
3.3.1 Introduction . . . 35
3.3.2 Rule 1: Listen to the Patient . . . 35
3.3.3 Rule 2: Fillers Are Only One Tool . . . 35
3.3.4 Rule 3: Talk About Money . . . 36
3.3.5 Rule 4: Talk About Possible Adverse Events . . . 36
3.3.6 Rule 5: Avoid Disturbed Patients . . . 36
3.3.7 Rule 6: Anesthesia (Treat with as Little Pain as Possible!) . . . 37
3.3.8 Rule 7: Position (Keep the Patient Upright) . . . 37
3.3.9 Rule 8: Use the Mirror/Digital Images . . . 37
3.3.10 Rule 9: Start with a Biodegradable Filler First . . . 38
3.3.11 Rule 10: Quantity of Filler (Do Not Inject Insufficient Amounts) . . . 38
3.3.12 Rule 11: Quantity of Filler (Do Not Inject Too Much) . . . 38
3.3.13 Rule 12: Use the Appropriate Depth of Injection . . 38
3.3.14 Rule 13: If Something Goes Wrong . . . 39
References . . . 39

4 Treatment Planning . . . 41
4.1 Introduction . . . 41
4.1.1 Product-Related Barrier . . . 42
4.1.2 Patient-Related Barrier . . . 43
4.1.3 Injector-Related Barrier . . . 45
4.1.4 Assessment . . . 46
4.1.5 The MdM 8-Point Lift . . . 52
4.2 Treatment Plan and Exponential Aging . . . 56
4.3 Cosmetic Investment Advisor . . . 58
References . . . 59

5 Anesthesia and Analgesia . . . 61
5.1 Introduction . . . 61
5.2 Evaluation Prior to Injection . . . 62

5.3 Local Anesthesia 62
5.4 Topical Anesthesia 62
5.5 Infiltrative Anesthesia 63
5.6 Nerve Block 63
5.6.1 The Supraorbital Nerve 64
5.6.2 The Supratrochlear Nerve 64
5.6.3 The Infraorbital Nerve 64
5.6.4 The Mental Nerve 65
5.6.5 The Zygomaticofacial Nerve 66
5.7 Adverse Events 67
5.8 Disadvantages of Local Anesthetics 67
5.9 Tips, Tricks and Key Points 68
References 68

6 The Most Common Indications 69
6.1 Forehead and Glabella 70
6.1.1 Introduction 70
6.1.2 Anatomy 70
6.1.3 Patient Evaluation and Selection 71
6.1.4 Techniques 71
6.1.5 Tips, Tricks and Key Points 74
6.2 Temples 74
6.2.1 Introduction 74
6.2.2 Anatomy 74
6.2.3 Patient Evaluation and Selection 74
6.2.4 Technique 75
6.2.5 Complications 75
6.2.6 Tips, Tricks and Key Points 75
6.3 Eyebrow 76
6.3.1 Introduction 76
6.3.2 Anatomy 76
6.3.3 Patient Evaluation and Selection 77
6.3.4 Technique 78
6.3.5 Complications 79
6.3.6 Tips, Tricks and Key Points 79
6.4 Epicanthal Fold and Sunken Upper Eyelid 80
6.4.1 Epicanthal Fold 80
6.4.2 Sunken Upper Eyelid 80
6.4.3 Tips, Tricks and Key Points 81
6.5 Infraorbital Hollow, Tear Trough, Cheekbones, and Cheek Reshaping 83
6.5.1 Introduction 83
6.5.2 Anatomy 84
6.5.3 Patient Evaluation and Selection 85
6.5.4 Tear Trough and Infraorbital Area 85
6.5.5 Cheekbones 89
6.5.6 Cheek 92
6.5.7 Complications 96
6.5.8 Tips, Tricks and Key Points 96

6.6 Nose Reshaping 97
6.6.1 Introduction 97
6.6.2 Anatomy 98
6.6.3 Patient Evaluation and Selection 100
6.6.4 Technique. 101
6.6.5 The Nasofrontal Angle 102
6.6.6 The Nasolabial Angle 102
6.6.7 The Tip and the Columella 102
6.6.8 Dorsum 103
6.6.9 Selection of Filler 105
6.6.10 Complications 105
6.6.11 Tips, Tricks and Key Points. 106
6.7 Nasolabial Folds 106
6.7.1 Introduction 106
6.7.2 Anatomy/Structure. 106
6.7.3 Patient Evaluation and Selection 108
6.7.4 Technique. 108
6.7.5 Touch-Up 109
6.7.6 Complications 110
6.7.7 Tips, Tricks and Key Points. 111
6.8 The Earlobe 112
6.8.1 Introduction 112
6.8.2 Anatomy/Structure. 112
6.8.3 Patient Evaluation and Selection 112
6.8.4 Technique. 113
6.8.5 Tips, Tricks and Key Points. 114
6.9 The Upper and Lower Lips 114
6.9.1 Introduction 114
6.9.2 Anatomy 114
6.9.3 Patient Evaluation and Selection 116
6.9.4 Technique. 117
6.9.5 Complications 120
6.9.6 Tips, Tricks and Key Points. 120
6.10 Marionette Lines 123
6.10.1 Introduction 123
6.10.2 Anatomy 123
6.10.3 Patient Evaluation and Selection 123
6.10.4 Technique. 123
6.10.5 Complications 123
6.10.6 Tips, Tricks and Key Points. 124
6.11 Jawline and Chin Reshaping 125
6.11.1 Introduction 125
6.11.2 Anatomy 125
6.11.3 Patient Evaluation and Selection 126
6.11.4 Technique. 127
6.11.5 Complications 128
6.11.6 Tips, Tricks and Key Points. 129

6.12 Other Facial Indications for Volumizers 131
6.12.1 Introduction 131
6.12.2 Facial Advancement. 131
6.12.3 Tips, Tricks and Key Points. 132
References. 132

7 Nonfacial Indications 135
7.1 Inverted Nipple 135
7.1.1 Introduction 135
7.1.2 Anatomy 135
7.1.3 Patient Evaluation and Selection 135
7.1.4 Techniques 136
7.1.5 Tips, Tricks and Key Points. 136
7.2 Hand Volume Replacement 137
7.2.1 Introduction 137
7.2.2 Anatomy 138
7.2.3 Patient Evaluation and Selection 139
7.2.4 Material to Be Used. 139
7.2.5 Anesthesia 139
7.2.6 Techniques 139
7.2.7 Potential Specific Adverse Events 141
7.2.8 Tips, Tricks and Key Points. 142
7.3 Penile Augmentation 143
7.3.1 Introduction 143
7.3.2 Anatomy 143
7.3.3 Patient Evaluation and Selection 143
7.3.4 Material to Be Used. 143
7.3.5 Procedure Prior to Injection. 145
7.3.6 Techniques 145
7.3.7 Tips, Tricks and Key Points. 147
References. 147

8 Safety: Assessment and Treatment of Adverse Reactions. . . . 149
8.1 Introduction 149
8.2 Epidemiology. 150
8.3 Identification of the Responsible Filler 150
8.4 Potential Risk Factors 150
8.4.1 The Doctor as a Risk Factor 151
8.4.2 The Product as a Risk Factor 151
8.4.3 The Patient as a Risk Factor 151
8.4.4 The Biofilm Theory 152
8.5 Treatment of Adverse Reactions 152
8.5.1 Bluish Discoloration 152
8.5.2 Hypersensitivity Reaction 153
8.5.3 Acute Vascular Reaction 153
8.5.4 Nodule Formation 154
8.5.5 Abscess Formation. 156
8.6 Guiding the Patient 157
References. 157

9 Combination Therapy 159
9.1 Introduction 159
9.2 Lasers and Fillers.................................. 159
9.3 Chemical Peels and Fillers.................................. 161
9.4 Botulinum Toxin and Fillers 162
9.5 Facial Plastic Surgery and Fillers 166
9.6 Topical Drugs in Combination with Fillers.................................. 167
9.7 Eye Rejuvenation as an Example for Combination Therapy 167
9.7.1 Step 1: Improvement of Eyelashes 167
9.7.2 Step 2: Restoration of Volume Loss 167
9.7.3 Step 3: Decreasing Muscular Activity by BoNT-A.... 169
9.7.4 Step 4: Develop a Plan for Maintenance Therapy .. 170
References.................................. 171

Index 173

Overview on Injectable Fillers: Efficacy and Safety

1

Berthold Rzany

Contents

1.1 **Introduction** ... 1

1.2 **Classification of Fillers** ... 1
1.2.1 Classification by Biodegradability ... 2
1.2.2 Classification by the Quality of Clinical Data ... 2

1.3 **Biodegradable Fillers** ... 2
1.3.1 Collagen ... 2
1.3.2 Hyaluronic Acid ... 5
1.3.3 Combination of Hyaluronic Acid with Other Substances ... 7
1.3.4 Alginates ... 8
1.3.5 Poly-l-lactic Acid ... 8
1.3.6 Calcium Hydroxylapatite ... 10

1.4 **Nonbiodegradable Fillers** ... 11
1.4.1 Silicone ... 11
1.4.2 Polyacrylamide ... 12
1.4.3 Polyalkylimide ... 13

1.5 **Combination of Nonbiodegradable and Biodegradable Fillers** ... 13
1.5.1 Polymethylmethacrylate and Collagen ... 14
1.5.2 Hydroxyethylmethacrylate and Hyaluronic Acid ... 15

1.6 **Combining Different Fillers in One Area** ... 15

1.7 **General Approach to New Fillers** ... 15

References ... 16

1.1 Introduction

In contrast to the USA, in most countries in Europe and South America, a great variety of injectable fillers are available. Therefore, not only for novices but also for experienced users it can sometimes be quite difficult to decide which filler to use. This chapter will give a brief overview on some of the most commonly used *present* and *past* injectable fillers. The selection of products reflects the interest of the authors and might appear arbitrary to someone familiar with other fillers.

FAQs

- Why should one show interest with fillers which are not on the market anymore?

  Even when fillers are not present on the market anymore, they may be important for two reasons: (1) they may be marketed again, and (2) permanent fillers will be always present as they will stay with the patient until the end.

1.2 Classification of Fillers

Basically there is no uniformly accepted classification of fillers. Injectable fillers may be grouped according to (1) the degree of degradability and (2) the quality of the clinical data behind them.

M. de Maio, B. Rzany, *Injectable Fillers in Aesthetic Medicine*,
DOI 10.1007/978-3-642-45125-6_1, © Springer-Verlag Berlin Heidelberg 2014

1.2.1 Classification by Biodegradability

Fillers can be grouped as biodegradable and non-biodegradable (permanent) products. There are also fillers where biodegradable as well as non-biodegradable materials are combined.

1.2.2 Classification by the Quality of Clinical Data

As the rules for marketing of fillers are quite relaxed in Europe, e.g., a clinical trial is not required, fillers can be grouped in those with and without clinical data. Those with clinical data can be grouped in those with good and less good clinical data.

What means good clinical data? Basically a randomized controlled clinical trial with a sufficient number of patients included (e.g., for a two-arm trial you want at least 50 patients). Based on such a trial simple but important questions as grade of correction that can be achieved, durability of the correction (e.g., efficacy), impact on quality of life, and safety (proportion of patients with swelling, etc.) can be answered.

1.3 Biodegradable Fillers

Biodegradable fillers are defined as having a limited life span usually ranging from a couple to several months, or even to a couple of years. They consist of purified dermal components from human, animal, or bacterial sources and can be divided into the following categories: xenografts (donor and recipient are from different species), autografts (donor and recipient are from the same individual), homografts (donor and recipient are from the same species), and synthetic materials (Table 1.1). Please note that in the last couple of years some of the most well-known biodegradable fillers were removed from the market.

1.3.1 Collagen

Collagens from various sources and with specific characteristics exist or better used to exist as most of the fillers discussed are not on the market anymore.

1.3.1.1 Collagen of Bovine Origin

Prior to the introduction of the hyaluronic acids, collagen was the most widely used filler and was

Table 1.1 Overview on biodegradable fillers

Material	Origin	Products[a]
Temporary injectable fillers		
Alginate	Nonanimal, algae	Novabel[b]
Collagen	Bovine	Zyderm[b], Zyplast[b]
	Porcine	Evolence[b]
	Human (cadaver derived)	Cymetra[b]
	Human (self-derived)	Isolagen[b]
	Human (cultivated)	Cosmoderm[b], Cosmoplast[b]
Hyaluronic acid	Avian	Hylaform[b]
	Nonanimal	Belotero[c], Emervel[c], Juvéderm[c], Restylane[c], Teosyal[c], Juvéderm Voluma[c]
Hyaluronic acid + dextran	Nonanimal	Reviderm
Poly-l-lactic acid (PLLA)	Nonanimal	Sculptra (former New Fill)
Calcium hydroxylapatite	Nonanimal	Radiesse

[a]Please note that this list is not intended to be complete
[b]Were removed or will be removed from the market
[c]HA product families with at least one product with good clinical trial data (RCTs), e.g. for the Emervel family we have good RCTs on E. deep and E. classic

considered the gold standard with which other dermal fillers were compared. However, the role of bovine collagen is declining. In the USA and in Europe, they are not available on the markets anymore. Nevertheless, bovine collagen still might be available in other parts of the world, and therefore we will give a brief overview on that substance. The classical bovine enzyme-digested collagen (95 % type I, 5 % type III) was available in several preparations, which were distinguished by the collagen content and the addition of glutaraldehyde for stabilization (Homicz and Watson 2004).

Depending on the collagen content and the degree of cross-linking, different products were designed for different levels of the dermis. For example, Zyderm 1 and Zyderm 2, which were built on noncross-linked collagen, were supposed to be injected into the superficial dermis. Zyplast, a cross-linked form, was supposed to be injected more deeply into the dermis. All of these products were easy to inject. In contrast to other products, overcorrection was recommended for Zyderm 1 and Zyderm 2.

Zyderm was cleared for marketing in 1981 by the Food and Drug Administration (FDA) after reviewing clinical data based on a large case series of 9,427 tested and 5,109 treated patients (Cooperman et al. 1985; Matti and Nicolle 1990). In addition to this case series, which focused mainly on safety issues, a further clinical trial showed that it was effective for at least several months (Cooperman et al. 1985; Matti and Nicolle 1990).

As collagen may elicit quite often hypersensitivity reactions, pretesting was mandatory. Pretesting consisted of an intradermal injection of Zyderm 1 collagen into the volar aspect of the forearm. A minimum of one skin test which was valuated after 28 days was required. The incidence of adverse reactions to collagen pretesting (here Zyderm I) was approximately 3 %. Of all test site reactions, 50 % occurred within the first 24 h. An additional 1.3 % of patients experienced adverse reactions despite a negative pretest. The observed reactions ranged from localized swelling to induration, erythema, and pruritus (Cooperman et al. 1985).

Key Points

- So far, bovine collagens are not available anymore in Europe and the USA. There might be two reasons for that: (1) the need of prior skin testing and (2) the decreased durability compared to the hyaluronic acid preparations.
- As bovine collagen was the comparator in the initial non-collagen filler trials, the evidence behind this group of products is good.

1.3.1.2 Collagen of Porcine Origin

Before Evolence there were only a very few reports on porcine collagen-based fillers in the literature (Saray 2003). Evolence, a novel porcine collagen filler, was introduced into the European market in 2004 and withdrawn from the markets in 2009. In contrast to other collagens, this product was cross-linked by glycation using D-ribose as the cross-linking agent. Unlike bovine collagen, no skin testing was necessary.

This porcine collagen was available in two preparations: Evolence and Evolence Breeze. Evolence Breeze was indicated for more superficial dermal injections and lip augmentation.

Being a new filler, efficacy was supported by a couple of good clinical trials (Monstrey et al. 2007; Narins et al. 2007, 2008). Furthermore, some smaller case series were reported focusing on specific areas as nonsurgical rhinoplasty (Cassuto 2009), tear trough correction (Goldberg 2009), cheek augmentation (Sadick and Palmisano 2009), and lip augmentation (de Boulle et al. 2009; Landau 2009).

The risk of hypersensitivity reactions for porcine collagen was much lower compared to bovine collagen. In an intradermal skin test study, no hypersensitivity reactions could be detected in a total of 519 subjects (Shoshani et al. 2007). Therefore, no skin testing was recommended. There are, however, a few reports on foreign body reactions inducing an abscess-like reaction (Braun and Braun 2008). As several thousands of patients had been treated before the withdrawal, this risk seemed to be comparable to other biodegradable fillers.

Porcine collagen was not as easy to inject compared to bovine collagen. By mixing lidocaine (0.2 ml) to the syringe, the injectability as well as the injection comfort (less pain!) could be increased. As for Like bovine collagen, the filler had a yellowish color which could be visible beneath the mucosal surfaces when the filler was injected too superficially. For this filler, a guideline is available (Rzany et al. 2010).

Key Points

- Evolence was a filler which was supported by good clinical data.
- With the withdrawal of the Evolence products, no porcine filler is at the moment available in Europe and the USA.
- Nevertheless, it cannot be ruled out that this or a comparable product will be reintroduced to the market again.

1.3.1.3 Collagen of Human Origin

Collagen of human origin can be of allogenous or autologous nature.

1.3.1.3.1 Collagen of Allogenous Nature (From Cadaver)

In addition to bovine or porcine sources, collagen can be derived from human cadavers. Data is available for two products: Dermalogen and Cymetra. Both products derive from pooled human cadaverous tissue from accredited tissue banks. Overcorrection is recommended by the manufacturer. Here again the available data on the efficacy and safety of the product are limited. Cymetra was tested against Zyplast in a small randomized controlled trial. A total of 47 patients were treated: 20 received Cymetra and 27 received Zyplast. Various photometric outcome measures were used in this study, which favored the new product over Zyplast (Sclafani et al. 2002a, b).

1.3.1.3.2 Collagen of Allogenous Nature (From Culture)

Later-generation noncadaverous collagen products are Cosmoderm and Cosmoplast (Baumann 2004). They were made from natural human collagen grown under controlled laboratory conditions. There was no need for a pretreatment skin test for these sterile devices, which were composed of highly purified human-based collagen that is dispersed in phosphate-buffered physiological saline containing 0.3 % lidocaine. Cosmoderm was a noncross-linked formulation that was used in the treatment of superficial lines, whereas Cosmoplast was cross-linked and was used primarily in the treatment of more pronounced wrinkles. A few clinical trials are available using Cosmoderm as a comparator. Based on these trials, the durability seems to be less as for other products (Man et al. 2008; Smith et al. 2007).

1.3.1.3.3 Collagen of Autologous Nature

The commercial preparation Autologon consists of dermal extracellular matrix, primarily collagen (types I, III, and VI), that has been harvested from the patient's own skin. It requires the excision of the patient's skin and is therefore mostly suitable for those undergoing surgical procedures. Here again, overcorrection is recommended by the manufacturer. The available data on the efficacy and safety of the product are limited (Sclafani et al. 2000).

Concerning the safety as said before, the number of studies for the above products is limited. Pretesting might reveal adverse self-limited local reactions (Moody and Sengelmann 2000). Adverse reactions after pretesting appeared only as mild, nontender erythema. Acute or severe reactions like allergic ulcerations or chronical granulomatous reactions were not reported in a nonsystematic review (Fagien 2000). Case reports describe acute choroidal infarction following the subcutaneous injection of allogenous collagen in the forehead region (Apte et al. 2003).

Key Points

- This overview is merely for academic reasons. The products to our knowledge are either not widely used or not available anymore.
- The quality of clinical data behind these products varied.

1.3.2 Hyaluronic Acid

After the bovine collagens, the emergence of different hyaluronic acid preparations revolutionized the injectable filler market for three main reasons: (1) no need for skin test, (2) better durability compared to the other available biodegradable fillers, and (3) the availability of antidote (hyaluronidase).

Hyaluronic acid, which belongs to the family of glycosaminoglycans, consists of repeated disaccharide units. The hydrophilic properties of hyaluronic acid attract water into the extracellular matrix and therefore increase the skin turgor. Hyaluronic acid is gradually degraded. In order to increase the durability of the various hyaluronic acid preparations, stabilization is usually obtained by cross-linking mostly with 1.4-butanediol diglycidyl ether (BDDE).

Hyaluronic acids can be derived from avian or bacterial sources; each product has its own, specific characteristics.

Key Points

- HA can be derived from different sources. Most HAs derive from bacterial origin.

1.3.2.1 Hyaluronic Acid of Avian Origin

Cross-linked hyaluronic acid of avian origin became the first non-collagen filler to be widely used. However, it is not available anymore. The Hylaform product family was based on hyaluronic acid derived from processed rooster combs. The Hylaform product family, with an average content of hyaluronic acid of 5.5 mg/ml, was easy to inject due to its good rheological properties and is less palpable than some products of bacterial origin (Manna et al. 1999).

In 2003, data from a clinical trial comparing Hylaform with Zyplast for the treatment of nasolabial folds was presented to the FDA. A total of 480 patients were included in this study which, to our knowledge, was never published. Based on the data that are available from the FDA, no difference between the products could be established. After 12 weeks the mean (±standard deviation) wrinkle severity score, which ranged from 0 to 5, was 3.3 ± 1.11 for Hylaform and 2.2 ± 1.12 for Zyplast (http://www.fda.gov/).

Key Points

- Hylaform is not available anymore.
- The product was based on good clinical data.

1.3.2.2 Hyaluronic Acid of Bacterial Origin

HA preparations of bacterial origin dominate the market. They are quite a heterogeneous group and sometimes quite confusing to differentiate as each company seems to have its specific wording to make it look more different from another one.

Basically they can be differentiated in products with good and in products with not-so-good or even nil clinical data.

1.3.2.2.1 Products with Good Clinical Data

The Q-Med Restylane Family

The Restylane family is the hyaluronic acid family with the best evidence behind it. The reason for that is as said before that after the bovine collagens it became the gold standard for comparative trials in the USA.

The first trial published was a randomized controlled clinical trial conducted to compare the efficacy and safety of Restylane and Zyplast. A total of 137 patients were included in the intention-to-treat analysis. After 6 months the authors concluded that Restylane was superior to Zyplast (based on the assessment of the Winkle Severity Rating Scale). The superiority of Restylane (i.e., where the investigator felt that Restylane was more effective) was observed in 56.9 % of their patients, compared to 9.5 % patients in whom the investigator felt that Zyplast was superior ($p < 0.0001$). Those patients in whom there was no difference between these products (33.6 %) were not included in the simple univariate statistics (Narins et al. 2003).

The Restylane family is sometimes described as biphasic HAs. What does biphasic mean? Basically it is a cross-linked HA product that is formed in particles which are enclosed by noncross-linked HA. As noncross-linked HA is degraded easily, the initial achieved correction might not be as good as this has been shown in the Emervel Deep and Teosyal Deep trials where the products were compared to Restylane Perlane (Nast et al. 2011; Rzany et al. 2011). The particle size determines the indication. The HA products with smaller particles are intended for more superficial use.

The Q-Med Emervel Family

The Emervel family is differently designed. All products have the same HA content with 20 ng/ml. The products, however, are specified for their designated indications by the degree of cross-linking and by the grade of calibration. Two good clinical trials exist comparing the efficacy and safety to the Restylane/Restylane Perlane products (Ascher et al. 2011; Rzany et al. 2011). Furthermore, there is a unique case series where patients could be treated for a variety of indications with a variety of the Emervel products (Rzany et al. 2012).

The Allergan Juvéderm Family

This is a very large family too, offering products for different wrinkles and volume indications. Like for the Q-Med products, the evidence for some of the products from the Juvéderm family is excellent (Baumann et al. 2007; Lupo et al. 2008; Pinsky et al. 2008).

The Allergan Voluma Family (aka Juvéderm Voluma Family)

These are the new products of Allergan. Compared to the Juvéderm products, the Voluma/Volbella/Volift fillers are cross-linked with shorter chains. Here we one good randomized clinical trials and some cases series (Callan et al. 2013; Jones et al. 2013). The Volbella case series is the case series on lip augmentation with the longest duration (e.g., 12 months) (Eccleston and Murphy 2012). Please note that as this is a newly designed HA filler, no final conclusion on the overall tolerability and safety can be made.

The Belotero Family

This is a product that was produced by Anteis and distributed by Merz, now with Merz having bought Anteis it is entirely in the hands of Merz. Like the abovementioned products, we have at least one good clinical trial here (Narins et al. 2010c).

The Teosyal Family

Again here we have a product with at least some clinical data behind it (Nast et al. 2011).

1.3.2.2.2 Products Without Good Clinical Data

Most available HA products in Europe do not have at least one good clinical trial in their background. They pretend to be as good as the products without clinical trials. However, caution is advisable.

1.3.2.2.3 Safety of HA Fillers

Hyaluronic acid is less allergenic than bovine collagen. Skin testing is not recommended. Although hyaluronic acids of human and of animal origins are identical in structure, immunological reactions in the recipient can be caused by residual proteins from the donor (avian or bacterial antigens) or from the cross-linking process.

For the products with good clinical trials besides the RCTs, several larger case series about safety are available. Lowe et al. (2001) reported 709 patients who were observed for a minimum of 1 year. Patients were treated with hyaluronic acid of avian or bacterial origin (patient cohort, follow-up study) between September 1996 and September 2000. The overall incidence of late inflammatory reactions (indurations, inflammation/erythema, abscess formation an average of 8 weeks after injection) is given as 0.42 % (3 out of 709 patients). Friedman et al. (2002) retrospectively reviewed the data of all unwanted effects of nonanimal hyaluronic acid from the Restylane family that were reported to the manufacturer between 1999 and 2000, worldwide (Europe, Australia, South America, and Asia). For 1999, based on 144,000 treatments, the incidence was calculated at 0.15 %; for 2000, based on approximately 262,000 treatments, the incidence of 0.06 % was given. Since the incidences reported by Lowe et al. (2001) and Friedman et al. (2002)

are based on either patients returning to their private practice or voluntary reports, the real incidence might be higher.

In 2004, Andre evaluated the incidence of adverse reactions with nonanimal, stabilized hyaluronic acid between 1997 and 2001 using a questionnaire-based survey. Out of 12,344 syringes sold and 4,320 treated patients, 16 cases of immediate hypersensitivity and 18 cases of delayed reactions were recorded. The global risk of sensitivity was calculated at 0.8 %. Since 2000, the amount of protein in the raw product was decreased and the incidence of hypersensitivity reactions has been reported to be around 0.6 %. As 50 % of these reactions were immediate and resolved within less than 3 weeks, the risk of a strong but transient, delayed reaction is around 0.3 %. Four cases of sterile abscess were reported (Andre 2004). Again, although the data were quite systematically assessed, an underestimation of the real incidence cannot be ruled out.

Further case reports that are available describe in detail adverse reactions such as erythema, pruritus, edema, urticae, and papulocystic nodules after injection with hyaluronic acid preparations of various origins. Arterial embolization and exudative granulomatous reaction after treatment with hyaluronic acid of avian origin have also been reported (Fernandez-Acenero et al. 2003; Lombardi et al. 2004; Lowe 2003; Lupton and Alster 2000; Micheels 2001; Raulin et al. 2000; Shafir et al. 2000). In rare cases, a bluish discoloration might occur. This bluish discoloration may reflect a Tyndall phenomenon.

Not every product is similar. There appear to be products there with an increased risk of adverse reactions. How are we able to detect these products? Only by communicating adverse reactions among colleagues and to the authorities! In the Netherlands the sales of Hyacorp H-S and H1000 were temporarily stopped after several cases occurred with two products of the family (Skipr. Tot nu toe 25 klachten over rimpelfiller. Online in the Internet: http://www.skipr.nl/actueel/id12523-tot-nu-toe-25-klachten-over-rimpelfiller.html [2012-10-25]). At the moment (August 2013), these cases are still investigated by the Dutch authorities. However, the company decided to withdraw Hyacorp H-S 500, H1000, and Hyacorp L from the European market (mailing to doctors using Hyacorp in August 2013).

Key Points

- Among the bacterial HAs, there is an easy way to distinguish between products with good clinical data and those without.
- If you use a product without good clinical data, the risk for a not-so-good efficacy or an increased risk of inflammatory reactions is with the patient and the treating physician.

1.3.3 Combination of Hyaluronic Acid with Other Substances

1.3.3.1 Combination with Dextrans

The combination of hyaluronic acid, hydroxpropylmethylcelluose and dextrans (dextranomers), marketed as Matridex, is thought to be more durable than other products. However, there is as yet no good clinical data on its efficacy and safety.

How safe is the addition of dextrans to an HA preparation? Or how safe are the HAs which are combined with dextrans? We do not have good clinical trials to answer these questions. However, we do have some case reports focusing on adverse reactions to these products (Huh et al. 2010; Massone et al. 2009). One patient developed after 5 weeks a delayed inflammatory reaction to Matridex injected in the glabellar fold that lasted more than a year. The patient was treated with oral doxycycline and intralesional injection of triamcinolone acetonide; this resulted in almost complete resolution of the lesion (Huh et al. 2010). The second patient was a 43-year-old woman who complained of multiple, painful, reddish, nonulcerated, hard nodules on both cheeks and periocular regions 4 weeks after the injection of Matridex. Histopathology showed a diffuse suppurative granulomatous reaction with the presence of multinucleate giant cells and many neutrophils involving the entire dermis (Massone et al. 2009).

1.3.3.2 Combination with Antioxidants

There are also HA products available where the HA is combined with, e.g., antioxidants. No good comparative trial data exists for these products. Therefore, it is not clear if these added substances have any clinically measurable effect at all.

Key Points
- We do not have good clinical data on HAs in a fixed combination with dextrans or antioxidants.
- Caution is therefore advisable as case reports of adverse reactions have been reported.

1.3.4 Alginates

At the end of 2009, a new filler, an alginate, which derives from brown algae was introduced to the market. Based on the results of the initial large cases series, the product looked very good. Erythema, swelling, and even hematomas seem to be less as for HA products (unpublished data presented at IMCAS Paris 2010).

In contrast to other filler, the alginate could be very easily injected. And this is probably what caused even experienced and trained injectors to inject too much in nonclinical investigated areas as the infraorbital hollow.

As some adverse events as nodule formation were reported specifically in areas as the infraorbital hollow and no antidote was available at that time, the filler was removed from the market (Schuller-Petrović et al. 2013).

Do's
- Watch out for this product. If reintroduced in the market, it could be (if an antidote is available) an interesting alternative in patients prone to erythema and edema after HA fillers.

Key Points
- The efficacy and safety of alginates were supported by a large case series.
- At the moment the filler is not available any more.

1.3.5 Poly-l-lactic Acid

Poly-l-lactid acid (PLLA) is a synthetic biodegradable material. It has an unique collagen stimulating quality. When injected into the dermis or subdermis, it gradually stimulates collagen formation and by this restructures the facial tissue, making it a facial volumizer. This is a gradual process, and the manufacturer recommends three initial treatment sessions, each approximately 6–8 weeks apart. After the three initial treatments, the results are supposed to last for up to 2 years and longer.

This product comes as a powder and needs to be diluted with sterile water several hours before injection. Although initially the recommended dilution for PLLA was 3 ml, the current recommendation is to dilute it in a volume of 5–9 ml or more. Most colleagues add an additional 2 ml of a local anesthetic to decrease injection pain. The correct recommendation from the SculpTraining Expert Group is 7 ml + 2 ml of a local anesthetic, making it a total of 9 ml. Furthermore, it is recommended to dilute the product at least 24 h before use. Even when administered using the correct injection technique and the higher dilution, in some cases the needle will block during the injection, at which point the syringe has to be withdrawn and the plunger retracted until the PLLA flows again.

Before 2010, studies on the efficacy and safety of PLLA were based mainly on the treatment of HIV patients with drug-induced lipoatrophy (Moyle et al. 2004; Perry 2004; Valantin et al. 2003). Only case reports and case series existed for the use of PLLA for aesthetic indications (Rzany et al. 2004; Woerle et al. 2004). In 2010 a large clinical trial was published comparing PLLA to human collagen (Narins et al. 2010a) ($n = 233$). In this trial, at 3 months already the superiority of this product was shown compared to human collagen. The mean number of treatment sessions required per subject was 3.2 in the injectable PLLA group compared with 2.6 in the collagen group. The mean (SD) volume of injectable PLLA used per session for both nasolabial folds was as follows: session 1, 4.1 (1.1) ml; session 2, 3.5 (1.2) ml; session 3, 3.3 (1.2) ml; and session 4, 3.5 (1.1) ml. For human collagen, the mean (SD) volume used per session was as follows: session 1, 3.1 (1.1) ml; session 2, 2.1 (1.1) ml; session 3, 1.9 (1.1) ml; and session 4, 1.7 (1.0) ml. Importantly the correction with PLLA lasted over 13–25 months. This is the reason why most patients preferred this product (Brandt et al. 2011). However, the correction that could be achieved was less than you would see in HA trials (approximately 0.66–0.85 on a six-point scale – compared to approximately 1 on a five-point scale in HA trials (see above)) (Narins et al. 2010a).

Nodule formation is the main adverse reaction of this filler. Based on the HIV-lipodystrophy data, granulomatous reactions, described as palpable but invisible subcutaneous micronodules, were observed in 22 out of 50 (44 %) patients. In 6 of these 22 patients, the nodules disappeared at week 96. In that particular study, one vial of PLLA was diluted in a volume of 3–4 ml (Valantin et al. 2003).

The prevalence of nodule formation seems to be associated with the volume that was used for dilution. We have some indirect evidence that nodule formation can be reduced when an increased volume for dilution is used (Rossner et al. 2009a; Schierle and Casas 2011). Nevertheless, nodule formation still occurs and was highest in the hands (12.5 %) and the cheeks (7.2 %) (Palm et al. 2010). There are case reports of large solitary nodular masses, e.g., in the temporal region (Avery and Clifford 2010) as well as abscess formation. However, nodule formation is in most patients temporary and will decrease over time (Sperling et al. 2010). Therefore, these nodules should not be too aggressively treated.

Do's

- Always dilute the PLLA with at least 5–7 ml at least 24 h before treatment.
- Add an additional 2 ml of a local anesthetic before injection.
- Patients with severe elastosis might benefit from a topical co-treatment with 0.05 % tretinoin.

Don'ts

- Do not inject PLLA too superficially in elastotic or naturally very thin skin as otherwise you might end up with small superficial bumps.
- Do not inject PLLA in hyperdynamic areas as the lips.
- Do not inject PLLA in patients with active autoimmune diseases as rheumatoid arthritis (see Chap. 8).
- Do not inject PLLA in patients which might be subject to interferon therapy (if foreseeable) – they might have an increased risk for nodule formation.

Key Points

- This is a product where we have at least a one good clinical trial and several case series available.
- PLLA needs to be injected several times to obtain a clinically relevant result. At least three treatment sessions should be planed, each session at least 4–6 weeks apart from the other.
- PLLA has a volumizing effect through its unique collagen stimulation properties and is ideal for the temples, the cheeks, and the restoration of the mandibular line.
- PLLA does not provide immediate gratification. Patients might be disappointed when they do not see an immediate result. In case patients want PLLA and in addition an immediate result before the PLLA sessions, an HA might be injected followed by the PLLA injections.

1.3.6 Calcium Hydroxylapatite

Calcium hydroxylapatite (CaHa) is made from synthetically formed calcium phosphate pearls, a procedure that is classified as bioceramics and involves the ionic bonding of calcium and phosphate ions. When injected, they form a foundation within a matrix that allows the local cellular infiltration of fibroblasts. The complex is available as a gel to allow easier application. The substance comes in 1.2-ml syringes and is injected through a 25- to 27-gauge needle.

Early studies focused on drug-induced lipoatrophy in HIV patients (Comite et al. 2004; Silvers et al. 2006). However, due to the quest for an aesthetic license in the USA, we do have now three randomized controlled clinical trials, one against collagen (Smith et al. 2007) and two against hyaluronic acid products (Moers-Carpi et al. 2007; Moers-Carpi and Tufet 2008) focusing on the correction of nasolabial folds. Not surprisingly CaHa was shown to be superior to human collagen in a 6-month study (Smith et al. 2007). For the comparison to the HAs, the picture is not as clear. The larger study of the two 12-month studies did not show a difference in the WSRS; the smaller study favored in the WSRS the CaHA-treated site (Moers-Carpi et al. 2007; Moers-Carpi and Tufet 2008). Patient preference and satisfaction with treatment favored CaHA (however, one has to note that neither study was double blind; therefore, a bias might favor the treatment under study). CaHa comes without lidocaine. In another RCT on 50 patients who received CaHa injections in the nasolabial folds, patients favored the site which was treated with a CaHA lidocaine mixture (Marmur et al. 2010; Grunebaum et al. 2010).

In contrast to the other fillers, CaHa is visible on x-rays. According to Feeney et al. (2009), hydroxylapatite is hyperattenuating on CT, hypermetabolic on FDG-PET imaging, of intermediate signal intensity on MRI, and by this a potential cause of a false-positive findings. Patients should be informed of this so that they can tell their doctors should they require an x-ray or another sophisticated radiological examination.

There is not much evidence for common adverse reactions to this filler. Sklar and White (2004) and Tzikas (2004) reported case series with 64 and 90 patients treated with CaHa for facial soft tissue augmentation. In addition to mild bruising and swelling, no immediate side effects were observed. Sklar and White (2004) reported five patients with complications after CaHa treatment. Three patients had palpable bumps, one had puffiness of the lower eyelid, and another patient developed a pink/white plaque. The two latter adverse events occurred when treating the tear trough area. The treatment period in that study was 6 months. In a 6-month nasolabial fold trial of CaHa compared to human collagen, patients treated with CaHa reported more edema (73.9 % compared to 56.4 %) and had more ecchymosis (63.2 % compared to 43.6 %) (Smith et al. 2007). Despite that, patients preferred CaHa compared to the human collagen. CaHa has been also studied in an open-label 6-month study in patients with skin types IV to VI (Marmur et al. 2009). No reports of keloid formation, hypertrophic scarring, hypo- or hyperpigmentation, or other clinically significant adverse events were recorded in this study comprising 100 patients.

The area where adverse reactions were quite frequently reported in the beginning is the lip area. In the study of Tzikas (2004), 7 out of 90 patients developed persistent visible mucosal lip nodules, 4 of whom required an intervention. The treatment period for this study was also 6 months. Furthermore, there are reports of CaHa causing arterial occlusion leading to local necrosis or even blindness (Kim and Choi 2013; Sung et al. 2010).

Do's

- Dilute CaHa with lidocaine before injection. Adding 0.2 ml of lidocaine hydrochloric acid (HCL) to the 1.2 ml of CaHa should be sufficient. This is done through a Luer Lock connector. On one side is the CaHA syringe and on the other side a syringe with 0.2 ml of HCl. In the next step, the content of both syringes will be mixed. N.B. in case a premixed combination of CaHA and a LA might become available the separate dilution of CaHa with lidocaine will not be necessary any more.

Don'ts

- Do not inject CaHa too superficially. If you do this, you will end up with visible lumps and an unhappy patient.
- Do not use this product for lip augmentation. Nodules due to the mechanical accumulation of the material have been reported.
- In case of severe pain, blanching, or visual disturbances, do not continue with the injection of CaHa. These might be signs of arterial occlusion.

Key Points

- CaHa is a biodegradable filler with a good scientific background on its efficacy and safety.
- It comes with a 25- to 27-gauge needle and needs to be injected deep dermal or subdermal.
- Diluting it with lidocaine will increase the injectability and decrease injection pain.
- For the first couple of weeks, it might feel a bit lumpy. Afterward, it will be nicely integrated in the surrounding tissue.
- Please do not forget that there is *no* antidote in case of overcorrection or arterial occlusion.
- Besides of the rate occurrence of arterial occlusion, the use of this product seems to be quite safe.

1.4 Nonbiodegradable Fillers

Several nonbiodegradable fillers are or were available (Table 1.2). As well as being expensive, frequent injections can be quite tiresome for both the patient and the physician, and so the application of a nonbiodegradable or permanent filler holds a certain attraction. Conversely, there are certain disadvantages that should be taken into account. First, patients of all ages can be treated in aesthetic medicine. It may therefore be quite uncertain how a permanent depot will appear after three or even four decades, by which time age and solar-induced elastosis has reduced the dermal and epidermal layers. Second, there is always a possibility of adverse reactions to fillers. The most common subacute or late reaction to permanent fillers is the development of a granuloma. Treatment of an adverse reaction to a filler material is much more difficult when the filler is nonbiodegradable because it will provide a permanent stimulus for the surrounding tissue.

Table 1.2 Nonbiodegradable fillers

Material	Origin	Products[a]
Silicone	–	ADATO SIL-ol 5000, Bioplastique, Biopolimero, Dermagen, SILIKON 1000 Silicex
Polyacrylamide	–	Amazingel, Aquamid, Argiform, Bioformacryl, Evolution[b], Outline
Polyalkylimide	–	Bio-Alcamid[b]

[a]Please note that this list is not complete
[b]Not on the market anymore

In order to ensure patient satisfaction, they should be thoroughly advised about the pros and cons of the suggested treatment with a nonbiodegradable product. We would not generally recommend the use of nonbiodegradable fillers at the first visit for patients who have never been treated before with a filler. Patients who are interested in being treated with a nonbiodegradable filler should first be preinjected with saline or a biodegradable filler to ensure that they are satisfied with the correction result.

1.4.1 Silicone

Injectable silicone is one of the oldest injectable filler materials used. Medical-grade silicon is a clear, oily, colorless liquid composed of long chains of polymerized dimethylsiloxane.

There are several methods of injection for this product. One of the recommended techniques is the microdroplet technique (Orentreich 2000; Webster et al. 1986). Fluid silicone is injected into the dermis as 0.01 ml microdroplets. Each mircodroplet is separated by 1 mm. Undercorrection is recommended as the main side effect is a foreign body (fibrotic) reaction.

Despite being touted by many authors as the ideal augmentation material, silicone – especially of questionable sources – has led to some disastrous local and systemic effects. In general, the inflammatory reaction surrounding injected silicone is self-limited; however, the extent of the reaction is unpredictable and in some cases can be quite severe. Local adverse reactions include chronic inflammation, migration, extrusion, ulceration, and silicone granuloma formation. Once these complications are recognized, removal of the injected silicone is quite difficult, necessitating wide tissue resections and complicated reconstructions (Homicz and Watson 2004).

Although the quality of the product in terms of purity has improved significantly in the last decades, a significant number of adverse events as granulomatous reactions, infection, ulceration, and migration have been published (Ersek et al. 1997; Ficarra et al. 2002; Rapaport et al. 1996; Requena et al. 2001). The frequency of these reactions is not known. In a chart review of 916 patients treated with 1,000-centistoke silicon oil, very few adverse events were documented. However, this was a retrospective chart review without contacting the treated patients (Hevia 2009). Therefore, the paper is only of limited help for assessing the real risk of this product. Nevertheless, silicone oil was and still is used inside and outside the USA. In a recent paper by Fulton and Caperton (2012), even a self-mixed HA-silicone filler was investigated in a larger case series. Again, as this was a small study, every conclusion on risk is limited.

Key Points

- The risk profile even of highly purified silicone is still not clear.
- Better clinical data is necessary for a final conclusion on this controversial product.

1.4.2 Polyacrylamide

Polyacrylamide (trade name, e.g., Aquamid) is composed of 97.5 % water and 2.5 % cross-linked polyacrylamide. It is recommended for folds, skin sculpturing, and facial atrophy. It is not effective for fine wrinkles. Aquamid should be injected deeply using the subcutaneous tunneling technique (Breiting et al. 2004; De Cassia Novaes and Berg 2003). In contrast to the last edition when the evidence was very limited, we can look back now to a couple of clinical trials on this substance (Narins et al. 2010a). This large trial ($n=315$) compared a polyacrylamide filler to an HA (NASHA) filler over a period of 12 months. In this study after 6 months and even 12 months, the degree of correction was comparable with approximately 2 points on a six-point scale.

Which adverse reactions can appear? In the small pilot study by De Cassia Novaes and Berg (2003), aside from mild to moderate immediate redness, swelling, and pain, which dissipated in less than 36 h, no long-term side effects were observed. In 2004, Breiting reported the results of a retrospective case series of 104 patients, from which 49 had undergone breast augmentation. Migration of the gel was demonstrated in three women who had their nasolabial folds treated. No long-term adverse effects were observed in this study, which reported an average observation time of 3.9 years (Breiting et al. 2004).

In 2003, Wang published a case series of 15 patients with adverse reactions assessed over 2 years and reported the following: nodules (80 %), pain (60 %), secondary deformity (20 %), discomfort (13 %), and long-lasting swelling (6.6 %). Pathologic examinations showed macrophagocyte infiltration (60 %), capsule formation (53.3 %), and granulomatous reactions (20 %; Wang et al. 2003).

At least by Christensen and colleagues these reactions are associated with biofilm formation, and antibiotic treatments are recommended (Bjarnsholt 2009).

Do's

- Before injections, disinfect the skin thoroughly.
- In case of an adverse reaction against polyacrylamide and a bacterial infection is suspected, there is no harm in following the therapeutic recommendations from Bjarnsholt et al. (2009), e.g., clarithromycin 500 mg and moxifloxacin 400 mg, twice daily for 10 days.

Don'ts

- Do not overcorrect.
- Do not inject polyacrylamides to superficially specifically in patients with elastotic skin. The injected material might look lumpy.

Key Points

- These are permanent products. For example, in case of overcorrection or adverse reactions, some difficulties might arise. For abscess-like reactions, a course of antibiotics is recommendable.
- In contrast to other filler, we do have at least some good clinical data here.

1.4.3 Polyalkylimide

Polyalkylimide was available as Bio-Alcamid. It consists of alkyl-imide group networks (approximately 4 %) and water (approximately 96 %). The product was available at two different viscosities for lip and facial augmentation and is used for folds, skin sculpting (including the lips), and facial atrophy, but not for the treatment of fine lines. The material must be injected subdermally and, according to the manufacturer's information, is supposed to be easily removable when injected in larger volumes (Protopapa et al. 2003).

In 2003 (Protopapa et al.), in 73 patients follow-up examinations were carried out for up to 3 years. No implant dislocation, implant migration, granuloma, allergic reaction, or intolerance was recorded. However, in a retrospective Dutch study on 3,194 patients, 154 complications were reported, the most common being inflammation, hardening, as well as migration (Schelke et al. 2009). The authors conclude that the prevalence of these reactions is too high and that the use of the product cannot be recommended. Similar conclusions were drawn from a British group of surgeons when reviewing 67 patients with HIV-drug-associated lipoatrophy who had all been treated with polyalkylimide where 50 % of the treated patients experienced at least one complication (migration, hardening, irregularity) (George et al. 2012). These results were supported by a Canadian group where in 19 % of 267 patients, infectious complications were noted (Nadarajah et al. 2012). At the moment, the product is not available in Europe anymore.

Key Point

- This is a product without good clinical data. It is not on the market anymore. The product was removed due to an increase risk of adverse reactions.

1.5 Combination of Nonbiodegradable and Biodegradable Fillers

Some fillers are a combination of nonbiodegradable (permanent) and biodegradable (temporary) materials. The purpose of the biodegradable material is to act as a carrier and to ensure an immediate effect until the fibrotic foreign body reaction induced by the nonbiodegradable filler leads to visible effects (Table 1.3).

Table 1.3 Combinations of permanent and temporary materials

Temporary	Permanent	Products[a]
Collagen (bovine)	Polymethylmethacrylate	Artecoll/ArteFill
Hyaluronic acid (from cell cultures)	Hydroxyethylmethacrylate	Dermalive, Dermadeep[b]

[a]Please note that this list is not complete
[b]Not on the market anymore

1.5.1 Polymethylmethacrylate and Collagen

The combination of polymethylmethacrylate (PMMA) and collagen (ArteFill (former preparation Artecoll)) was introduced at the end of the 1980s and is the oldest available combination preparation. PMMA beads are suspended in a solution of 3.5 % bovine collagen (as a carrier) and 0.3 % lidocaine (for pain relief). While the collagen resorbs over a period of 2–3 months, the PMMA spheres become encapsulated by fibrotic material.

ArteFill should be injected into the lower third of the dermis with a 26- to 27-gauge needle using the tunneling technique. The material should not be injected too superficially; the needle should never be visible through the skin. Careful massage with a fingertip after application helps to distribute the material more evenly. Overcorrection is not advisable; however, a second implantation may be necessary after 3 months (Lemperle et al. 2003). Although the preparation contains collagen, in Europe, a skin test is not mandatory.

This is the only permanent filler that has been subject to a large clinical trial (Cohen and Holmes 2004). Based on this clinical trial data, the efficacy and safety have been proven for a 12-month period.

Granulomatous reactions are well-known complications for this filler (Alcalay et al. 2003). The retrospective case series by Lemperle et al. (1998) is based on 515 questionnaires from 290 patients treated between 1993 and 1994. Immediately after PMMA implantation, swelling, redness, and itching were reported. Late reactions such as erythema, transparency, unevenness, and dislocation have also been documented. Longer-lasting redness after Artecoll implantation was reported in 6.1 % of reported cases in 1993 and in 0.5 % of reported cases in 1994. The overall complication rate in 1994 was 3 % (6 out of 201 patients). In addition, an acute allergic reaction was reported in one woman. Based on data from the manufacturer, the rate of granulomatous reaction was given as 1 in 1,000 patients. Nodules did arise 6 months to 2 years after treatment. Again, as this data relies on spontaneous reports, underreporting is likely to have occurred.

This product is under the name of ArteFill, the only permanent product available in the USA so far. Based on the clinical study that led to the approval of that product and comprised 251 patients who were followed over 1 year, the risk for adverse reactions in the observed period is low (Cohen and Holmes 2004). Even when followed over further 4–5 years, the risk remained low (Cohen et al. 2006). However, as the product is permanent, adverse reactions might develop after years (Zielke et al. 2008). Furthermore, 251 patients are not enough to detect rare events. Therefore, the product still needs to be closely monitored.

Do's

- Be careful when you inject this product. Disinfect the skin thoroughly and do not inject too much in one spot.

Key Points

- This is one of the few permanent products that have been subject to a clinical trial.
- Be aware that this product as other permanent products has a risk of increased foreign body reactions. Patients should be aware of that.

1.5.2 Hydroxyethylmethacrylate and Hyaluronic Acid

Hydroxyethylmethacrylate (HEMA) and ethylmethacrylate microspheres suspended in hyaluronic acid were available in Europe as Dermalive since the end of the 1990s until 2007. This product consisted of 40 % bacterial hyaluronic acid and 60 % acrylic hydrogel particles (diameter of 45–65 μm). A similar formulation with larger-sized particles (about 85–110 μm) and a somewhat higher hyaluronic acid content was marketed as DermaDeep and was intended to be injected deeper.

Dermalive was supposed to be injected with a 27.5-gauge needle into the deeper layers of the dermis, at the junction between the dermis and the hypodermis, with the tunneling technique, while DermaDeep was supposed to be injected with a slightly bigger needle (26.5 gauge) deeper into the subperiosteal layer or the hypodermis. Overcorrection was to be avoided. At least 3 months should be left between two injection sessions (Bergeret-Galley et al. 2001).

This product was probably the product with the highest risk of adverse reactions to injectable fillers (Rossner 2009b). Early after the introduction to the market, case reports became known focusing on nodule formation to HEMA (Requena et al. 2001; Waris 2003). Besides nodule formation, abscesses as well as ulcerations are part of the adverse reactions spectrum of this product (Zielke et al. 2008). In 2001, Bergeret-Galley published an overview in which the overall incidence of late side effects and complications (nodules, swelling, and erythema, on average 6 months after injection) based on data from the manufacturer is given as <1.2 per 1,000 patients (Bergeret-Galley et al. 2001). As the data from the manufacturer is based on spontaneous reports and with this being an early study, e.g., with a limited observation period, the real incidence will be higher.

Although this product is not produced anymore, we will very likely see further adverse reactions to this permanent product.

Don'ts
- We would not recommend using this or a similar product in patients.

Key Points
- This product had a bad efficacy/safety ratio. Adverse events as nodule formation were not infrequent and very difficult to treat (see Chap. 8).
- Although the product is not on the market anymore, we still do see adverse reactions against it. Therefore, it is still important to know the product.

1.6 Combining Different Fillers in One Area

Nonbiodegradable and biodegradable products may be combined by the injector in one area, but should this be done? This question raises some controversy. For example, with PLLA, where the onset of efficacy may be delayed, combination with another biodegradable filler such as hyaluronic acid might improve the patient's satisfaction. On the other hand, if an adverse event occurs, the culprit filler might be much more difficult to identify. Nevertheless, the combination of different fillers in one area does not necessarily increase the risk. Only 8.9 % of patients with adverse reactions to injectable fillers from the Berlin registry reported an individual combination therapy. Nevertheless, since good epidemiological data is lacking, we would recommend using extreme caution when combining fillers of different origin for the same indication.

1.7 General Approach to New Fillers

Especially in Europe, South America, and Asia, new injectable fillers are popping up like daisies. CE certification is the official way to introduce a new product onto the European market, but data from clinical trials are not required for a new filler if comparable filler substances are already on the market. As such, no clinical data on efficacy and safety exist for most of the new injectable fillers.

Users should thus be cautious in embracing new products. Marketing approaches tend to include claims of durability and safety for biodegradable and nonbiodegradable products that may not stand the scrutiny of a clinical trial or postmarketing safety studies. Good data on efficacy and safety should be requested by every user to prevent patients being used as guinea pigs for companies that are reluctant to invest in clinical trials.

Fortunately there is a tendency for improvement, although at the moment most studies are being carried out in the USA. In general, it is advisable not to conduct studies in only one country but to place clinical trials in Europe or South America, for example, to acknowledge cultural differences and provide a broader and better base for regulatory decisions.

Do's

- If a new filler is introduced to you, ask for clinical data. A randomized controlled clinical trial against an established HA would be the best base. However, a large case series, e.g., 50 and more patients, can also give you some important information on efficacy and safety.

Don'ts

- Do not believe everything the marketing guys from the company will tell you. Ask yourself if being "made in Germany" or "Switzerland" is enough to make it a good filler.
- Do not start to treat tricky areas with a new filler, e.g., the tear trough and lips are the second step.

Key Points

- Ask for good clinical data before you use a new filler. As good as Restylane or Juvéderm is not enough. You should ask for clinical data depicting efficacy (does the filler do the job?), durability (how long does it last?), and patient's perception (did the patient like the product?).

References

Alcalay J et al (2003) Late-onset granulomatous reaction to Artecoll. Dermatol Surg 29(8):859–862

Andre P (2004) Evaluation of the safety of a non-animal stabilized hyaluronic acid (NASHA – Q-Medical, Sweden) in European countries: a retrospective study from 1997 to 2001. J Eur Acad Dermatol Venereol 18(4):422–425

Apte RS et al (2003) Acute choroidal infarction following subcutaneous injection of micronized dermal matrix in the forehead region. Retina 23(4):552–554

Ascher B, Bayerl C, Brun P, Kestemont P, Rzany B, Poncet M, Guennoun M, Podda M (2011) Efficacy and safety of a new hyaluronic acid dermal filler in the treatment of severe nasolabial lines – 6-month interim results of a randomized, evaluator-blinded, intra-individual comparison study. J Cosmet Dermatol 10:94–98

Avery C, Clifford N (2010) Foreign body granulomatous reaction of the temporal region following dermal filler administration. Br J Oral Maxillofac Surg 48(6):488, Epub 2010 Jul 7

Baumann L (2004) CosmoDerm/CosmoPlast (human bioengineered collagen) for the aging face. Facial Plast Surg 20(2):125–128

Baumann LS, Shamban AT, Lupo MP, Monheit GD, Thomas JA, Murphy DK, Walker PS, Juvéderm vs. Zyplast Nasolabial Fold Study Group (2007) Comparison of smooth-gel hyaluronic acid dermal fillers with cross-linked bovine collagen: a multicenter, double-masked, randomized, within-subject study. Dermatol Surg 33(Suppl 2):S128–S135

Bergeret-Galley C et al (2001) The value of a new filler material in corrective and cosmetic surgery: Dermalive and Dermadeep. Aesthetic Plast Surg 25(4):249–255

Bjarnsholt T, Tolker-Nielsen T, Givskov M, Janssen M, Christensen LH (2009) Detection of bacteria by fluorescence in situ hybridization in culture-negative soft tissue filler lesions. Dermatol Surg 35(Suppl 2):1620–1624, Epub 2009 Aug 26

Brandt FS, Cazzaniga A, Baumann L, Fagien S, Glazer S, Kenkel JM, Lowe NJ, Monheit GD, Narins RS,

Rendon MI, Rohrich RJ, Werschler WP (2011) Investigator global evaluations of efficacy of injectable poly-L-lactic acid versus human collagen in the correction of nasolabial fold wrinkles. Aesthet Surg J 31(5):521–528
Braun M, Braun S (2008) Nodule formation following lip augmentation using porcine collagen-derived filler. J Drugs Dermatol 7(6):579–581
Breiting V et al (2004) A study on patients treated with polyacrylamide hydrogel injection for facial corrections. Aesthetic Plast Surg 28(1):45–53
Callan P, Goodman GJ, Carlisle I, Liew S, Muzikants P, Scamp T, Halstead MB, Rogers JD (2013) Efficacy and safety of a hyaluronic acid filler in subjects treated for correction of midface volume deficiency: a 24 month study. Clin Cosmet Investig Dermatol 6:81–89
Cassuto D (2009) The use of Dermicol-P35 dermal filler for nonsurgical rhinoplasty. Aesthet Surg J 29:S22–S24
Cohen SR, Berner CF, Busso M, Gleason MC, Hamilton D, Holmes RE, Romano JJ, Rullan PP, Thaler MP, Ubogy Z, Vecchione TR (2006) ArteFill: a long-lasting injectable wrinkle filler material–summary of the U.S. Food and Drug Administration trials and a progress report on 4- to 5-year outcomes. Plast Reconstr Surg 118(Suppl 3):64S–76S
Cohen SR, Holmes RE (2004) Artecoll: a long-lasting injectable wrinkle filler material: report of a controlled, randomized, multicenter clinical trial of 251 subjects. Plast Reconstr Surg 114(4):964–976; discussion 977–9
Comite SL et al (2004) Treatment of HIV-associated facial lipoatrophy with Radiance FN (Radiesse). Dermatol Online J 10(2):2
Cooperman LS et al (1985) Injectable collagen: a six-year clinical investigation. Aesthetic Plast Surg 9(2):145–151
De Boulle K, Swinberghe S, Engman M, Shoshani D (2009) Lip augmentation and contour correction with a ribose cross-linked collagen dermal filler. J Drugs Dermatol 8:1–8
De Cassia Novaes W, Berg A (2003) Experiences with a new nonbiodegradable hydrogel (Aquamid): a pilot study. Aesthetic Plast Surg 27(5):376–380
Eccleston D, Murphy DK (2012) Juvéderm Volbella™ in the perioral area: a 12-month prospective, multicenter, open-label study. Clin Cosmet Investig Dermatol 5:167–172
Ersek RA et al (1997) Bioplastique at 6 years: clinical outcome studies. Plast Reconstr Surg 100(6): 1570–1574
Fagien S (2000) Facial soft-tissue augmentation with injectable autologous and allogeneic human tissue collagen matrix (autologen and dermalogen). Plast Reconstr Surg 105(1):362–373; discussion 374–375
Feeney JN, Fox JJ, Akhurst T (2009) Radiological impact of the use of calcium hydroxylapatite dermal fillers. Clin Radiol 64(9):897–902, Epub 2009 Jul 5
Fernandez-Acenero MJ et al (2003) Granulomatous foreign body reaction against hyaluronic acid: report of a case after lip augmentation. Dermatol Surg 29(12):1225–1226
Ficarra G et al (2002) Silicone granuloma of the facial tissues: a report of seven cases. Oral Surg Oral Med Oral Pathol Oral Radiol Endod 94(1):65–73
Friedman PM et al (2002) Safety data of injectable non-animal stabilized hyaluronic acid gel for soft tissue augmentation. Dermatol Surg 28(6):491–494
Fulton J, Caperton C (2012) The optimal filler: immediate and long-term results with emulsified silicone (1,000 centistokes) with cross-linked hyaluronic acid. J Drugs Dermatol 11(11):1336–1341
George DA, Erel E, Waters R (2012) Patient satisfaction following Bio-Alcamid injection for facial contour defects. J Plast Reconstr Aesthet Surg 65:1622–1626
Goldberg DJ (2009) Correction of tear trough deformity with novel porcine collagen dermal filler (Dermicol-P35). Aesthet Surg J 29:S9–S11
Grunebaum LD, Elsaie ML, Kaufman J (2010) Six-month, double-blind, randomized, split-face study to compare the efficacy and safety of calcium hydroxylapatite (CaHA) mixed with lidocaine and CaHA alone for correction of nasolabial fold wrinkles. Dermatol Surg 36(S1):760–765
Hevia O (2009) Six-year experience using 1,000-centistoke silicone oil in 916 patients for soft-tissue augmentation in a private practice setting. Dermatol Surg 35(Suppl 2):1646–1652
Homicz MR, Watson D (2004) Review of injectable materials for soft tissue augmentation. Facial Plast Surg 20(1):21–29
Huh SY, Cho S, Kim KH, An JS, Won CH, Chang SE, Lee MW, Choi JH, Moon KC (2010) A case of complication after matridex(r) injection. Ann Dermatol 22(1):81–84
Jones D, Murphy DK (2013) Volumizing hyaluronic acid filler for midface volume deficit: 2-year results from a pivotal single-blind randomized controlled study. Dermatol Surg. 2013 Oct 4. [Epub ahead of print]
Kim YJ, Choi KS (2013) Bilateral blindness after filler injection. Plast Reconstr Surg 131(2):298e–299e
Landau M (2009) Lip augmentation and rejuvenation using Dermicol-P35 30G: personal experiences from my clinic. Aesthet Surg J. 29(3 Suppl):S12–15
Lemperle G et al (1998) PMMA-Microspheres (Artecoll) for long-lasting correction of wrinkles: refinements and statistical results. Aesthetic Plast Surg 22(5): 356–365
Lemperle G et al (2003) Soft tissue augmentation with artecoll: 10-year history, indications, techniques, and complications. Dermatol Surg 29(6):573–587; discussion 587
Lombardi T et al (2004) Orofacial granulomas after injection of cosmetic fillers. Histopathologic and clinical study of 11 cases. J Oral Pathol Med 33(2): 115–120
Lowe NJ (2003) Arterial embolization caused by injection of hyaluronic acid (Restylane). Br J Dermatol 148(2):379; author reply 379–380

Lowe NJ et al (2001) Hyaluronic acid skin fillers: adverse reactions and skin testing. J Am Acad Dermatol 45(6):930–933

Lupo MP, Smith SR, Thomas JA, Murphy DK, Beddingfield FC 3rd (2008) Effectiveness of Juvéderm Ultra Plus dermal filler in the treatment of severe nasolabial folds. Plast Reconstr Surg 121(1): 289–297

Lupton JR, Alster TS (2000) Cutaneous hypersensitivity reaction to injectable hyaluronic acid gel. Dermatol Surg 26(2):135–137

Man J, Rao J, Goldman M (2008) A double-blind, comparative study of nonanimalstabilized hyaluronic acid versus human collagen for tissue augmentation of the dorsal hands. Dermatol Surg 34:1026–1031

Manna F et al (1999) Comparative chemical evaluation of two commercially available derivatives of hyaluronic acid (hylaform from rooster combs and restylane from streptococcus) used for soft tissue augmentation. J Eur Acad Dermatol Venereol 13(3):183–192

Marmur E, Green L, Busso M (2010) Controlled, randomized study of pain levels in subjects treated with calcium hydroxylapatite premixed with lidocaine for correction of nasolabial folds. Dermatol Surg 36:309–315

Marmur ES, Taylor SC, Grimes PE, Boyd CM, Porter JP, Yoo JY (2009) Six-month safety results of calcium hydroxylapatite for treatment of nasolabial folds in Fitzpatrick skin types IV to VI. Dermatol Surg 35(Suppl 2):1641–1645

Massone C, Horn M, Kerl H, Ambros-Rudolph CM, Giovanna Brunasso AM, Cerroni L (2009) Foreign body granuloma due to Matridex injection for cosmetic purposes. Am J Dermatopathol 31(2):197–199

Matti BA, Nicolle FV (1990) Clinical use of Zyplast in correction of age- and disease-related contour deficiencies of the face. Aesthetic Plast Surg 14(3):227–234

Micheels P (2001) Human anti-hyaluronic acid antibodies: is it possible? Dermatol Surg 27(2):185–191

Moers-Carpi M et al (2007) A multicenter, randomized trial comparing calcium hydroxylapatite to two hyaluronic acids for treatment of nasolabial folds. Dermatol Surg 33(Suppl 2):S144–S151

Moers-Carpi MM, Tufet JO (2008) Calcium hydroxylapatite versus nonanimal stabilized hyaluronic acid for the correction of nasolabial folds: a 12-month, multicenter, prospective, randomized, controlled, split-face trial. Dermatol Surg 34(2):210–215

Monstrey SJ, Pitaru S, Hamdi M, Van Landuyt K, Blondeel P, Shiri J, Goldlust A, Shoshani D (2007) A two-stage phase I trial of Evolence30 collagen for soft-tissue contour correction. Plast Reconstr Surg 120:303–311

Moody BR, Sengelmann RD (2000) Self-limited adverse reaction to human-derived collagen injectable product. Dermatol Surg 26(10):936–938

Moyle GJ et al (2004) A randomized open-label study of immediate versus delayed polylactic acid injections for the cosmetic management of facial lipoatrophy in persons with HIV infection. HIV Med 5(2):82–87

Nadarajah JT, Collins M, Raboud J, Su D, Rao K, Loutfy MR, Walmsley S (2012) Infectious Complications of Bio-Alcamid Filler Used for HIV-Related Facial Lipoatrophy. Clin Infect Dis 55:1568–1574

Narins RS et al (2003) A randomized, double-blind, multicenter comparison of the efficacy and tolerability of Restylane versus Zyplast for the correction of nasolabial folds. Dermatol Surg 29(6):588–595

Narins RS, Baumann L, Brandt FS, Fagien S, Glazer S, Lowe NJ, Monheit GD, Rendon MI, Rohrich RJ, Werschler WP (2010a) A randomized study of the efficacy and safety of injectable poly-L-lactic acid versus human-based collagen implant in the treatment of nasolabial fold wrinkles. J Am Acad Dermatol 62(3):448–462

Narins RS, Brandt FS, Lorenc ZP, Maas CS, Monheit GD, Smith SR (2008) Twelve-month persistency of a novel ribose-cross-linked collagen dermal filler. Dermatol Surg 34(Suppl 1):S31–S39

Narins RS, Brandt FS, Lorenc ZP, Maas CS, Monheit GD, Smith SR, McIntyre S (2007) A randomized, multicenter study of the safety and efficacy of Dermicol-P35 and non-animal-stabilized hyaluronic acid gel for the correction of nasolabial folds. Dermatol Surg 33(Suppl 2):S213–S221; discussion S21

Narins RS, Coleman WP 3rd, Rohrich R, Monheit G, Glogau R, Brandt F, Bruce S, Colen L, Dayan S, Jackson I, Maas C, Rivkin A, Sclafani A, Spivak JC (2010b) 12-Month controlled study in the United States of the safety and efficacy of a permanent 2.5 % polyacrylamide hydrogel soft-tissue filler. Dermatol Surg 36(Suppl 3):1819–1829

Narins RS, Coleman W, Donofrio L, Jones DH, Maas C, Monheit G, Kaur M, Grundy SL, Pappert EJ, Hardas B (2010c) Nonanimal sourced hyaluronic acid-based dermal filler using a cohesive polydensified matrix technology is superior to bovine collagen in the correction of moderate to severe nasolabial folds: results from a 6-month, randomized, blinded, controlled, multicenter study. Dermatol Surg 36(1):730–740

Nast A, Reytan N, Hartmann V, Pathirana D, Bachmann F, Erdmann R, Rzany B (2011) Efficacy and durability of two hyaluronic acid-based fillers in the correction of nasolabial folds: results of a prospective, randomized, double-blind, actively controlled clinical pilot study. Dermatol Surg 37:768–775

Orentreich DS (2000) Liquid injectable silicone: techniques for soft tissue augmentation. Clin Plast Surg 27(4):595–612

Palm MD, Woodhall KE, Butterwick KJ, Goldman MP (2010) Cosmetic use of poly-l-lactic acid: a retrospective study of 130 patients. Dermatol Surg 36:161–170

Perry CM (2004) Poly-L-lactic acid. Am J Clin Dermatol 5(5):361–366; discussion 367–368

Pinsky MA, Thomas JA, Murphy DK, Walker PS, Juvéderm vs. Zyplast Nasolabial Fold Study Group (2008) Juvéderm injectable gel: a multicenter, double-blind,

randomized study of safety and effectiveness. Aesthet Surg J 28(1):17–23. doi:10.1016/j.asj.2007.09.005
Protopapa C et al (2003) Bio-Alcamid in drug-induced lipodystrophy. J Cosmet Laser Ther 5(3–4):226–230
Rapaport MJ et al (1996) Injectable silicone: cause of facial nodules, cellulitis, ulceration, and migration. Aesthetic Plast Surg 20(3):267–276
Raulin C et al (2000) Exudative granulomatous reaction to hyaluronic acid (Hylaform). Contact Dermatitis 43(3):178–179
Requena C et al (2001) Adverse reactions to injectable aesthetic microimplants. Am J Dermatopathol 23(3):197–202
Rossner F, Roßner M, Hartmann V, Erdmann R, Wiest LG, Rzany B (2009a) Decrease of reported adverse events to injectable polylactic acid after recommending an increased dilution: eight year results from the Injectable Filler Safety-Study (IFS-Study). J Cosmet Dermatol 8(1):14–18
Rossner M, Roßner F, Bachmann F, Wiest L, Rzany B (2009b) Increased risk of severe adverse reactions towards an injectable filler composed of a fixed combination of methacrylate particles and hyaluronic acid (Dermalive®). Dermatol Surg 35(Suppl 1):367–374
Rzany B et al (2004) Anwendung von Polymilchsäure (New-Fill) in der Ästhetischen Medizin: Ergebnisse des ersten deutschen Konsensustreffens an der Charité. Ästhetische Dermatologie 3
Rzany B, Hilton S, Prager W, Hartmann V, Brandl G, Fischer TC, Gekeler O, Glöckner S, Gramlich G, Hartmann M, Lederman K, Luckner-Neugebauer J, Pavicic T, Stangl S, Walker T, Zenker S, Wolters M (2010) Expert guideline on the use of porcine collagen in aesthetic medicine. J Dtsch Dermatol Ges 8:210–217
Rzany B, Bayerl C, Bodokh I, Boineau D, Dirschka T, Queille-Roussel C, Sebastian M, Sommer B, Poncet M, Guennoun M, Podda M (2011) Efficacy and safety of a new hyaluronic acid dermal filler in the treatment of moderate nasolabial folds: 6-month interim results of a randomized, evaluator-blinded, intra-individual comparison study. J Cosmet Laser Ther 13:107–112
Rzany B, Cartier H, Kestemont P, Trevidic P, Sattler G, Kerrouche N, Dhuin JC, Ma YM (2012) Full-face rejuvenation using a range of hyaluronic acid fillers: efficacy, safety, and patient satisfaction over 6 months. Dermatol Surg 38(7 Pt 2):1153–1161
Sadick NS, Palmisano L (2009) Cheek augmentation with Dermicol-P35 27G. Aesthet Surg J 29:S5–S8
Saray A (2003) Porcine dermal collagen (Permacol) for facial contour augmentation: preliminary report. Aesthetic Plast Surg 27(5):368–375
Schelke LW, van den Elzen HJ, Canninga M, Neumann MH (2009) Complications after treatment with polyalkylimide. Dermatol Surg 35(Suppl 2):1625–1628
Schierle CF, Casas LA (2011) Nonsurgical rejuvenation of the aging face with injectable poly-L-lactic acid for restoration of soft tissue volume. Aesthet Surg J 31(1):95–109
Schuller-Petrović S, Pavlović MD, Schuller SS, Schuller-Lukić B, Neuhold N (2013) Early granulomatous foreign body reactions to a novel alginate dermal filler: the system's failure? J Eur Acad Dermatol Venereol 27(1):121–123
Sclafani AP et al (2000) Autologous collagen dispersion (Autologen) as a dermal filler: clinical observations and histologic findings. Arch Facial Plast Surg 2(1):48–52
Sclafani AP et al (2002a) Rejuvenation of the aging lip with an injectable acellular dermal graft (Cymetra). Arch Facial Plast Surg 4(4):252–257
Sclafani AP et al (2002b) Homologous collagen dispersion (dermalogen) as a dermal filler: persistence and histology compared with bovine collagen. Ann Plast Surg 49(2):181–188
Shafir R et al (2000) Long-term complications of facial injections with Restylane (injectable hyaluronic acid). Plast Reconstr Surg 106(5):1215–1216
Shoshani D, Markovitz E, Cohen Y, Heremans A, Goldlust A (2007) Skin test hypersensitivity study of a cross-linked, porcine collagen implant for aesthetic surgery. Dermatol Surg 33(Suppl 2):S152–S158
Silvers SL, Eviatar JA, Echavez MI, Pappas AL (2006) Prospective, open-label, 18-month trial of calcium hydroxylapatite (Radiesse) for facial soft-tissue augmentation in patients with human immunodeficiency virus-associated lipoatrophy: one-year durability. Plast Reconstr Surg 118(Suppl 3):34S–45S
Sklar JA, White SM (2004) Radiance FN: a new soft tissue filler. Dermatol Surg 30(5):764–768; discussion 768
Smith S, Busso M, McClaren M, Bass LS (2007) A randomized, bilateral, prospective comparison of calcium hydroxylapatite microspheres versus human-based collagen for the correction of nasolabial folds. Dermatol Surg 33(Suppl 2):S112–S121
Sperling B, Bachmann F, Hartmann V, Erdmann R, Wiest L, Rzany B (2010) The current state of treatment of adverse reactions to injectable fillers. Dermatol Surg 36(Suppl 3):1895–1904
Sung MS, Kim HG, Woo KI, Kim YD (2010) Ocular ischemia and ischemic oculomotor nerve palsy after vascular embolization of injectable calcium hydroxylapatite filler. Ophthal Plast Reconstr Surg 26(4):289–291
Tzikas TL (2004) Evaluation of the Radiance FN soft tissue filler for facial soft tissue augmentation. Arch Facial Plast Surg 6(4):234–239
Valantin MA et al (2003) Polylactic acid implants (New-Fill®) to correct facial lipoatrophy in HIV-infected patients: results of the open-label study VEGA. AIDS 17(17):2471–2477
Wang YB et al (2003) Clinically analyzing the possible side-effects after injecting hydrophilic poly-acrylamide gel as a soft-tissue filler. Zhonghua Zheng Xing Wai Ke Za Zhi 19(5):328–330
Waris E (2003) Alloplastic injectable biomaterials for soft tissue augmentation: a report on two cases with complications associated with a new material (Dermalive)

and a review of the literature. Eur J Plast Surg 26:350–355

Webster RC et al (1986) Injectable silicone for facial soft-tissue augmentation. Arch Otolaryngol Head Neck Surg 112(3):290–296

Woerle B et al (2004) Poly-L-lactic acid: a temporary filler for soft tissue augmentation. J Drugs Dermatol 3(4):385–389

Zielke H, Wölber L, Wiest L, Rzany B (2008) Risk profiles of different injectable fillers: results from the Injectable Filler Safety Study (IFS Study). Dermatol Surg 34(3):326–335; discussion 335

Selection of Patients 2

Mauricio de Maio

Contents

2.1 **Introduction** 21
2.2 **General Rules** 22
2.3 **The First Consultation** 24
2.4 **The Facial Thirds System** 25
2.5 **The Ideal Patient** 25
2.6 **The Aging Patient** 25
2.7 **The Patient with Facial Imperfections** 26
2.8 **The Patient You Do Not Want to Treat** 27
2.9 **The Dysmorphic Patient** 28
References 28

2.1 Introduction

Patients' perception of their needs and medical diagnosis differs much more than we imagine. One important reason is that patients usually look at themselves at the mirror in frontal view while the observers (including the doctor) look at them mainly in the oblique view. Differences in position and angles result in differences in prioritization of aesthetic needs for both patients and doctors. We also find differences in treatment planning among doctors which may lead to confusion to patients if they happen to consult more than one injector for the same indication. Differences in experience, problems in communication, and to a large extent limitation in injector's technical skills represent the main reasons for discrepancy in treatment planning among different doctors. For example, the reasons that some injectors will *not* suggest volume replacement in a patient with severe sunken temples include (a) the unawareness of the patient of this indication which therefore remains unrequested and/or (b) the doctor's inability to give a proper diagnosis, technical deficiency, and lack of experience to predict whether the diagnosis, technique, and product will lead to a result that will finally make the patient happy! Cultural aspects, poor training in medical/patient communication, and lack of time or patience to educate patients are further barriers to obtain more efficient results (see also Chap. 4).

Technical ability is fundamental for good medical practice, but the correct selection of

M. de Maio, B. Rzany, *Injectable Fillers in Aesthetic Medicine*,
DOI 10.1007/978-3-642-45125-6_2, © Springer-Verlag Berlin Heidelberg 2014

patients is mandatory. Physicians who would like to successfully practice aesthetic medicine must understand that the vast majority of patients are unaware of what they really need (see above). They know (hopefully) what they want; however, it is the physician who has the knowledge of the anatomical base and the aging process and who has to find a compromise between the expectations of the patient and what is feasible.

Do's

- Do take time to educate your patient about the benefits of the treatments that you believe are important to them.
- Do try to overcome the barriers that block you to obtain more efficient treatments. Long-term patient retention will depend on that.

Don'ts

- Do not automatically deliver what the patients are asking for. They may have a wrong perception of their needs.

Key Points

- All injectors will sooner or later be able to deliver a satisfactory technical result. Long-term patient retention does not rely on delivering patients' request only.

FAQs

- Why are some doctors reluctant to be more active in indicating a procedure that the patient is unaware of?

  Cultural aspects, problems in communication, lack of time or patience to educate patients, the inability to perform proper diagnosis, technical deficiency, and lack of experience to predict whether the diagnosis, technique, and product are the main reasons that prevent injectors from being more active and efficient in treating cosmetic patients.

Patients are prone to ask for procedures that they have heard of or read about in lay magazines. For example, it is quite common for patients to request treatment of nasolabial folds with botulinum toxin A (BoNT-A) only because this product is widely advertised. In most cases, however, injection of BoNT-A into the nasolabial fold would result in an unhappy patient because this would have little effect on the depth of the fold. Understanding patients' complaints and educating them according to their needs will minimize patient dissatisfaction and increase patient retention.

Patients with multiple needs and requesting immediate results are legendary. The first consultation is very important, as it gives the physician the opportunity to establish the kind of patient he will be treating. Uncompromising patients, for example, are best avoided. Dissatisfaction with prior aesthetic procedures is one of the most important points to be evaluated. It is therefore mandatory to conduct a thorough examination of their past history, which should include any prior cosmetic procedure, and how the result was perceived by the patient. Depending on the answer, the practitioner can evaluate the patient's perception. Unrealistic expectations are another important factor to be analyzed before starting with any treatment. Experience shows that sometimes it is preferable not to treat a specific patient because, whatever is done, dissatisfaction will invariably result.

2.2 General Rules

As mentioned before, the first consultation is very important for both the patient and the physician. Before the advent of the digital camera, the physician would make a communicative effort to make the patient understand the limits of treatments and, in particular, the limits of a specific treatment for a specific patient. The lack of knowledge of the vast majority of patients would often make it difficult for them to truly understand what the physician is telling them. Showing some before and after pictures could be useful in some cases but may be disastrous in others. Only the best cases would be shown, and patients may gain an unreasonably positive impression of the results, since these results may not be achievable in their case.

Without the digital camera, it is particularly hard to make patients understand the physical limitations of certain procedures. Patients often do not look at themselves in the mirror in the proper way (they perceive themselves in a more frontal view). Patients unconsciously correct any defects by smiling or changing the angle when facing the mirror. It is quite difficult for human beings to face differences in beauty and accept the aging process. If a woman was quite beautiful when she was young, it is even harder to accept that she cannot become that beautiful again, even after an invasive cosmetic procedure.

After many years working with cosmetic patients and also teaching injectors worldwide, it became evident that there is a "blind spot" for both patients and injectors when it comes to the evaluation of facial features. Basically, cosmetic practitioners aim to beautify, correct, or prevent aging signs. When assessing a patient, we may use a simple quantitative scale that almost everybody in the world is familiar with: 0–10. We may deliberately say that 0 (zero) is the worst that someone may look at that specific age, ethnicity, and gender and 10 (ten) is the top, the most desirable, and perfect human being that exists on the planet. We dare say that no one will be a zero or 10! But we can exercise and assess a patient and roughly and subjectively give a grading in this scale. Even more interesting is to evaluate what upgrades and downgrades the overall grading. For instance, a 50-year-old woman may have a beautiful nose according to the beauty pattern of that specific community but may have an unfavorable lip. We may then say that her nose upgrades her but her lips downgrades her. Facial shape, proportion, eyebrows, cheekbones, and so forth should receive the same rule.

As discussed previously, patients are mostly aware of problems that they see in the frontal view and basically the signs that come with the aging process. So, a patient that was born with a distracting nose but is used to it since she was born will most likely complain about the nasolabial fold that became more prominent with aging (and in the frontal view!). So, her nose is in the "blind spot" of self-perception. This is so true that when a doctor, a relative, or a friend uncovers it, patients become aware and may decide to have that area treated. The "blind spot" also affects the doctors' ability to assess patients unbiased. These blind spots might be ethnic related. For a Caucasian doctor, wide, low, and flat noses may be considered distracting because he understands that noses are expected to be high and narrow as commonly found in Caucasians. That means that low noses should be included in the treatment plan of a patient. Some noses that are in the "blind spot" for Asian doctors are not for Caucasian doctors. The same is found for the lack of chin projection, mid-cheek deficiency, or prominent ears in Asians. In contrast, Caucasians are happy when they have only three to five wrinkles in the crow's feet area (where they may have 15!) compared to a single wrinkle in a young Asian female patient (that she considers distracting) which may be in the "blind spot" for a Caucasian doctor when prioritizing the treatment for that patient.

Do's

- Do analyze the structural and aging signs of your patient before establishing the treatment plan.
- Do take a mirror and/or digital photographs when communicating with the patient.
- Take sufficient time for yourself and your patients when analyzing the facial structures.

Don'ts

- Do not disregard yours and your patient's ethnic background.

Key Points

- Remember the "blind spot": patients usually complain about aging signs and they are blind to structural problems or deficiencies.
- Patients see what is in the frontal view, while observers mainly see the oblique view.
- If you want to give a "WOW" look to your patients, try to enhance the facial aspects that are seen mainly in the oblique view. Make a test!
- Ask your patients to look at the mirror or to look at their photos and ask them to describe what they see. You will be impressed by the complete absence of self-perception that most of them have. On the other hand, you may also find some that are extremely accurate and help you see details that were in the injector's blind spot!

2.3 The First Consultation

When patients come into the office, they usually complete a consultation form in which they are asked what they would like to be treated. In the next step, a complete past history should be obtained and pictures taken in several positions (frontal, oblique, profile), from both the static and dynamic points of view. Before the consultation, the photographs are downloaded onto a computer, and the physician and the patient go through the consultation form and finally the photographs themselves. It is important to tell the patients before the pictures are shown that nobody likes this phase of the consultation but that it is the most effective way of getting straight to the point and that it will be helpful to make them understand their needs. By following this procedure, the consultation becomes more objective and time is not wasted.

It is impressive how difficult it is for patients to see themselves exposed in this way, particularly when it is the own body that is being analyzed, and as such the practitioner should be very sensitive towards their potential feelings.

It is interesting that it is usually the patient him- or herself who points out what treatment is required rather than the practitioner. It is also at this point that some patients quickly change their mind about what they want to treat and discrepancies that arise with regard to what was noted on the consultation form and what is desired now can be pointed out. This is the best opportunity to enlist the patient's trust and when we can begin to point out what we can do to help the patient improve.

The first consultation is also an important moment to get in contact with the patient's personality. Anxious and very talkative patients may affect our judgment and influence our decision. It is also the moment to reflect the patients' and injectors' blind spots. Initially, the patient's motivation has to be verified, followed by a systematization of the diagnosis process and the design of a consistent treatment plan.

Do's

- Do take time to listen and observe your patient in the first consultation. It is one of the most important moments to build up a long-term relationship with your patient.
- Do have time to think and design your treatment plan for your patient before you both decide what is the best option for them.

Don'ts

- Do not let yourself be contaminated or influenced negatively by your patients' anxiety or misperception of their needs.

Key Points

- The first consultation is the ideal opportunity to identify both patients' and injectors' "blind spots."

2.4 The Facial Thirds System

To ensure that patients understand their aesthetic problems, the face is divided didactically into the classical three thirds: superior, medial, and inferior. The patient will be informed that in the process of the consultation, all of the positive and less positive aspects of their face will be discussed (it is recommendable that physicians avoid the use of any *negative* word during the consultation). Any possible negative aspect should be balanced by some positive aspect in the face. The physician should point out what must be treated and whether it is a surgical or nonsurgical procedure that should be performed. In general, saggy skin is treated with surgery, peels, or fractionated lasers, dynamic wrinkles with BoNT-A, and wrinkles, folds, and volume loss with fillers. Patients start to realize what can be treated with these different types of procedures and what is needed to promote a real improvement. Some patients cannot be subjected to all procedures due to either social or economic reasons. Depending on specific circumstances, the intended procedures need to be discussed and their limitations pointed out. It is very important to tell patients directly about the benefits and limitations of each procedure that they will be subject to.

The facial thirds system is very helpful to structure the consultation so that no important aspect on the face is overlooked (see also Chap. 4).

Do's

- Do use the facial thirds system to structure the consultation and to bring awareness about the potential of the areas to be treated.

Don'ts

- Do not forget to observe every detail during the facial thirds analysis. It will be helpful for the treatment plan.

2.5 The Ideal Patient

The ideal patient is happy to listen to what the physician has to say. This patient is able to point out what is bothering him or her and is willing to understand what steps must be taken in order to reach the desired aesthetic improvement. The ideal patient is able to balance the positive and negative outcomes and therefore is able to make the most suitable choice. It is clear to him or her that even minimum invasive procedures must be handled by experienced physicians. The ideal patient discusses the type of product to be injected and is concerned about adverse effects. When it comes to the duration of the fillers, the ideal patient can understand perfectly differences in degrees of permanence when informed about the internal and external factors that may influence filler duration. The ideal patient is willing to learn what can be done to maintain good results and what should be avoided. It is perfectly understandable to him or her that the aging process is a continuing process and that there will be a need to return for other procedures to maintain the aesthetic result.

2.6 The Aging Patient

The aging process happens to all people who live long. This does not mean, however, that our patients are prepared for that. Women, in general, are more likely to feel depressed by age-related changes to their body. Saggy skin, deep folds, wrinkles, and aging spots are some of the major signs that develop during this phase. It is hard to look at the mirror and at previous photographs and realize that time has passed. It is important to explain to patients that the aging process is complex and it results from various factors. If that is understood, patients may admit that a single procedure is not enough to solve all of the disturbances that accompany the aging process. It is easier if it is explained to the patients that the aging process derives from intrinsic and extrinsic reasons. Extrinsic aging results from environmental influences such as sun exposure, smoking, and climate. Intrinsic aging is influenced mainly by genetics. Asking the patients what their parents look like makes them aware of the fact that what is happening to them is natural. The most important information that patients must be given is that nothing can stop the aging process but that something can always be done to smooth the signs of aging. The better they are, the better they can get. The sooner they start, the less invasive the procedure will be. It happens very often with fillers. The deeper the fold is, the greater the number of injections must be given. When I am asked about duration, I advise patients that they are starting a recovery process and that they should not let the wrinkles or folds get that deep again. Patients must be told that when they are starting a new procedure, they will have to come more frequently during the first year and that it is possible that the intervals between visits will increase if they are to be properly treated. They must be told that even with very good fillers, there is no permanent miracle. The aging process is dynamic, and so, therefore, must be the procedures.

Do's

- Do remind yourself and your patients that the sooner the treatment is started, the better the results will be.

Don'ts

- Do not ignore the external and internal factors that might have influenced the aging process.

Key Points

- Aging is a continuous process that starts from mild to moderate and may end up severe or even finally very severe.
- We do not go to sleep looking young and wake up looking old the following day.

FAQs

- Why should we start treating our patients early when the problems are still mild?

  Firstly, because at an early stage, mild problems are easier to handle from a technical point of view; secondly, the quantity of product used and the total number of procedures to achieve satisfactory results are lower when compared to severe cases.
- Why do older patients seem to be happier than younger patients with the results?

  Younger patients may become very happy with our results, but some younger patients in contrast will be more demanding and are much less tolerant to any not-so-perfect result. This might be even a barrier for some injectors who finally may end up avoiding treating younger and/or very attractive patients.

2.7 The Patient with Facial Imperfections

We are all quite asymmetric, and yet beauty is defined by balance and symmetry. The vast majority of patients that search for cosmetic improvement may be neither symmetric nor balanced. Before initiating the consultation, it is important to define as objectively as possible the evaluation of the patient's physical attributes. The patient should be examined in the anterior, posterior, oblique, and profile positions. Static and dynamic analyses are also important. A patient's imperfections may only be observed during dynamic analysis. It is usually quite impolite for the practitioner to start pointing out all the imperfections that patients present. Here, a digital camera may play a fundamental role in protecting the physician against being unkind to the patient. As it is often said, a picture or a short video in case of dynamic asymmetries says more than 1,000 words. It is the patient who, when looking at the picture, will see and describe what he or she sees. This may be very difficult for patients, and the physician again should be gentle and lead them to understand what can be done to improve their facial imperfections. It is not uncommon that patients feel depressed when they look at their pictures.

The dialogue starts and the patient's wishes and expectations are evaluated. Patients with imperfections may say they want everything changed; they feel themselves distorted, old, and imperfect. Dividing the face into the aforementioned three thirds is useful for the physician to focus on specific areas and ask the patient questions such as: What do you see in your forehead? Is there anything that bothers you there? Questions like these help the physician to indicate either surgical or nonsurgical methods. It is also important to determine whether or not the patient is open to a surgery or a nonsurgical procedure. Depending on the patient's answer, the physician may explain what result is achievable by surgical or nonsurgical methods. A patient's dissatisfaction arises mainly from promises made by the physician that remain unfulfilled after the procedure.

Patients should be told that there are imperfections that arise from the osseous structures and that it is hard to treat these with noninvasive methods. The practitioner should be experienced enough to establish whether the imperfections are from soft or hard tissues or from skin, fat, or muscle. The combination of BoNT-A and fillers may solve many imperfections in the skin, fat, and muscle. It is advisable to treat the imperfections step by step to perceive the gradual improvement. The physician may, based on experience, start with the procedures that will produce the most benefit for the patient. The patient's confidence grows and so will continue to allow other procedures. It is important to point out that balancing both the static and dynamic aspects of the face involves more than simply filling a wrinkle or fold. It is very rewarding for a physician to realize that the patients with unusual cosmetic imperfections that they have treated feel much better after the procedure.

Do's

- Do remember that with accurate assessment and proper technique, we may help with injectables many patients with facial imperfections that are not eligible for surgery or do not desire surgery.

Don'ts

- Do not promise anything that you cannot or are uncertain to deliver to patients with facial imperfection. They may already be a victim of an inexperienced or unethical injector.

2.8 The Patient You Do Not Want to Treat

Bad candidates for cosmetic procedures may come from different economic, social, and ethnic backgrounds. The physician must be able to see the red flags behind some patients at the first consultation. At this time the physician must evaluate whether it is worthwhile recommending the procedure or not. Patients with unrealistic expectations will invariably be dissatisfied with the results of cosmetic procedures. Extreme expectations may lead to poor results. For the cosmetic practitioner, some results may be considered excellent, but the patient may consider them extremely poor. Patients may believe that a cosmetic procedure will solve their personal problems, such as the expectation of looking 30 years younger, getting a new job, and improving their love life. Patients who have suffered any acute extreme psychological stress (e.g., the loss of a spouse) should also be avoided until they recover from it. Cosmetic procedures should not be considered as a compensation for life's disappointments. Both the physician and the patient must agree with the expected final result; if not, it is advisable to avoid the procedure.

Patients are sometimes reluctant to hear what they are being told; they are considered poor listeners. Patients with deficient communication skills are also undesirable candidates. The understanding of possible adverse events and complications is very important. Poor listeners do not tend to hear topics like these. They must be encouraged to repeat what the likely result is and the risks of any procedure. Care should also be taken with manipulative, indecisive, impulsive, and hysterical patients. Other patients to be avoided are those who are obsessively concerned with some aspects of their appearance; they may be dysmorphic.

Do's

- Do give yourself the right NOT to treat a patient that you are not comfortable with. There will always be the right patient for the right injector. Refer them!

Don'ts

- Do not treat patients that have suffered from an acute psychological stress until they have recovered.

2.9 The Dysmorphic Patient

Patients with dysmorphism are those obsessively preoccupied with real or imaginary defects. They may even take the mirror to point out a defect that has not been noted by the physician. In general, those defects are minor but are perceived by them to be disfiguring. The inability to deal with unavoidable scars is also a warning that dissatisfaction may arise after the cosmetic procedure. Some patients do have a real psychiatric or emotional disorder. Patients with depression, borderline personality, obsessive-compulsive, and narcissistic disorders should be avoided (Fig. 2.1).

The physician should decline any patient that they consider to be a poor candidate, telling them objectively, but, in a compassionate way, that the result they are looking for cannot be obtained by him.

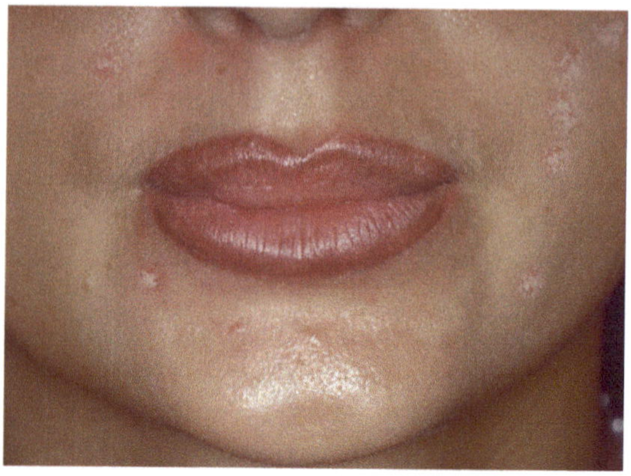

Fig. 2.1 Dysmorphic patient. The patient perceived her lips as too small and requested a touch up. Please note the small excoriations on the patient's cheek, which are consistent with the features of acne excoriée, a neurotic skin disease

Don'ts

- Do not try to compensate dysmorphic patients with cosmetic procedures. It will usually not work well.

Key Points

- If your assessment differs considerably from the assessment of a patient (e.g., the lip looks normal to you; for the patient the lips looks disastrously wrong), be very careful. It might be a patient who suffers from dysmorphism. You will very unlikely be able to make this patient happy.

References

Adamson PA, Kraus WM (1995) Management of patient dissatisfaction with cosmetic surgery. Facial Plast Surg 11(2):99–104

Baker TJ (1978) Patient selection and psychological evaluation. Clin Plast Surg 5(1):3–14

Katez P (1991) The dissatisfied patient. Plast Surg Nurs 11(1):13–16

Lewis CM et al (1983) Patient selection and patient satisfaction. Clin Plast Surg 10(2):321–332

Sarwer DB (1997) The "obsessive" cosmetic surgery patient: a consideration of body image dissatisfaction and body dysmorphic disorder. Plast Surg Nurs 17(4): 193–197, 209

Vuyk HD, Zijlker TD (1995) Psychosocial aspects of patient counseling and selection: a surgeon's perspective. Facial Plast Surg 11(2):55–60

Requirements and Rules

3

Berthold Rzany and Mauricio de Maio

Contents

3.1 **General Requirements** 31
3.1.1 Introduction 31
3.1.2 Documentation 31
3.1.3 Charts 31
3.1.4 Photographs 32
3.1.5 Consent 33
3.1.6 Treatment Plan 33
3.1.7 Staff 33

3.2 **Technical Requirements** 34
3.2.1 Room 34
3.2.2 Chair 34
3.2.3 Mirror 34
3.2.4 Small Things 34
3.2.5 First Aid Kit 34
3.2.6 Tips, Tricks and Key Points 35

3.3 **The 13 General Rules** 35
3.3.1 Introduction 35
3.3.2 Rule 1: Listen to the Patient 35
3.3.3 Rule 2: Fillers Are Only One Tool 35
3.3.4 Rule 3: Talk About Money 36
3.3.5 Rule 4: Talk About Possible Adverse Events 36
3.3.6 Rule 5: Avoid Disturbed Patients 36
3.3.7 Rule 6: Anesthesia (Treat with as Little Pain as Possible!) 37
3.3.8 Rule 7: Position (Keep the Patient Upright) 37
3.3.9 Rule 8: Use the Mirror/Digital Images 37
3.3.10 Rule 9: Start with a Biodegradable Filler First 38
3.3.11 Rule 10: Quantity of Filler (Do Not Inject Insufficient Amounts) 38
3.3.12 Rule 11: Quantity of Filler (Do Not Inject Too Much) 38
3.3.13 Rule 12: Use the Appropriate Depth of Injection 38
3.3.14 Rule 13: If Something Goes Wrong 39

References 39

3.1 General Requirements

3.1.1 Introduction

To ensure a safe and efficient procedure, several requirements must be met. The following list is not intended to give a complete overview, but to give some tips on preparations that might be helpful.

3.1.2 Documentation

A thorough documentation of all treatment-related data is highly recommended. This not only is advisable for legal and billing reasons but will help to improve your own performance and consequently the patient's satisfaction.

3.1.3 Charts

The patient's chart should include all necessary information. It does not matter if the chart is paper based or electronic. The only thing that counts is that the information in the chart is complete and accurate.

As with every chart, the patient's identification data, gender, and age need to be documented first. In the next step, the reason for the patient's visit should be documented. Furthermore, at this step, the history of relevant concomitant diseases (e.g., autoimmune diseases), present relevant drug intake (e.g., the

M. de Maio, B. Rzany, *Injectable Fillers in Aesthetic Medicine*,
DOI 10.1007/978-3-642-45125-6_3, © Springer-Verlag Berlin Heidelberg 2014

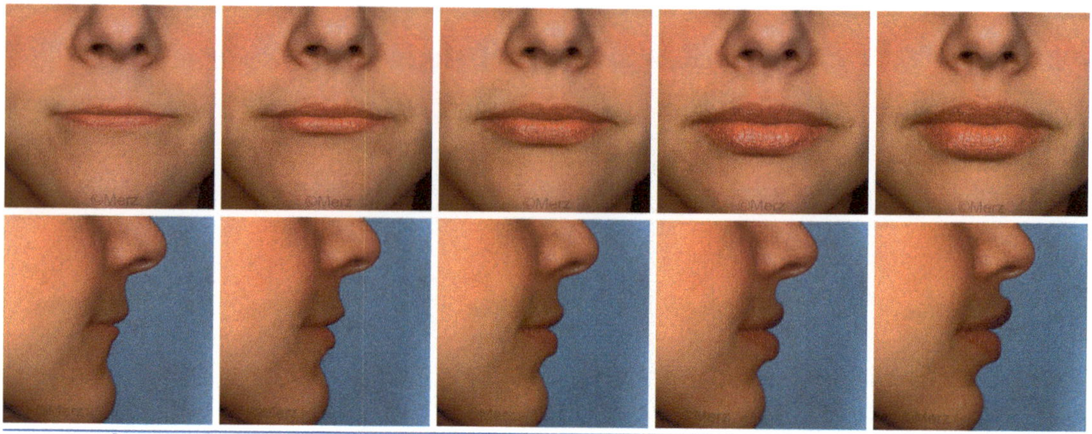

Fig. 3.1 Validated Lip Fullness Grading Scale (Carruthers et al. 2008d; © Merz)

intake of acetylsalicylic acid!), and previous aesthetic procedures should be documented. In particular, all previous injections of fillers should be thoroughly assessed.

Patients must be thoroughly examined. Clinical severity can be assessed by using clinical wrinkles and volumes scales as the Merz Aesthetics Scales™ (Carruthers et al. 2008a, b, c, d, e (several publications) and 2012; Flynn et al. 2012) (Fig. 3.1).

Besides that, the treatment itself needs to be documented. The product used, the dilution (if any), the injected areas, the depth of injections, and the injected volumes should be logged. A graphical sketch might be helpful, too. Special attention should be given to the "lot" number of the filler used because this identifies the production batch and, in the event of adverse effects, might allow the manufacturer to trace an entire batch.

Last but not least, the chart should always include the informed consent of the patient. If you use electronic medical records, the consent should be scanned. For legal reasons, however, it might be necessary to keep the original in a specific binder.

3.1.4 Photographs

It is advisable to document the status of the patient before the treatment. If possible, the photographs should be standardized. Patients should be photographed frontal and at 90° and/or 45°. Standardization requires some effort, such as using a fixed setting or following standard procedures. In addition to being useful as legal documentation, these photographs will help to improve your communication with the patient (see Chaps. 2 and 4).

If you already have incorporated standardized photographs in your practice, you may also consider taking the full set of photos in selected cases. There are five traditional positions as described above (frontal view, right and left oblique, right and left full profile) in variable situations such as angry, surprised, kissing, full smile, chin down, and chin up depending on the type of treatment that is being carried out on the patient (Fig. 3.2).

Do's

- Do take photographs! You need them anyway for the first consultation when the first steps of the treatment plan are laid out.

Don'ts

- Do not worry if the photographic quality is not as good as you want it to be. This is not a photography contest but a tool for patient communication and documentation. A photo from your smartphone might be sufficient enough.

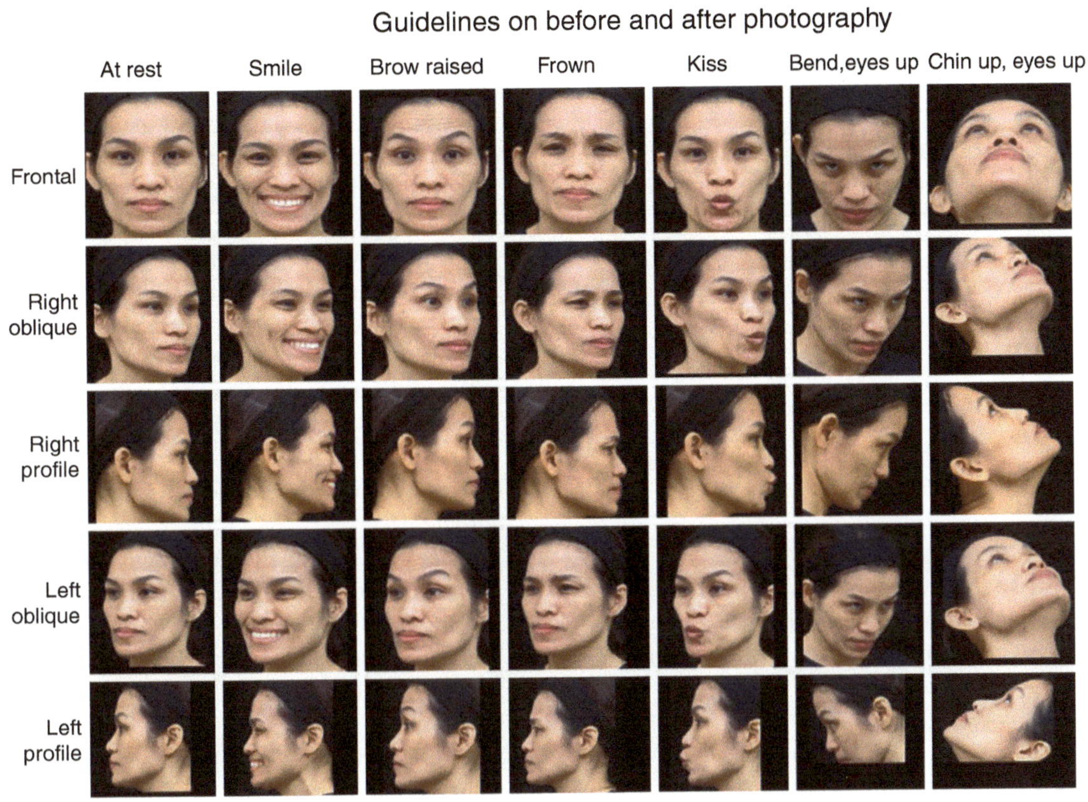

Fig. 3.2 Ideal baseline documentation of a patient's full face (© de Maio and Allergan)

3.1.5 Consent

The consent of each patient should be thoroughly documented. Patients should date and sign a consent form for each new filler substance. A patient information brochure that includes all of the necessary information on the estimated efficacy and possible adverse events should accompany the consent form.

Don'ts

- Do not forget to also get the photographic consent if you would like to use the photos for educational purposes.

3.1.6 Treatment Plan

When using fillers, which ususally require repeated injections, a treatment plan is highly recommended. A treatment plan allows realistic planning, taking into account the patient's and the doctor's perspectives (see Chaps. 2 and 4).

3.1.7 Staff

Staff needs to be trained in marketing, quality control, and assistance. They should be aware of the aesthetic procedures offered and should be able to provide some information about the fillers used. They are responsible for monitoring the patient's chart and for ensuring that all necessary documents are available and signed by the patient. And finally, the staff may help to apply topical anesthesia, massage the area after the injection of the filler, or add cooling before or after the injection to reduce pain and swelling. Staff might also assist with, makeup after the treatment, so that the patient leaves the clinic with no or little visible signs of the procedure performed.

3.2 Technical Requirements

3.2.1 Room

The procedure room should be brightly lit. Light from above might be helpful to detect even the tiniest areas to be corrected.

Do's

- Do provide good light for result evaluation. Make sure your patient leaves the office assured that expectations have been met.

Key Points

- It is not uncommon that patients complain about results when they evaluate themselves at home under improper light conditions.

3.2.2 Chair

For most procedures, patients should have a relaxed upright position to ensure that optimal correction of the facial lines or volume deficits can be achieved. However, a more reclined position might be helpful when treating more painful areas such as the upper lip. In case of a vasovagal syncope – which occasionally might happen – the chair should be adjustable, allowing an elevation of the legs.

3.2.3 Mirror

Like the patient's baseline digital photography, a mirror should be provided to ensure that patient–doctor communication is optimal from the start. The doctor should use the mirror to ensure that patient and doctor are discussing exactly the same areas to be treated and the grade of correction that is desired. When using the mirror, ask the patient to point at the area where he or she wants the correction. This will reduce the risk of misinterpretations.

3.2.4 Small Things

A standard setting can prove useful to ensure that all tools required are available. All required tools, listed below, should all be within reach.

- Patient information and consent forms
- Documentation material for source data (electronic or conventional charts)
- Handheld mirror
- Camera (conventional or digital) for photographic documentation (an iPad or another tablet computer might prove to be very helpful here – or even an iPhone or another smartphone)
- Gloves (unsterile gloves are usually sufficient)
- Topical local anesthetic or syringe, cannulas, and/or needles with appropriate local anesthesia
- Topical disinfectant (octenidine-containing solutions will be fine)
- Compresses
- The injectable filler, appropriate syringes, cannulas and/or needles
- Cool packs or precooled saline to soak the compresses
- Cosmetic powder makeup powder to decrease the visible redness after the filler injections (this works for men too!)
- Emergency kit (in case of an anaphylactic reaction towards the local anesthetic). Please note for some procedures such as high-volume replacement (e.g., penile enlargement) more sterile conditions apply.

Do's

- Do not forget to stack make up or cosmetic powder. Your patients will be thankful if they can cover post-injection redness before leaving your practice.

3.2.5 First Aid Kit

Most injectable fillers have zero risk for systemic reactions. However, local anesthesia might cause anaphylactic reactions (fortunately very rarely), and it is possible for patients to collapse due to circulatory imbalance, for example, when treating the upper lip area with insufficient local anesthesia (Berkun et al. 2003). The first aid kit should also include hyaluronidase which needs to be used immediately after an inadvertent arterial occlusion after an HA injection.

Do's

- Do include hyaluronidase in your first aid kit in case you are treating with HAs.

3.2.6 Tips, Tricks and Key Points

Most complaints from unsatisfied patients can be attributable to insufficient communication between the doctor and the patient. So please take your time to listen to the patient and make sure that you understand what the patient actually wants and not what you want to understand (see also Chaps. 2 and 4).

3.3 The 13 General Rules

3.3.1 Introduction

Working with injectable fillers can be extremely rewarding for both the patient and the treating physician if some simple rules are followed. These rules will be discussed more in depth in other chapters of this book.

3.3.2 Rule 1: Listen to the Patient

Patients and doctors are prone to the same verbal misunderstandings as everybody else. In aesthetic medicine, the results may be disastrous if the doctor misunderstands the patient. It is therefore very important to listen to the patient, to try to understand what the patient really wants. If possible, use a digital photograph of the patient as the basis for your discussions and also introduce realistic pre- and post-photos of patients that have been treated in a similar way. However, try to make it clear that every patient presents different responses and the patient must understand that the very same result is not applicable and it is used mainly for patient education.

Do's

- Do explain the potential of treatment of areas that are not primarily requested by your patient, but are important to aesthetic balance of the face. Most of the time, patients' dissatisfaction results from wrong perception or lack of proper medical advice (see Chap. 4).

Key Points

- Check the legal aspect in your country regarding showing other patients' results. This may be seen as a "promise" of result and may lead to legal issues when not obtained.

3.3.3 Rule 2: Fillers Are Only One Tool

Even when you are very enthusiastic about fillers, do not forget that fillers are only one tool in aesthetic medicine. Do not treat indications with fillers that might better be treated with another method. For example, BoNT-A is the first-line treatment for wrinkles of the glabella; biodegradable injectable fillers should come as a second step in this area (see also Chap. 9).

Key Points

- Some patients are reluctant to the use of botulinum toxin due to negative media information. Proper patient's education is mandatory.
- Aging process is multifactorial and a single tool cannot cope with the complexity of it.

3.3.4 Rule 3: Talk About Money

The patient should have a clear understanding of what he will have to pay for which treatment. If you use biodegradable fillers, make it clear that for most patients, one treatment will not be enough and that subsequent treatments will be necessary to ensure a good result. It might be helpful to include the subsequent treatments in the first cost estimation for the patient. Tell the patient, for example, "If you start with this procedure (and you like it), you will need to have at least two to three treatments over the following 12 months, which will cost you approximately this amount of money per month."

Do's
- Do explain to your patients what the benefits are of starting the treatments when the problems are mild to moderate.
- Do make realistic estimations. If the final bill is somewhat less than the initial estimate, patients will appreciate that.

Don'ts
- Do not lure patients with unrealistically cheap prize calculations. They will be disappointed when they discover at some time point that they will need far more money to achieve satisfying results.

Key Points
- Most of the difficulties when dealing with patients' budgets derive from the inability of the injector to thoroughly explain the benefits of the investment.
- The sooner we start, the less amount of product is needed and the lower the cost will be.
- Aesthetic financial planning is as much an art as it is to inject properly!

3.3.5 Rule 4: Talk About Possible Adverse Events

Adverse events can occur with all fillers (see Chap. 8). Make sure that patients understand what might occur without frightening them.

Key Points
- With the advent of longer-lasting biodegradable fillers, the proportion of patients suffering from adverse reactions to nonbiodegradable fillers will decrease as nonbiodegradable filler will be used less and less. However, adverse events will be always present.
- Adverse events might be patient related, product related, and/or injector related. The triad of an inexperienced injector, products not evaluated in good clinical trials, and patients with present risk factors might multiply the risk of adverse or an unwanted reaction.
- Patients need to be aware of a certain risk without being unnecessarily frightened.

3.3.6 Rule 5: Avoid Disturbed Patients

Dysmorphia (see Chap. 2) exaggerates the negative implications of certain bodily features for a patient. The patient shown in Fig. 2.1, for example, felt her lips to be particularly small and requested a touch up to make the lips even bigger. Patients with a dysmorphic disorder can make a physician's life miserable. Therefore, be very careful if there is a disproportion between what the patient sees and what you can see. If you have doubts, talk the patient out of the procedure (or your office).

Don'ts
- Don't try to apply the very same recipe to all patients. Patients must be analyzed correctly in order to understand their motivation.

Key Points

- Most of the time, dysmorphic patients are impossible to please because their complaints are not realistic.

3.3.7 Rule 6: Anesthesia (Treat with as Little Pain as Possible!)

You do not want a patient with tears running down the cheeks. Using a filler which is premixed with lidocaine (as most of the HA fillers are now [Monheit et al. 2010]) or mixing lidocaine to a filler which otherwise might be painful (as hydroxylapatite) will reduce pain considerably (Marmur et al. 2010). Pain can be further reduced by topical anesthetics or local anesthesia (see Chap. 5).

Do's

- Use lidocaine-containing fillers or add a local anesthetic to the filler.
- Usually a topical local anesthetic will be sufficient when a lidocaine-containing filler is used.
- For very pain-sensitive patients, a nerve block might be considered.

Key Points

- Patients may be reluctant to undergo cosmetic procedures due to bad experiences related to pain.
- Cosmetic experience must be pleasant and not a nightmare due to pain.
- Be especially cautious with novice patients.

3.3.8 Rule 7: Position (Keep the Patient Upright)

You might treat the patient in a supine position. However, when gravity is likely to influence the depth of the wrinkles, for example, in the case of volume deficiencies or deep folds, the patient should be seated in the upright position. If not, the deficits or folds will be under- or even over corrected.

Some injectors feel more comfortable to inject the patient lying down than in an upright position. This is helpful in reducing a vasovagal syncope. But the evaluation of results is preferably performed with the patient in an upright position where the effect of gravity can be verified.

Do's

- Do evaluate your patient in the upright position to check if the treatment with fillers or volumizer was effective.

Key Points

- Do not forget to evaluate the patient not only in upright position but also in the leaning forward position (chin down – eyes up). If there is loss of correction in these positions, patients might not be satisfied for a long time.

3.3.9 Rule 8: Use the Mirror/Digital Images

Using mirror and/or digital images will help your communication with the patient: to plan the procedure appropriately, to increase the patient's understanding of the nature and the possibilities of the procedure, and to ensure that the final effect is what the patient wants. Although most patients do not want to watch the procedure itself, they are usually very interested in taking a look at the preliminary results. Showing the patient the half-treated status will ensure that they acknowledge the difference. The frequency of sentences like "I do not see any difference" may be reduced by this.

Do's

- Do encourage the patients to look at the mirror/digital images before starting the

treatment and do ask them to clearly point out the areas that they consider to be treated.
- With a small quantitiy of the the product left in the syringe hand the patient the mirror again and ask them what in their eyes still needs correction. It is a disaster if the patient has the final look in the mirror and sees something that, with an additional 0.1 ml, could have been corrected.

Key Points
- Women and mirrors are interesting to watch! They are likely to start fixing the hair and pursuing before they can really focus and point out the distracting areas. Another habit is to put down the mirror and avoid looking at it. Be aware of this and guide them gently back on track.

3.3.10 Rule 9: Start with a Biodegradable Filler First

If you have a patient who comes for a nonbiodegradable filler, start with a biodegradable filler first. Injecting a nonbiodegradable filler at the first visit can lead to very unhappy patients, e.g., if the results are not what the patient expected.

Key Points
- The use of nonbiodegradable fillers was frequent in the past due to the short duration of biodegradable fillers. Nowadays, high performance and long duration of biodegradable fillers have made "permanent" fillers much less opted both by injectors and patients.

3.3.11 Rule 10: Quantity of Filler (Do Not Inject Insufficient Amounts)

Injection of insufficient filler will leave you with an unhappy patient. Make sure that the patient understands that if he wants an optimal result, he must make the according investment.

Key Points
- One of the trickiest topics with injectable fillers is the proper evaluation of the amount of product that patients may need to obtain optimal results. Duration is also affected by the quantity of fillers injected. The patient's satisfaction is directly influenced by immediate performance and duration of results.

3.3.12 Rule 11: Quantity of Filler (Do Not Inject Too Much)

Too much filler is not a good idea either. You do not want a patient with large lumps of injectable filler that can be seen or felt for weeks or even months.

Key Points
- Over-injected patients are unpleasant to look at especially on animation.
- Cheekbones and lips are two areas of frequent overtreatment.

3.3.13 Rule 12: Use the Appropriate Depth of Injection

Not all fillers are intended for superficial injections. You can end up with very unhappy patients if you inject a material that is designed for deep injections such as hydroxylapatite too superficially. This will result in papules and nodules that will take a very long time to go away.

Key Points
- In the past, we basically had "dermal fillers." Nowadays, a greater variety of products are available on the market and injectors must know beforehand what the correct level to inject is.

3.3.14 Rule 13: If Something Goes Wrong

If something goes wrong, for example, the patient is overcorrected or the patient has an adverse reaction to the injectable filler, be accessible and understanding. Most lawsuits arise when the doctor/patient relationship is dysfunctional.

Key Points
- When something goes wrong, we must not add distance and lack of care to patients. They have already the complication to carry on their shoulders.

References

Berkun Y, Ben-Zvi A, Levy Y et al (2003) Evaluation of adverse reactions to local anesthetics: experience with 236 patients. Ann Allergy Asthma Immunol 91(4):342–345

Carruthers A, Carruthers J, Hardas B et al (2008a) A validated grading scale for crow's feet. Dermatol Surg 34(2):S173–S178

Carruthers A, Carruthers J, Hardas B et al (2008b) A validated grading scale for marionette lines. Dermatol Surg 34(2):S167–S172

Carruthers A, Carruthers J, Hardas B et al (2008c) A validated lip fullness grading scale. Dermatol Surg 34(2):S161–S166

Carruthers A, Carruthers J, Hardas B et al (2008d) A validated grading scale for forehead lines. Dermatol Surg 34(2):S155–S160

Carruthers A, Carruthers J, Hardas B et al (2008e) A validated brow positioning grading scale. Dermatol Surg 34(2):S150–S154

Carruthers J, Flynn TC, Geister TL et al (2012) Validated assessment scales for the mid face. Dermatol Surg 38(2):320–332

Flynn TC, Carruthers A, Carruthers J et al (2012) Validated assessment scales for the upper face. Dermatol Surg 38(2):309–319

Marmur E, Green L, Busso M (2010) Controlled, randomized study of pain levels in subjects treated with calcium hydroxylapatite premixed with lidocaine for correction of nasolabial folds. Dermatol Surg 36(3):309–315

Monheit GD, Campbell RM, Neugent H et al (2010) Reduced pain with Use of proprietary hyaluronic acid with lidocaine for correction of nasolabial folds: a patient-blinded, prospective, randomized controlled trial. Dermatol Surg 36(1):94–101

Treatment Planning

4

Mauricio de Maio

We do not go to sleep looking young and wake up in the following morning looking old. Aging is a continuous process that starts from mild aging signs to moderate that become severe and lead to very severe aesthetic problems. The sooner we start to correct them, the better!

Maurício de Maio

Contents

4.1 **Introduction** 41
4.1.1 Product-Related Barrier 42
4.1.2 Patient-Related Barrier................................ 43
4.1.3 Injector-Related Barrier 45
4.1.4 Assessment.. 46
4.1.5 The MdM 8-Point Lift 52

4.2 **Treatment Plan and Exponential Aging** 56

4.3 **Cosmetic Investment Advisor** 58

References.. 59

4.1 Introduction

Treatment planning for medical cosmetic procedures is a challenge. When we compare it with the medical interventions, one becomes aware of the difference. One reason is that minimal invasive cosmetic procedures are relatively new when compared with cardiology where commonly used interventions such as cardiovascular stent applications have a much longer history of use. Another difference is the different input of the patient. When a patient sees a cardiologist for high blood pressure, for example, the treatment planning is usually done by the doctor and not by the patient. There may be slight different approaches among cardiologists, but when following existing guidelines, we might assume quite consistent and reproducible treatment suggestions. But when it comes to aesthetics and cosmetic procedures, the rules are different. Patients are more likely to take responsibility for the treatment planning. They might even try to be the decision makers of what should be treated and – what is even worse – with what kind of product should be injected! For some mostly less experienced injectors, this might be even welcome because they find themselves relieved from designing an accurate treatment plan for their patients. For the experienced injector, however, this might pose a challenge.

Although the use of fillers in aesthetics is not new and if we think about collagen, silicone, or even paraffin, which goes back several decades, so far we have not succeeded in establishing a

M. de Maio, B. Rzany, *Injectable Fillers in Aesthetic Medicine*,
DOI 10.1007/978-3-642-45125-6_4, © Springer-Verlag Berlin Heidelberg 2014

consented strategy for a treatment plan. In this chapter we will try to help our readers with the treatment planning of their patients, but before that we will briefly describe the barriers that may interfere with accomplishing this task.

4.1.1 Product-Related Barrier

Since our first edition of the book *Injectable Fillers in Aesthetic Medicine*, we have pointed out in the first chapter by "At the moment new injectable fillers are popping up like daisies" that we have an abundance of fillers. Specifically for Europe and Latin America, the situation is not much different by now. Fortunately for some products we do know now at least something about their clinical behavior. Nevertheless, there are still unanswered questions even for those specifically when it comes to the understanding of the long-term behavior.

We started with silicone, PMMA, methyl methacrylates, polyacrylamides, collagens (bovine and later porcine), poly-l-lactic acid, hydroxylapatite, and HAs. Lately we seem to be focusing mostly on HA-based fillers and HA-based volumizers. However, within the HAs themselves it is easy to get confused as industry gives us different names (all the brands), types (mono- and biphasic), as well as cross-linkers that initially made us curious but finally ends up making us more and more confused. We have now products for fine lines, folds, lips, cheekbones, jawline, etc., with and without lidocaine. These products have helped us to achieve many incredible results in an individual patient but also make it sometimes difficult for us to position a specific product. For example, can we or can we not use a product that was designed to be used in lips and nasolabial folds? The answers are not so simple.

There are indeed products that perform well in different areas and are very much versatile when it comes to different indications. There are other products that are obviously only suitable for a specific area such as a fine line product (i.e., low-density HA) which does not make a lot of sense to be injected into the chin area for projection and volumization as well as a volumizer (i.e., high-density HA) to be used in the fine lines of the lower eyelid – which might end up in an aesthetic challenge (e.g., a very visible HA roll).

Table 4.1 De Maio/Rzany rough classification for the clinical use of HA fillers and volumizers

Degree 0	Very-low-density HA: to be used preferably intradermally or high subdermally
Degree 1	Medium- or high-density HA: to be used in any layer except intradermally
Degree 2	Very-high-density HA: to be used ONLY in deep planes close to the bone

Sometimes a specific product is designed and clinically investigated by good trials for a specific indication in a specific way, and we discover in our practice that there is another way to inject it (e.g., with a cannula instead of a needle) or that a different indication can be treated (e.g., a volumizer that was designed to be injected down deep to the bone and found useful in treating folds in a more superficial, e.g., subcutaneous mode) (Table 4.1). If we are working with a versatile HA product, we may obtain an accurate response of this product regardless of the area we are injecting it as long as we respect its limits. If we are working with a less versatile product, there might be still some variability. We may use a volumizer (degree 1) to treat a prominent nasolabial fold as long as they are injected subdermally. By using such a filler, less volume compared to a standard filler might be needed. On the other side a very-low-viscosity product (degree 0) may also be injected into a deep fold but with the certain disadvantage of using more volume and a shorter durability.

The performance of a product also depends on the experience that we develop by injecting it over the years. The same product may perform differently in different patients and among different injectors. So, it is basically quite important to keep a clear and critical mind to be aware of the *product as well as the injection technique* for the benefit of the patients and us.

We will be constantly invited to try different products and requested by patients to inject new areas. We have to remember that respecting the science behind the products and our learning

Table 4.2 A practical reminder to deal with new challenges of areas and/or products

	New area	Known area
New product	High risk	Intermediate risk
Known product	Intermediate risk	Low risk

Colleagues should be aware that the risk may differ depending on the combination of factors

curve is of utmost importance to protect our patient and also us against avoidable reactions from both products and techniques. We have to try to be as good as possible when it comes to new challenges, and we have to be very careful with new products specifically when treating new areas (Table 4.2).

Do's
- Do try to understand what product you are using and check the performance in different areas and in different patients.

Don'ts
- Do not try a new product in area which is new for you (e.g., an area where you have little or no experience). The result can be frustrating if not a disaster.

Key Points
- If possible stay with products where there is at least one good clinical trial available (this will give you at least a good idea on the expected common adverse events).
- If you are interested in injecting a completely new area, use a product that you are familiar with.
- If you are interested in trying a new product, inject into an area that you are familiar with and observe for consistent results compared to the product you are used to.

FAQs
- Why should an injector be interested in clinical data?

  If good clinical data (e.g., randomized controlled trials or at least large case series) are available, you have a pretty good idea about the efficacy and common adverse events for the investigated areas.
- Why should an injector link a product to a technique?

  For example, use in a new area only a product you are familiar with. Just to give you a picture: imagine you were a horse jumper; in a competition a successful horse jumper will not jump obstacles with a horse that he had never tried before. We should do the same with our patients.

4.1.2 Patient-Related Barrier

Another barrier to overcome when putting a treatment plan together may be the patient-injector relationship. As discussed before, when it comes to aesthetic procedures, patients have a stronger influence on treatment decision when compared to other medical fields. Sometimes one may wonder if medical aesthetics is not closely associated to buying/selling a car than to health care.

There are patients that are very much aware of their needs and open to listen to advice. These are considered the ideal patients. But unfortunately it is not the rule. There are many patients that will not listen to the physicians' opinions and only see the injector as a "deliverer" of their wishes. That would be acceptable if the patients' perceptions were always accurate – which is of course not always the case. Patients usually tend to look at themselves in the mirror in the frontal view and their complaints are usually focused on the glabella, tired eyes, and nasolabial folds. They only see what can be seen in the frontal view and this is not necessarily what makes them look more exhausted or older (Rzany et al. 2012). In society, however, we do not look at each other frontal to frontal – which is considered confronting – but instead we look at each other more in the oblique view which is softer and nicer. Only by this can we see a discrepancy of analysis and perception between patient and physician.

The "blind spot" definition presented in the chapter "Patient Selection" is another important aspect to be considered. We defined "blind spot" as the area/areas that untreated worsen the patients' appearance. Usually the patients are unaware of these areas – that are mainly determined by the patients' genetics, for example, very small chin, sunken eyes, and asymmetries. Patients usually complain and request treatment of the areas that worsen with aging. So patients may be biased toward aging signs and will disregard their "blind spots" completely. In fact this would be adequate if these patients only want to look younger but not more attractive. Bringing awareness to the "blind spots" must be handled with care as it may lead up to the patient's frustration especially when we cannot or can only with great difficulties or expenses improve or solve the underlying defects. A careful way to help patients discover their "blind spots" is to show their pictures in different positions (frontal, oblique, profile, leaning forward) in different situations (at rest, full smile, angry, kissing, etc.) and ask them what they like and dislike when they see their pictures. At this moment we may find people that will get frightened by their look and even patients that are really becoming distressed. For those patients that feel severely impaired and depressed with their looks, we advise to stop the photo analysis and proceed to treatment options, and for those patients that are completely blind and cannot establish an adequate analysis, we should try to help them see their aesthetic problems and monitor and control their reaction.

The interaction between patients and injectors may also be a challenge and may differ depending on cultural aspects. We may separate those patients that are aware of what they want and seek for advice and those patients that are unaware of what they want and seek for advice and in whom the injector is unable to promote a treatment plan (Table 4.3).

Table 4.3 Barriers between patients and injectors

Barrier 1	Patients with misperceptions and which are not open for advice
Barrier 2	Patients with coherent different requests for which the injector is unable to technically deliver the treatment
Barrier 3	Patients that do not know what they want and seek for advice and in whom the injector is unable to promote a treatment plan

Female patients might be highly influenced by the media and celebrities. It is not uncommon to have a patient asking an injector for Angelina Jolie's lips. But what she is unaware of is that those lips will only be suitable on her face if she has similar facial structure as Angelina. As a result of this misconception, many distracting lips are seen in real life as well as on TV. Some other patients feel that they become a more accentuated look when they have their lips injected. The problem is that they request further injections to make their lips even more pronounced and by this (in their view) more attractive. The result is that (in case they find an injector and of course they will) they will do get more attention but not because they look more attractive but because they look weird. Patient education about proportion and beauty is very important to avoid distracting results. A very important rule must be observed here: "the posttreatment photo must be more pleasant to look at than the before-treatment photo." Obvious as it can be, we might surprise ourselves with the opposite.

Do's

- Do deliver patients' request if you agree with their perception. You will make the patient happy.

Don'ts

- Do not inject a patient with misperception of his/her needs. It is quite likely that you will be creating a future problem for yourself.

Key Points

- If you only treat the aging signs of your patients, they may look better, sometimes younger but not necessarily more attractive. We also need to pay attention to structural or genetic flaws and improve them (the so-called blind spots).

Table 4.4 The three important questions to answer to understand our *status quo* as an injector

Question 1	Am I aware of and have I solved my technical deficiencies? Or do I still have technical deficiencies?
Question 2	Can I properly assess the patient by identifying the main needs?
Question 3	Am I able to build up a coherent treatment plan for that patient?

4.1.3 Injector-Related Barrier

This is the most difficult area because injectors also have their "blind spots." Many aspects may hinder the injector to deliver an accurate treatment plan for their patients. The Greek proverb "In the kingdom of the blind, the one-eyed man is king" teaches us that this is more an opportunity than a barrier. The more we are aware of our abilities and limits, the faster we may try to solve them (Table 4.4).

Technical deficiency is the barrier number one that we have to overcome to evolve as an injector especially if we are interested in delivering a global approach with injectables. The first step it is to be aware of our deficiencies. As otherwise we might continue overtreating an area that we are confident to treat (e.g., the nasolabial folds) instead of treating the area that poses a challenge for us. We may be able to make the proper diagnosis, i.e., sunken temples, but avoid discussing it or indicating it as a treatment option for the patient because of our technical deficiency. In some cases, patients themselves might request such a treatment and we may find us saying that "treating your temples is not important."

If we are not prepared to successfully inject into an specific area, we should either search for adequate training or refer the patient to a more experienced injector. Sooner or later, all injectors will be able to inject the commonest facial areas. The easiest way to learn is to start by writing down the areas and types of patients that we have difficulty treating and secondly to check if someone is obtaining good results for this indication. Be aware that sometimes, what is difficult for you is difficult for everybody!

Accurate patient assessment and the judgment if that product or technique will work are much more difficult than overcoming technical deficiencies – as incredible as it may seem. Injectors that are not familiar with exercising the assessment process and usually are only used to delivering patients' requests (usually glabella with BoNT-A and nasolabial fold with dermal fillers) should be aware that patients' needs are not restricted to these two areas and they may end up suffering from low patient retention. Assessing patients does take time and the speed that we can reach a final conclusion will vary according to our experience and the type of patient we are dealing with. It is also a longtime learning curve and requires exercise.

After solving the two first barriers (technique and assessment), we can really assume that we are now prepared to tackle the last barrier: to build up the treatment plan. The treatment plan is to be programmed according to patients' social and economic situation, and that is a tremendous opportunity for us to become a long-term trusted *cosmetic investment advisor* (CIA) for the patient. A CIA is someone that is able to build up consistent treatment plans for their patients along the years and is able to work efficiently with the patients' budget. One of the biggest challenges of the cosmetic business is patients' retention. They are looking for someone that is able to help them look better, increase their self-esteem, or rejuvenate. Regardless of their initial request, they will be happy to find an aesthetic physician that they can trust and guide them. That is the gap in the market. Hence, there is the opportunity!

Do's

- Do try to be aware of our skills, try to up-skill yourself, and overcome your technical deficiencies. Both your patient and you will benefit from that.
- Do try to assess your patients without knowing what motivated them to visit

your office then contrast their opinion with yours. You will have a surprising experience!

Don'ts

- Do not deny the benefit of the treatment to your patient of an area that you are not trained yet. You may refer this patient to a colleague who is more experienced with this indication.
- Do not forget to benchmark your technical abilities and assessment skills – it is for the good of your patients and yourself.

Key Points

- There are difficult areas to treat only with injectables because results will be limited. If you are not sure, check with experts if that is the case. Differentiating what is easy from what is technically difficult is a huge step in the learning curve.
- It is not only the technical skill that makes a top injector.

FAQs

- What is a cosmetic investment advisor (CIA)?

  A CIA is someone that has surpassed technical and diagnosis deficiencies and is able to build up a coherent treatment plan, working efficiently with patients' budget over a long time period.

4.1.4 Assessment

A systematic approach is recommended when assessing the aesthetic patients. This approach might be quite individual and might differ from injector to injector. Some important aspects, however, should always be considered as, e.g., facial shape, proportion, symmetry, and facial units.

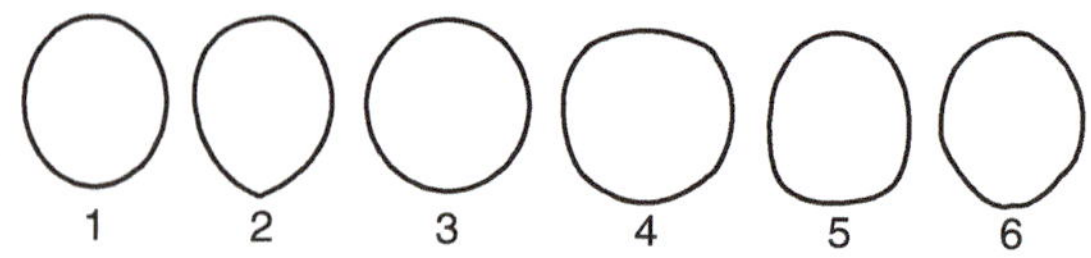

Fig. 4.1 Facial shape according to Terino and Flowers (2000)

The first aspect that should be analyzed is the facial shape (Figs. 4.1 and 4.2, Table 4.4) because it will give us important information regarding how close or far we are to the oval shape which is considered the most attractive for females (Terino and Flowers 2000).

Facial proportion is an important aspect for facial balance and harmony. The proportions of the three facial thirds need to be analyzed to get an idea if volumization of any of the thirds is required. The evaluation should include always the profile where we need to establish if it is straight, convex, or concave. Usually, patients with a straight profile are easier to treat. Severe concavities or convexities may limit the results with injectables.

Another important aspect is symmetry. Symmetry is beauty but we are all asymmetrical and correction of asymmetries should follow a reasonable rule. Slight natural asymmetries are acceptable and sometimes do bring even charm to the patient's appearance. Injectors, however, are not expected to produce asymmetry and definitely prohibited to enhance it. If the asymmetry is mild, acceptable, or even charming, no specific treatment planning is needed. Please observe the following example: imagine a patient whose right side contains a total of 100 ml of volume and whose left side is somewhat bigger and contains 110 ml. The percent difference is 10 %. Now let us suppose that we decide to add the same amount of volume in both sides and add 100 ml for each. The right side has 100 ml + 100 ml, which will end up with 200 ml of total volume, and the left side has 110 ml + 100 ml, which will result in 210 ml. The percent difference is now 5 %. This simple mathematical explanation shows that only by adding the same volume, a reduction in asymmetry is obtained (Table 4.6).

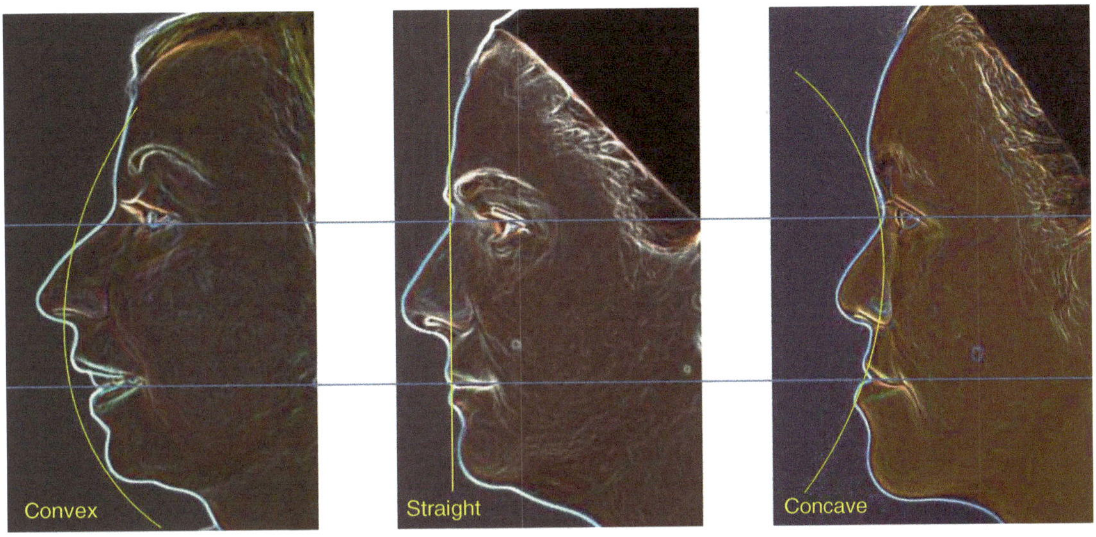

Fig. 4.2 Facial profile according to Terino and Flowers (2000)

Table 4.5 Facial shape according to Terino and Flowers (2000)

1	Oval
2	Heart-shaped
3	Round
4	Square
5	Round head and square jaw
6	Round head and oval jaw

Table 4.6 The effect of volumization on the improvement of asymmetry

	Right side (ml)	Left side (ml)	Percent difference (%)
Baseline differences	100	110	10
Volume replacement	100	100	
Final difference	200	210	5

Just by adding the same volume, the asymmetry will improve

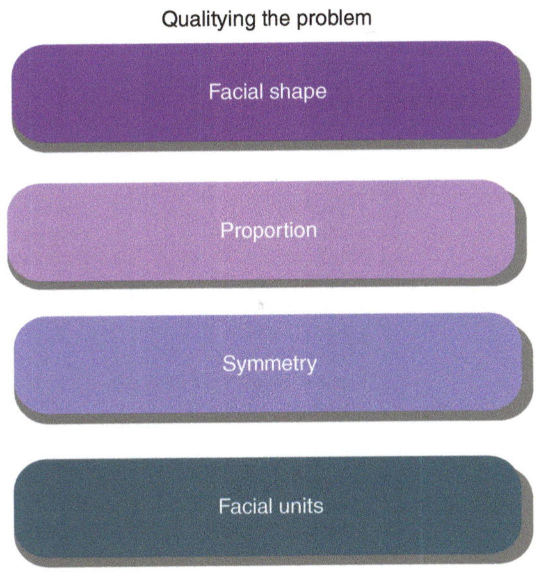

Fig. 4.3 Qualifying the problem by analyzing facial shape, proportion, symmetry, and facial units

4.1.4.1 Step 1: Qualify the Problem!

After assessing facial shape, proportion, and asymmetry, the injector should analyze the facial units. It is important to analyze the face at rest, on animation, and in a forward position to qualify the important points. For example, when assessing the upper third, we may start by the forehead and verify if the shape is adequate, if there is a volume loss at frontal view and profile, and if there are static and/or dynamic forehead lines (Fig. 4.3). Treatment planning might be facilitated by a chart (Table 4.7).

The treatment plan chart is a guide to help injectors to include all important areas during the patient assessment. After filling up the chart, the top part is completed with the areas to be treated, the products to be used, and the prioritization. Below there is an example of *qualifying the problems* (Fig. 4.4).

Table 4.7 Chart for treatment planning

	Treatment Area / Indication	Products	Priority Ranking
Treatment Plan			1st
			2nd
			3rd
			4th
			5th

Facial Assesments

Facial Shape	Frontal View 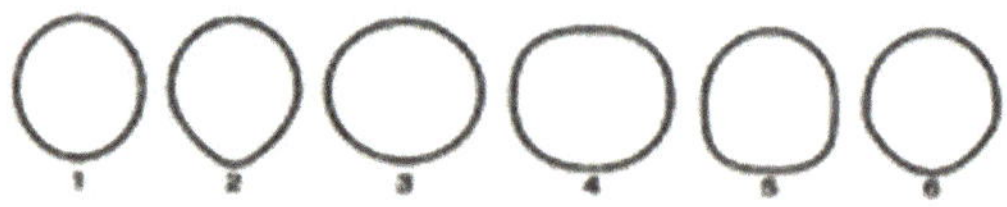
	Profile View 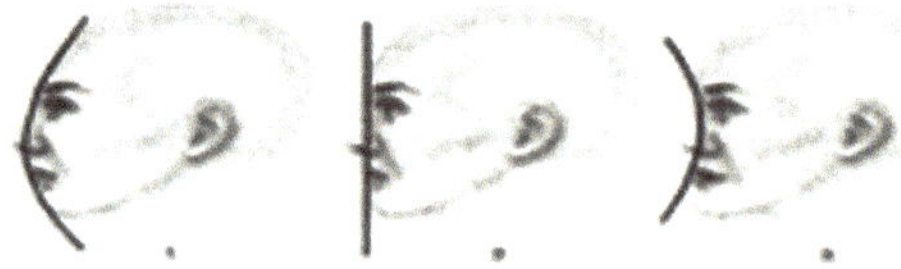 ( ) Convex ( ) Straight ( ) Concave

Proportion	Upper third: Mid Third: Low third (Ratio 1: 1: 1)	Width of Nose: Mouth (1: 1.618)	Upper lip: Lower lip (1: 1.618)
Asymmetry	( ) Yes ( ) No		

	At Rest		On Animation	Chin down/eyes up
	Frontal View	Profile View		
Upper Third	( ) Asymmetry ( ) Forehead shape ( ) Forehead lines ( ) Glabellar lines ( ) Crow's feet ( ) Brow drooping ( ) Temporal hollows ( ) Sunken upper eyelid ( ) Eye-bags	( ) Forehead concavity ( ) Forehead bossa ( ) Forehead volume loss	( ) Asymmetry ( ) Forehead lines ( ) Glabellar lines ( ) Crow's feet	( ) Asymmetry ( ) Forehead volume loss
Mid Third	( ) Asymmetry ( ) Bunny lines ( ) Nasolabial folds ( ) tear-trough ( ) elongated lid-cheek junction ( ) Mid cheek deficiency ( ) Flat cheekbone ( )Low nasal bridge ( ) Nasal flare widening ( ) Cheek volume loss	( ) Low nasal bridge ( ) Nose hump ( ) Nose tip drooping ( ) Round nose tip ( ) Retruded columella ( ) Wide nasal base	( ) Asymmetry ( ) Bunny lines ( ) Nasolabial folds ( ) Nasal flare widening ( ) Nasal tip drooping ( )Gummy Smile	( ) Asymmetry ( ) Tear trough ( ) Mid cheek deficiency ( ) Flat cheekbone ( ) Cheek volume loss ( ) Skin laxity
Lower Third	( ) Asymmetry ( ) Flat philtrum column ( ) Long upper lip ( ) Lip lines ( ) Thin upper lip/ volume ( ) Lack of lip definition ( ) Mouth angle drooping ( ) Marionette lines ( ) Jowls ( ) Prejowl sulcus ( )Masseter hypertrophy ( ) Mental crease / cobblestone chin	( ) Lack of chin projection ( ) Short chin ( ) Loss of mandible ( ) Marionette lines ( ) Jowls ( ) Prejowl sulcus	( ) Asymmetry ( ) Lip wrinkling ( ) Mentalis ( ) Masseter ( ) Platysma bands ( ) Loss of mandible definition	( ) Marionette lines ( ) Jowls ( ) Prejowl sulcus ( ) Skin laxity

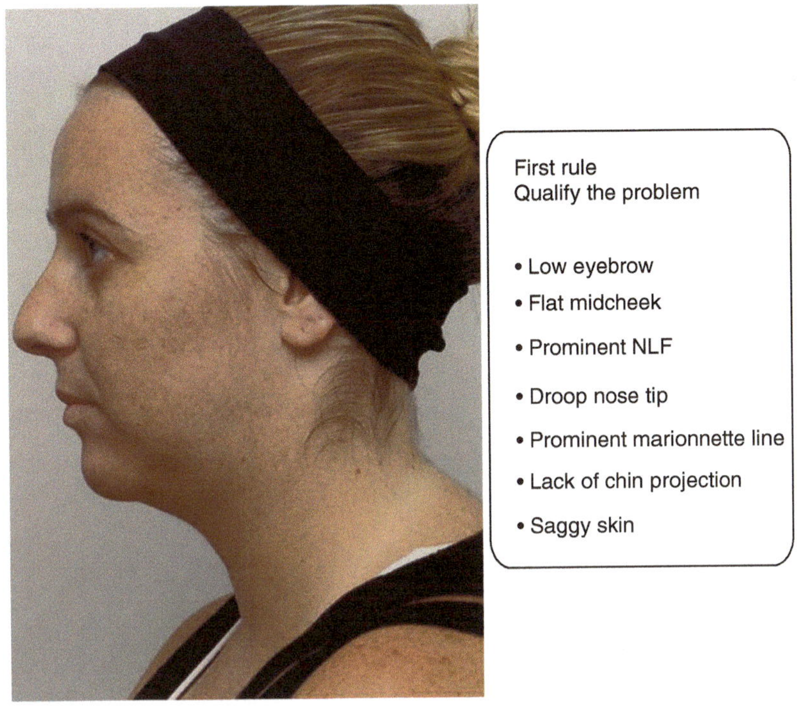

Fig. 4.4 First rule: qualify the problems!

4.1.4.2 Step 2: Quantify the Problem!

After a detailed qualification of the problems, the next step is quantifying them. There are many validated 4- or 5-point scales that can be used and simple work with classifications of none, mild, moderate, severe, and very severe/extreme (Carruthers et al. 2008a, b, c, d, e; Rzany et al. 2012). These scales come quite handy. Another very simple way to document the present status of the patient is to work with crosses (+) (Table 4.8). For example, a prominent nasolabial fold may be mild (+) or mild to moderate (+/++).

Culturally, patients and cosmetic surgeons tend to decide for treatment when the problems are severe. Facelifts are performed when saggy skin has become intolerable! Unfortunately, the same happens with injectables. Patient and injector may only decide to treat when the problems become severe and sometimes when the solution is better handled by surgery or another intervention and not by injectables.

Table 4.8 Quantifying the problem with a simple scale using crosses to evaluate the degree of severity

Number of crosses	Degree of severity
+	Mild
++	Moderate
+++	Severe
++++	Very severe

The correct approach for minimal invasive procedures such as the use of injectables should be "the sooner, the better," not only from a financial point of view but also from a technical point of view. Despite the injector's philosophy, mild problems are easier to improve than severe problems, and that is unquestionable.

The sequence of deficits that may be found during the aging process is easily diagnosed when we analyze patients' photos or if we happen to know someone for a long time but only see this person from time to time. As mentioned before, we do not age in a single night. It takes years to move from mild to very severe deficiencies. The problem is that patients' and injectors' perception seems to be more sensitive when the exponential aging has started. Below there are examples of different patients in different degrees of severity for the same area (Fig. 4.5). After

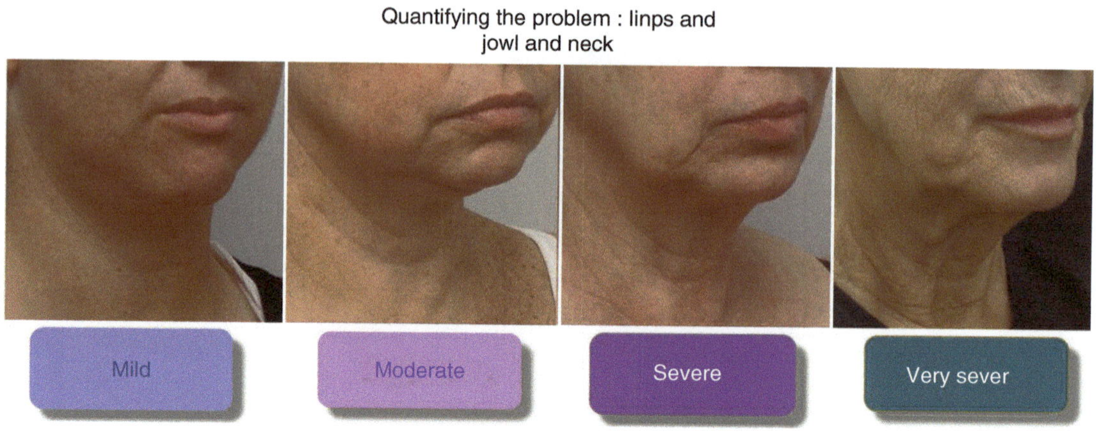

Fig. 4.5 Quantify the problem! We do not go to sleep with mild problems and wake up in the following morning with very severe deficiencies. How can someone develop a severe problem if we never let it become moderate?

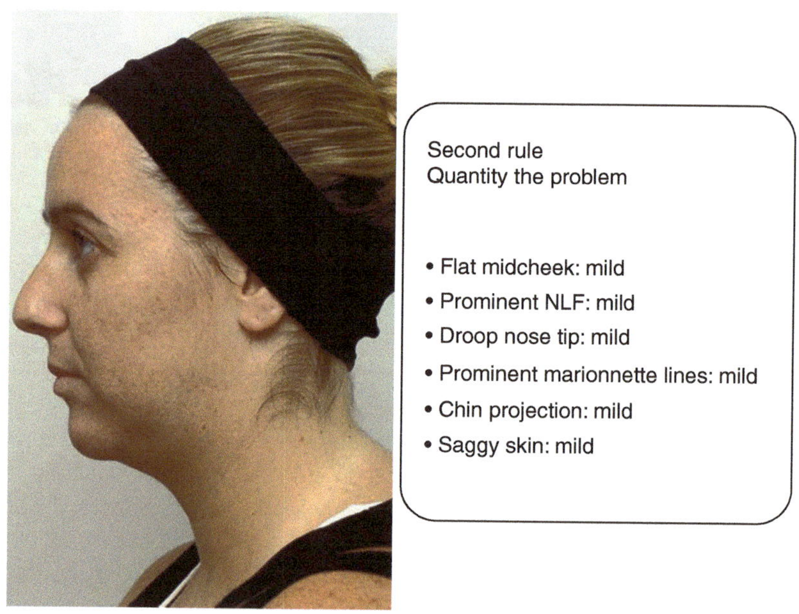

Fig. 4.6 Quantifying the problems for this patient demonstrated that they are still mild, and that means high probability of successful outcomes

qualifying the problem, it is time to quantify them according to the degree of severity as follows (Fig. 4.6).

Do's
- Do start to correct problems when they are still mild.
- Do educate your patients about the benefits of starting the treatment at an early stage.

Don'ts
- Do not forget to qualify then quantify the problems to build up an efficient treatment plan.

Key Points
- Mild problems are easier to improve than severe problems.
- The sooner we start to correct, the better.

> **FAQs**
>
> - How can someone develop a severe problem if we never let it become moderate?
>
>   They will not and that is the importance of creating an efficient treatment plan. We can and we should slow down aging process as soon as possible.

4.1.4.3 Step 3: Create a Treatment Plan!

After qualifying and quantifying the problems, the next step is to build up the treatment plan. Depending on the patient, multiple diagnoses might be made and the next step is to prioritize and include them in the treatment timeline. After finishing the treatment plan, one step further is to contrast the technical evaluation with the patients' request. At this time, we may discuss different possibilities finding in the extremes either total agreement or complete disagreement. In the latter situation good communication skills are mandatory. A treatment plan is only efficient when there is synchronicity between the injector's and the patient's beliefs. Here communication is everything! Please find below some possibilities that may arise when patients' and injectors' opinions are contrasted and suggestions (Table 4.9).

When patients present mild problems, we should try to correct them so that they maintain always the status of mild degree. The patient will continue aging but in a slower speed (Fig. 4.7).

Table 4.9 Different assessment situations for patients and injectors and possible solutions

Possibilities	Comparison	Suggestion to injectors
1	Patient's request is in agreement with injector	Proceed with the treatment
2	Patient's request is in agreement with injector but prioritization is different	Discussion on prioritization tends to come easily into agreement between both parts
3	Patient's request is different and *better* than injector's opinion	Deliver patient's request and *learn* with patients
4	Patient's request is different and does not make sense according to injector's opinion	Take time to educate your patient. It will be good for you, for the patient, and for the next injector if you are able to convert the patient

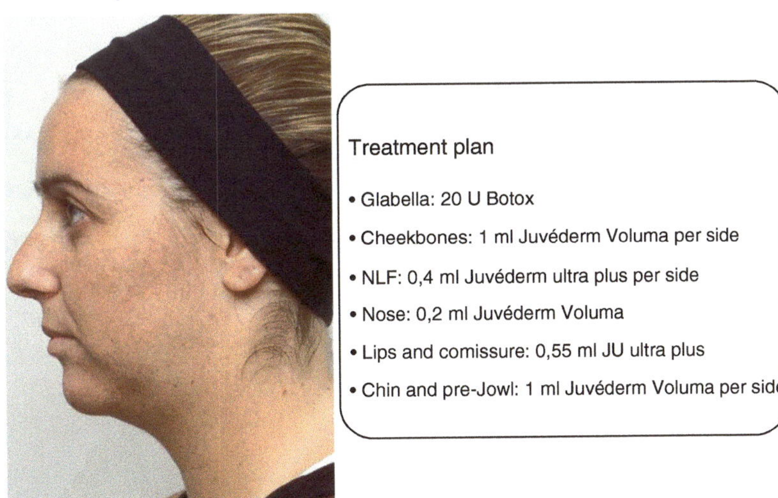

Fig. 4.7 Both structural and aging problems were improved in this patient. Her aging process will be slower now

Do's

- Be open. Contrast your opinion with the patients' opinion. Sometimes we learn a lot from them.
- Do invest time for creating a treatment plan for your patients.

Don'ts

- Do not let patients confuse or contaminate your therapeutic concept and try to develop your communication skills to guide them.

Key Points

- It is also the injectors' responsibility to educate and guide patients when they have misperception of their needs. To invest time in communication is an important aspect to increase treatment success and patient retention.

4.1.5 The MdM 8-Point Lift

Patients with mild or moderate problems may present some technical challenges, but those deficiencies are expected to be solved and longer-lasting results are expected. However, there are some patients that already present severe and very severe problems and may not be open for surgery or present a medical condition that contraindicates the surgical option (Fig. 4.8).

The challenge to treat patients that present formal surgical indication is higher than treating mild to moderate deficiencies with injectables. Before volumizers such as Juvedérm Voluma got to the market, treatments with injectable fillers for this kind of patients were often not really satisfying. Besides, the product in complex cases requires a technical strategy as important questions should be asked before the treatment starts (Table 4.10).

If an injector injects this patient in the traditional way, a large amount of product may be required and the lifting effect may not be achieved. We decided to describe *the MdM (Mauricio de Maio) 8-point lift* to cope with this

Table 4.10 For complex cases, a more refined strategy needs to include also the injection sequence

Questions	Important aspects to consider
1	Where to inject?
2	What to inject?
3	How to inject?
4	*What sequence to inject?*

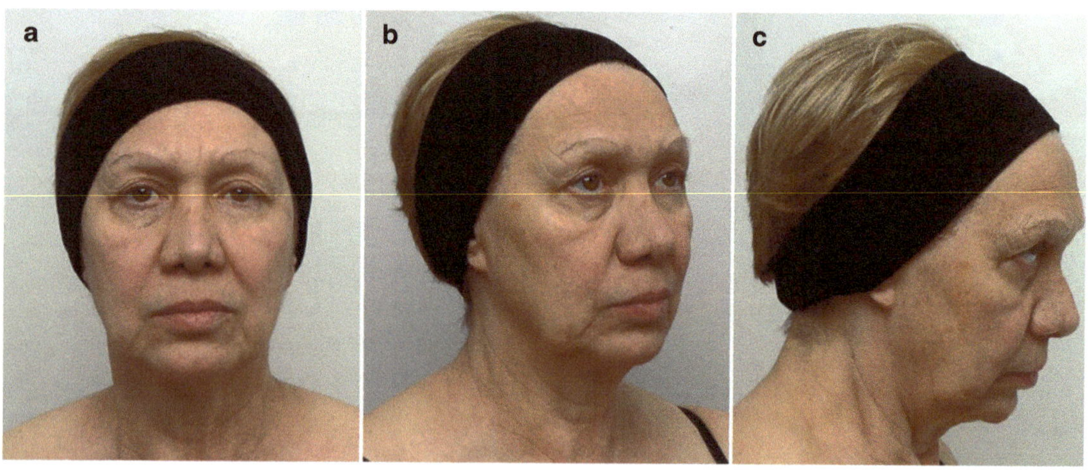

Fig. 4.8 (**a–c**) This is a typical surgical patient that presents severe to very severe problems on the face including extensive saggy skin

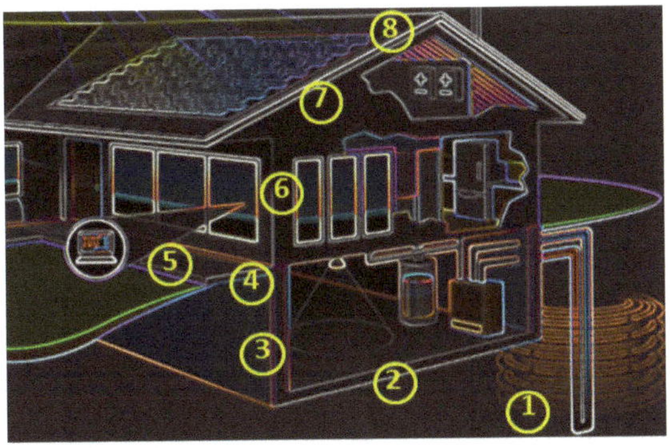

Fig. 4.9 To build a house there is a sequence of events that should be respected. We all understand pretty well that to reach the ceiling (point 8), we must have started by point

kind of patients. For better understanding, please follow the illustration below where respecting the sequence is mandatory (Fig. 4.9).

It should not be forgotten that faces are composed as a mechanical structure with hard and soft tissues that need support to cope with gravity. As described in Chap. 6, the treatment of the cheekbone area with volumizers may improve the appearance of the nasolabial fold and the lid-cheek junction. That clearly means that there is an improvement of an area that was not injected only by injecting in the neighborhood. Let us apply the 1st (qualify the problem!) and the 2nd (quantify the problem!) rules for the following patient that will be submitted to *the MdM 8-point lift* (Table 4.11).

As it could be noticed above, the lower third presents more and more severe challenges than the mid-third. Starting the treatment in the lower third is not the best technical approach even if the patient is requesting only the treatment of marionette lines. Results are limited if only a direct approach to this area is undertaken (Fig. 4.10). *The MdM 8-point lift* follows a multiple region strategy (Table 4.12).

Patients with very severe saggy skin should be injected with caution. Any product injected into the NO GO! area may lead to worsening of the fold or sagginess. Represented in the illustration are the GO! areas (in blue) and the NO GO! areas (in red), which must be avoided (Fig. 4.11). With not much quantities used, the results with the MdM 8-point lift may be amazing (Figs. 4.12, 4.13, and 4.14).

Table 4.11 Qualifying and quantifying steps for the patient with severe (+++) and very severe (++++) problems

Mid-third	*Qualify the problem!*	*Quantify the problem!*
	Infraorbital hollow	+++
	Volume loss in mid-cheekbone	+++
	Volume loss in lateral cheekbone	+++
	Prominent nasolabial fold	+++
Lower third	*Qualify the problem!*	*Quantify the problem!*
	Marionette lines	++++
	Pre-jowl sulcus	+++
	Jowls	++++
	Jawline loss of definition	++++
	Parotid area volume loss	++++

These steps are important before creating the treatment plan

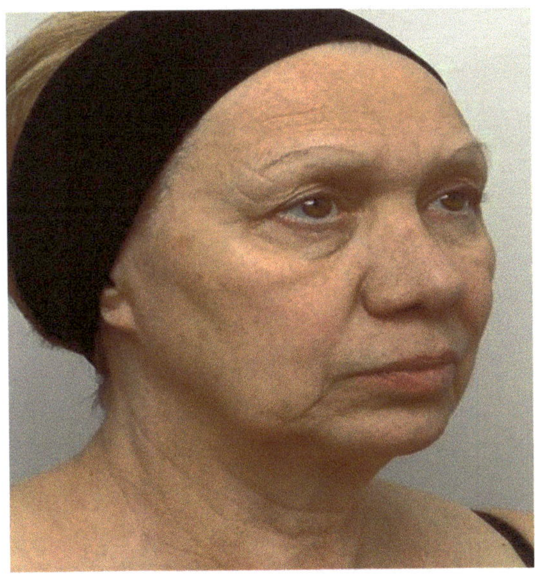

Fig. 4.10 The MdM 8-point lift: note that 8 areas are to be injected with small bolus technique and massage. By respecting this sequence, the volume requirement along the jawline will be lower. Area number 9 represents chin projection when improvement of area 6 (pre-jowl sulcus) is still needed

Table 4.12 *The MdM 8-point lift*: the areas, regions, and comments

Point	*Region*	*Comments*
1	Zygomatic region	Lifting point of lateral cheekbone
2	Intermediate infraorbital region	Projection of cheek bones and improvement of elongated lid-cheek junction
3	Medial infraorbital region	Improvement of tear trough
4	Canine fossa and upper part of nasolabial fold	Less volume requirement is needed after areas 1, 2, and 3 were treated
Lower third	*Region*	*Comments*
5	Marionette lines	Start from top to bottom by strengthening the oral commissure
6	Pre-jowl sulcus	Small bolus or retrograde techniques are suitable here. *Do not inject the jowls!*
7	Jawline	Linear and retrograde technique is preferable at this level
8	Parotid region	When volume loss is replaced here, lifting effect is obtained

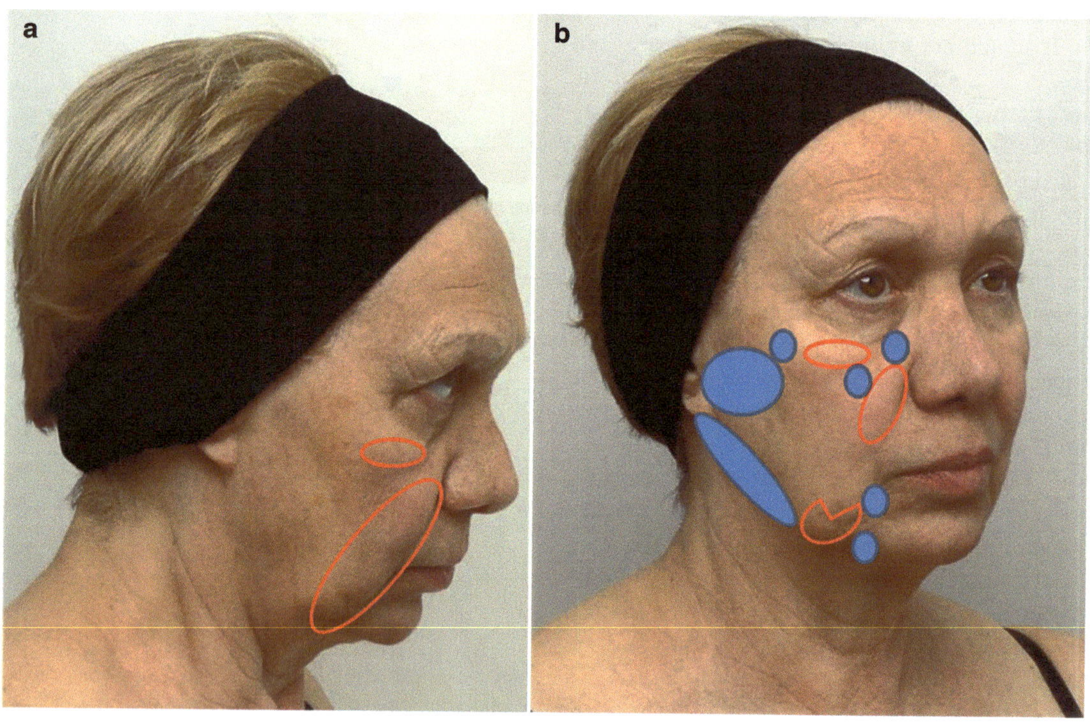

Fig. 4.11 (**a**, **b**) It is very important to demarcate the GO! (*blue*) and NO GO! (*red*) areas before starting. Note that the NO GO! areas must also be evaluated with the patient with "eyes up and chin down"

It must be reinforced that the amount per point will vary from patient to patient depending on the volume loss, bone structure, and degree of laxity. Younger patients with moderate saggy skin usually require 1 ml of Juvedérm Voluma or a comparable product per side.

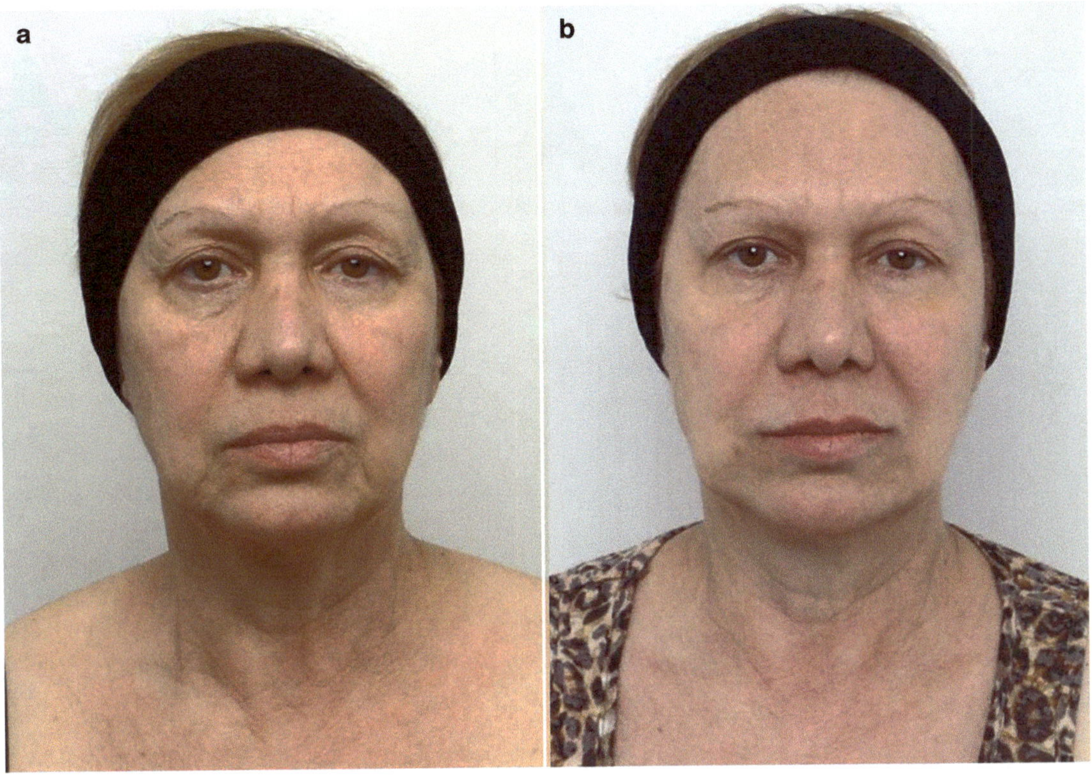

Fig. 4.12 (a, b) Before and after frontal view photos from the patient that was treated with "the MdM 8-point lift." Note that it seems that the patient was submitted to eye surgery and a light surgical lift

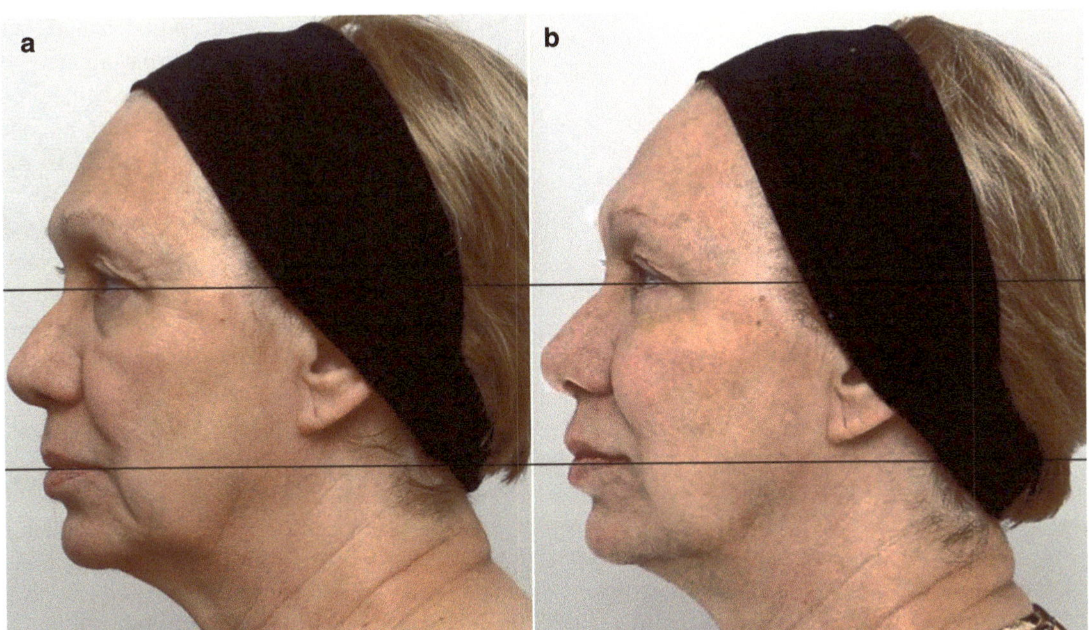

Fig. 4.13 (a, b) Profile view of the pre- and post-photos after the MdM 8-point lift. Note the shortening of the lid-cheek junction, projection and lifting of the cheekbones, and improvement of the marionette lines, pre-jowl area, jowls, and jawline definition. The overall saggy skin was also improved. A total of 2.7 ml of Juvedérm Voluma was injected per side and 20 U of Vistabel in the glabella

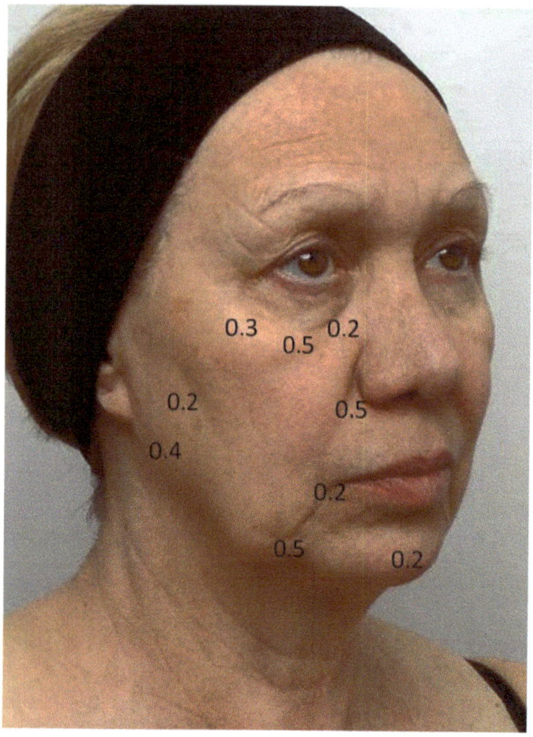

Fig. 4.14 Quantity of Juvedérm Voluma and Juvedérm smile (points 4 and 5, Marionette lines and nasolabial folds) injected per point in ml. Note that point 9 was also injected to increase chin projection and enhance the pre-jowl sulcus

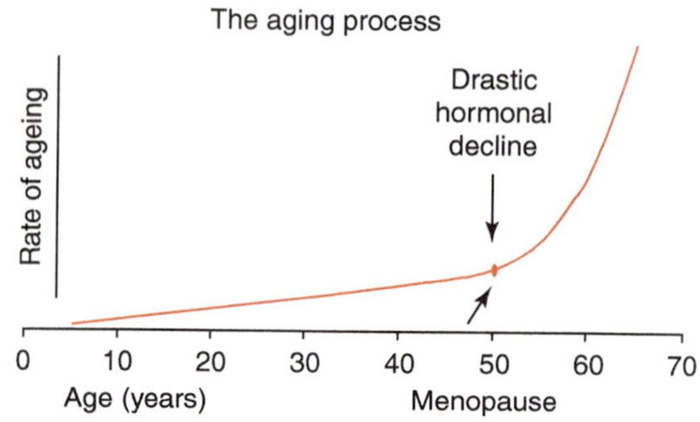

Fig. 4.15 The aging curve in females: aging is linear and becomes exponential with hormonal decline especially for women but also for men

> **Key Points**
>
> - As a conclusion, *the MdM 8-point lift* may be considered an important ally and an alternative in facial rejuvenation for patient's signs of severe aging that are not eligible for the surgical option for variable reasons.

4.2 Treatment Plan and Exponential Aging

As stated in the beginning of this chapter, aging is a continuous process that goes from mild to very severe deficiencies. Aging obeys the linear rule of the domino effect, but at a certain point, it becomes exponential. Please find bellow the definition:

"The domino effect is a chain reaction that occurs when a small change causes a similar change nearby, which then will cause another similar change, and so on in linear sequence. The term is best known as a mechanical effect, and is used as an analogy to a falling row of dominoes. It typically refers to a linked sequence of events where the time between successive events is relatively small. It can be used literally (an observed series of actual collisions) or metaphorically."

An injector that only delivers what the patients request will not help the patient to prevent or combat aging and properly risk patients' long-term retention. It is important to understand that it is not the injection technique that makes the difference but the understanding of the aging process and at what point of that curve the patient stands. Aging occurs in early stages in a linear ascendant curve, and at a certain point (e.g., menopause/andropause), the deflection of the curve changes and the speed of aging becomes exponential. The conclusion is simple: the worse we are, the worse we get; the older we are, the older we get (Fig. 4.15)!

So if we understand that there is a moment where the speed of aging becomes exponential, then we should ask ourselves two questions (Table 4.13).

The next curve shows a possibility of slowing down the aging process by medical intervention, and that is the importance of creating an effective treatment plan for the patients. By controlling the worsening of aging signs, which means avoiding problems to go from mild to moderate then to severe, there will be a reduction in the speed of

Table 4.13 Important questions that injectors should be aware of

Questions		Answer
Question 1	Can we slow down the aging process?	Yes
Question 2	Are patients technically prepared to decide how to slow down aging?	No

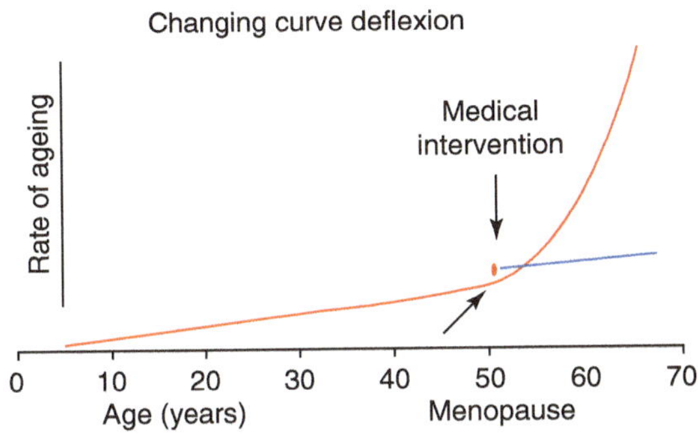

Fig. 4.16 Medical intervention is of utmost importance to postpone the exponential aging and keep the aging linear

aging and the exponential aging will be postponed more as possible (Fig. 4.16).

Many treatment options exist to slow down aging at different stages. Injectables such as fillers and BoNT-A are powerful tools to prevent and correct aging signs. The performance of many different types of treatments is influenced by adequate hormonal condition especially longevity of results. Premenopausal phase does present better results than long postmenopausal treatments do. It is important to understand that several interventions need to be employed to get the best results (Fig. 4.17).

To effectively achieve the desirable outcomes with our patients, a treatment plan timeline should be incorporated into the injectors' daily practice. We will not be young forever and we become each year more and more complex to treat due to three aspects that may be seen below (Table 4.14).

It is becoming clearer and clearer that injectors need to reflect if they want to be technical deliverers of patients' requests or if they want to combat the aging process more effectively by creating a long-term treatment plan for their patients.

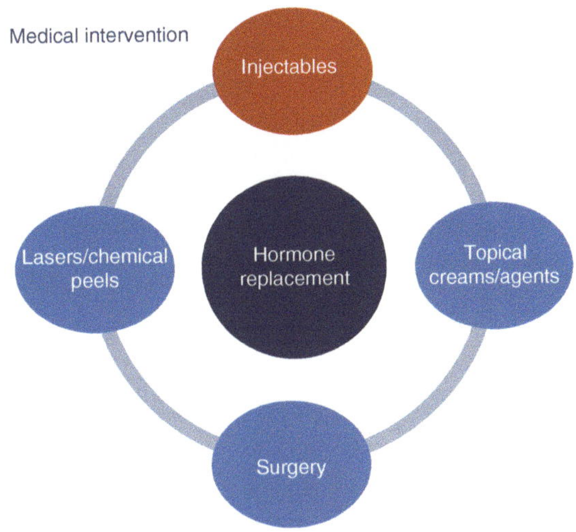

Fig. 4.17 Treatment options to combat and slow down aging process

Table 4.14 Three aspects that should be taken into consideration for cosmetic practice

		Comments
Step 1	Qualify the problems!	Each year the number of aging signs tends to increase
Step 2	Quantify the problems!	Each year the degree of severity of the aging signs will increase
Step 3	Create a treatment plan!	Each year lost will lead to more complexity in treatment planning

Depending on the age that our patients come to visit us, there is more or less time to be effective in slowing down aging process. A patient under 40s may have their requests satisfied although we do believe that we should have started earlier to correct aging signs or intrinsic cosmetic deficiencies – even before 40s. However, a patient in her/his 40s, who still has 10 years before exponential aging, is the best candidate to "prepare for the impact!" of menopause/andropause. Female patients are usually asked about their first period and the age their mother entered menopause to estimate the average number of years we have to work with them. This knowledge will also influence the prioritization as well as the effort that will be given to educate them during this crucial phase for prevention. Menopause changes will be affected by the presence or absence or hormonal

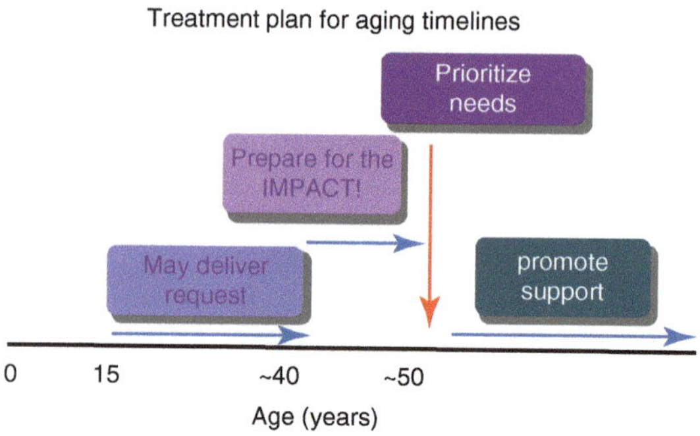

Fig. 4.18 Treatment plan for aging timelines

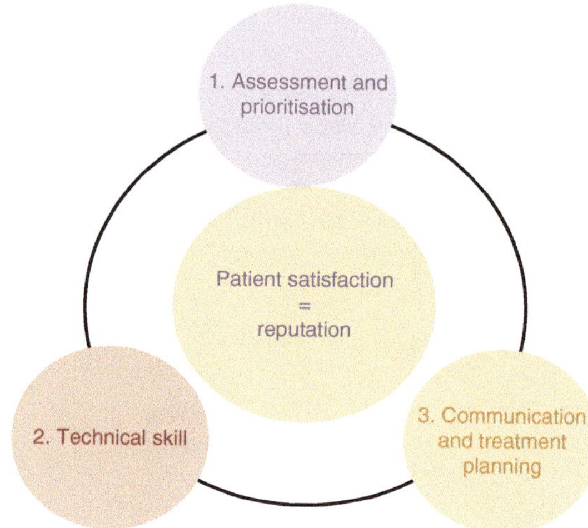

Fig. 4.19 The power of three: the important pillars that lead to patient satisfaction and reputation

replacement therapy and is not the scope of this book. But if there is no formal contraindication to it, patients should be motivated to have a second opinion of a hormone specialist on this topic because the performance of surgical and nonsurgical cosmetic treatments may be influenced positively by hormone replacement therapy (oral as well as topical). Regardless of that, menopause is a moment to prioritize needs and choose which treatment should start first, and the follow-up plan is mandatory to maintain results. Postmenopausal patients that were never treated before are a challenge for injectables. The further they are from the 50s, the more formal indications are found. Promoting support with volumizers become mandatory because more superficial fillers may have very little effect if deep tissue support is not provided (Fig. 4.18).

4.3 Cosmetic Investment Advisor

To become a cosmetic investment advisor (CIA), it is important to develop skills that are beyond technique. The first pillar is the ability to do proper assessment and prioritization. The second pillar is the appropriate injection technique. An appropriate injection technique is the base for an efficient treatment, and deficiencies at this level will pose as a barrier for the injectors – that when one is aware of those should be solved as soon as possible. The third pillar is the communications skills which are necessary to teach and convert patients if they present misperception of their needs. These three pillars will finally lead to a treatment plan which will reflect best practice in aesthetic medicine (Fig. 4.19).

As a final conclusion, we would like to present an illustration with the *standards of 8* that include important topics that an injector should observe and develop to become an expert in this field (Fig. 4.20).

Do's

- Do verify at which stage your patient is in the aging curve and try to identify the time point when the exponential aging will start.
- Do postpone the exponential aging with appropriate interventions to avoid the domino effect.

Don'ts

- Do not wait too long to put your patients in the best aesthetic condition before the exponential aging occurs.
- Do not forget that fillers are only one intervention. Other interventions as botulinum toxin, topical (e.g., retinoids), hormone replacement therapy, peels, and laser need to be taken into account, too.

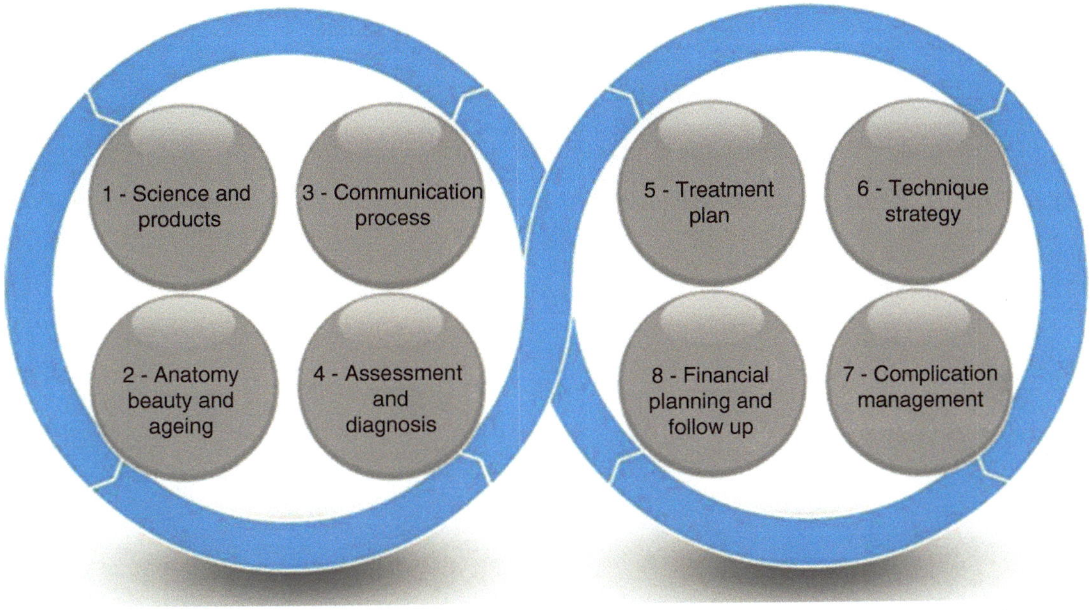

Fig. 4.20 The standards of eight: injectors should recognize their strengths and weak points that need improvement based on the eight important aspects that are found in real-world clinical practice

Key Points

- The older we are, the older we get.
- It is important to correct all unfavorable signs (including genetic and aging) before the exponential aging occurs.

FAQs

- What is the advantage of becoming an efficient cosmetic investment advisor?

  It is based on increased patient satisfaction which will along the years ultimately lead to increased patient retention and an increased reputation among your patients.

References

Carruthers A, Carruthers J, Hardas B, Kaur M, Goertelmeyer R, Jones D, Rzany B, Cohen J, Kerscher M, Flynn TC, Maas C, Sattler G, Gebauer A, Pooth R, McClure K, Simone-Korbel U, Buchner L (2008a) A validated hand grading scale. Dermatol Surg 34 (Suppl 2):S179–S183

Carruthers A, Carruthers J, Hardas B, Kaur M, Goertelmeyer R, Jones D, Rzany B, Cohen J, Kerscher M, Flynn TC, Maas C, Sattler G, Gebauer A, Pooth R, McClure K, Simone-Korbel U, Buchner L (2008b) A validated grading scale for crow's feet. Dermatol Surg 34(Suppl 2):S173–S178

Carruthers A, Carruthers J, Hardas B, Kaur M, Goertelmeyer R, Jones D, Rzany B, Cohen J, Kerscher M, Flynn TC, Maas C, Sattler G, Gebauer A, Pooth R, McClure K, Simone-Korbel U, Buchner L (2008c) A validated grading scale for marionette lines. Dermatol Surg 34(Suppl 2):S167–S172

Carruthers A, Carruthers J, Hardas B, Kaur M, Goertelmeyer R, Jones D, Rzany B, Cohen J, Kerscher M, Flynn TC, Maas C, Sattler G, Gebauer A, Pooth R, McClure K, Simone-Korbel U, Buchner L (2008d) A validated lip fullness grading scale. Dermatol Surg 34(Suppl 2):S161–S166

Carruthers A, Carruthers J, Hardas B, Kaur M, Goertelmeyer R, Jones D, Rzany B, Cohen J, Kerscher M, Flynn TC, Maas C, Sattler G, Gebauer A, Pooth R, McClure K, Simone-Korbel U, Buchner L (2008e) A validated grading scale for forehead lines. Dermatol Surg 34(Suppl 2):S155–S160

Rzany B, Carruthers A, Carruthers J, Flynn TC, Geister TL, Görtelmeyer R, Hardas B, Himmrich S, Jones D, de Maio M, Mohrmann C, Narins RS, Pooth R, Sattler G, Buchner L, Merito M, Fey C, Kerscher M (2012) Validated composite assessment scales for the global face. Dermatol Surg 38(2 Spec No):294–308

Terino EO, Flowers RS (eds) (2000) The art of alloplastic facial contouring. Mosby, St. Louis

Anesthesia and Analgesia

5

Mauricio de Maio

Contents

5.1 **Introduction** 61

5.2 **Evaluation Prior to Injection** 62

5.3 **Local Anesthesia** 62

5.4 **Topical Anesthesia** 62

5.5 **Infiltrative Anesthesia** 63

5.6 **Nerve Block** 63
5.6.1 The Supraorbital Nerve 64
5.6.2 The Supratrochlear Nerve 64
5.6.3 The Infraorbital Nerve 64
5.6.4 The Mental Nerve 65
5.6.5 The Zygomaticofacial Nerve 66

5.7 **Adverse Events** 67

5.8 **Disadvantages of Local Anesthetics** 67

5.9 **Tips, Tricks and Key Points** 68

References 68

5.1 Introduction

Do we really need a chapter on local anesthesia? We have good topical anesthetics and by now a large amount of new preparations of HA-based fillers and volumizers containing lidocaine (0.3 %). Both measures have helped to decrease injection pain considerably. Furthermore, preparations with lidocaine have an additional advantage as we can go back to the treated area as many times as needed to enhance the results. The longer it takes to retouch the area, the more efficient the numbness will be – e.g., our results will be better as we no longer have to be afraid of inflicting more pain to the patient.

Although the products with lidocaine are here to stay, topical anesthetics or ice bags continue to play a part in reducing pain during the penetration of the needle through the skin, especially for sensitive patients.

Cannulas are becoming ever more popular. The gauge may vary from 30 to 18. Even when cannulas are to be used with products with lidocaine, some injectors still perform nerve blocks to minimize patients' discomfort during the injection. This chapter should help those colleagues less familiar with these procedures to understand and perform local anesthesia properly, as the main goal should be to make the procedure as comfortable as possible.

M. de Maio, B. Rzany, *Injectable Fillers in Aesthetic Medicine*,
DOI 10.1007/978-3-642-45125-6_5,

Do's

- Do try to avoid pain for your patients. For example, they may like the results but never undergo a lip treatment again if the overall experience (nice lips, too much pain) was unpleasant.

5.2 Evaluation Prior to Injection

The evaluation prior to injection helps to determine the type of anesthetic procedure to be used as well as the need for any analgesic after the treatment. Simple procedures rarely require the use of adjunctive agents, except for very anxious patients. Be aware that a medical history must be taken and a physical examination performed prior to the use of any medication (Snow 1982). Preexisting medical conditions such as hypertension and heart diseases may influence the use of anesthetics in combination with epinephrine. A history of alcohol consumption, use of sedatives, and problems with anesthetics during dental procedures may indicate that extra care should be taken with these patients. It is important to ask the patients if they have had any undesirable experience with topical, infiltrative, or blocking procedures. Patients should also be asked about the use of any illegal drugs before the administration of any anesthetic medication.

Do's

- Do make it clear to patients that they must report any use of recreational drugs before anesthetic procedures.

Key Points

- Be aware that the usage of recreational drugs such as cocaine might interfere with the anesthesia.

5.3 Local Anesthesia

Local anesthetics decrease or completely block sensory, autonomic, and motor functions. They act by blocking sodium channels at the cell membrane and interrupting the excitation-conduction process (Carvalho and Mathias 1997). The systemic absorption of local anesthetics depends upon the vascular flow at the injection site, the chemical and physical characteristics of the agents, and the adjunctive use of vasoconstrictors such as epinephrine. Vasoconstrictors will decrease the absorption and enhance the availability of the local anesthetic to the nerve cells, thus prolonging the duration of action and decreasing possible systemic effects. Care should be taken not to inject local anesthetics with epinephrine into areas of terminal circulation, due to an increased risk of necrosis.

5.4 Topical Anesthesia

In most cases, the level of anesthesia achieved with a topical anesthetic will be sufficient to alleviate discomfort during the injection of dermal fillers. There are basically two groups of topical agents: the ester group (cocaine, tetracaine, and benzocaine) and the amide group (lidocaine and prilocaine).

The stratum corneum is a strong barrier to the absorption of drugs through the skin. The skin should be cleaned with antiseptics before applying the topical anesthetic cream, as this will allow better permeation of the topical agents. The effect may also be enhanced by rubbing dry gauze onto the surface to remove dead cells and grease. The vasodilatation that results from this rubbing of the skin may also increase the permeation of the drug.

One of the most common topical anesthetics is a eutectic mixture of 2.5 % lidocaine and 2.5 % prilocaine, which is marketed as EMLA cream. It is a nontoxic mixture which use results in very low plasma levels. The usual dose is 1 g for each 10 cm^2 of intact epidermis. The cream should be in contact with the skin for approximately 45 min to 1 h with occlusive dressing (Hallen and

Uppfeldt 1982). There is a new lidocaine and tetracaine mixture on the market which is marketed in Europe as Pliaglis. So far (Summer 2013) the experience with this product, which is quite different from EMLA (more a paste than a cream), is limited (Cohen 2013).

Cryoanesthesia is another method of inducing topical anesthesia. The simple application of ice bags may enhance the anesthetic effect. In fact, for some patients, the use of ice bags alone will provide enough anesthesia. Other topical freezing agents include ethyl chloride or dichlorotetrafluoroethane sprays, but these are unlikely to be used when the treatment involves dermal fillers.

Key Points

- Skin permeation of topical anesthetic may be enhanced by rubbing dry gauze on the skin.
- When you use topical anesthetics, make sure that the topicals are applied a sufficient time before the injection.

5.5 Infiltrative Anesthesia

Direct inhibition of nerve ending excitation may be achieved by infiltrative anesthesia. The drug of choice is generally 1 % lidocaine, which is injected intradermally or subcutaneously. Intradermal injection results in a rapid onset and longer duration of anesthesia, but it has the disadvantage of being painful and causing tissue distortion. Subcutaneous injection is less painful but has a shorter-lasting effect (Arndt et al. 1983). During infiltrative anesthesia, patients usually feel a prick when the needle pierces the skin and a burning sensation with infusion of the anesthetic itself. Pain results from rapid tissue distention. Therefore the use of smaller volumes is advised to avoid discomfort. The combination of freshly prepared solutions with epinephrine or bicarbonate can greatly reduce the pain during infiltration (McKay et al. 1987). For very anxious patients, it may be useful to apply topical anesthetics before administering the infiltrative anesthesia.

Key Points

- Infiltrative anesthesia is not commonly used before injectable fillers because it can distort the analysis of the treatment area.

5.6 Nerve Block

Nerve block anesthesia is performed by an injection of a small amount of local anesthetic around a nerve, resulting in anesthesia within the area supplied by that nerve. The volume of anesthetic used in these procedures is small. Therefore, the risk of systemic toxicity is low. In contrast to the infiltrative method, there is almost no imbalance with nerve blocks, and they are associated with less discomfort. However, this method requires good technical and anatomical knowledge to obtain optimal results with few injections and to avoid adverse events. There is the possibility of inadvertent laceration of the nerve and blood vessel injuries. Long-lasting dysesthesia and hematoma or ecchymosis may occur in a few patients, which may be quite distressing (Laskin 1984). The sensitivity and motion of the face depend on the fifth pair of cranial nerves (Fig. 5.1). The main trigeminal branches have independent exits from the skull. The ophthalmic branch is more superior and passes inside the orbit, forming the frontal branch, which bifurcates into the supraorbital and supratrochlear nerves. The other two branches are the maxillary nerve, which produces the infraorbital nerve, and the mandibular nerve, which is the largest, the only one to contain motor fibers, and which produces the mental nerve. Nerve block is usually achieved with 1 or 2 % lidocaine. A combination of epinephrine and lidocaine is preferable when a quicker and longer-lasting anesthetic response is required. Care should be taken not to inadvertently inject this into the blood vessels. Epinephrine should also be avoided in patients with hypertension or cardiovascular diseases. Pain results from tissue expansion during the injection, and irritation from the anesthetic itself. Gentle injections are preferable and provide a quite tolerable nerve block.

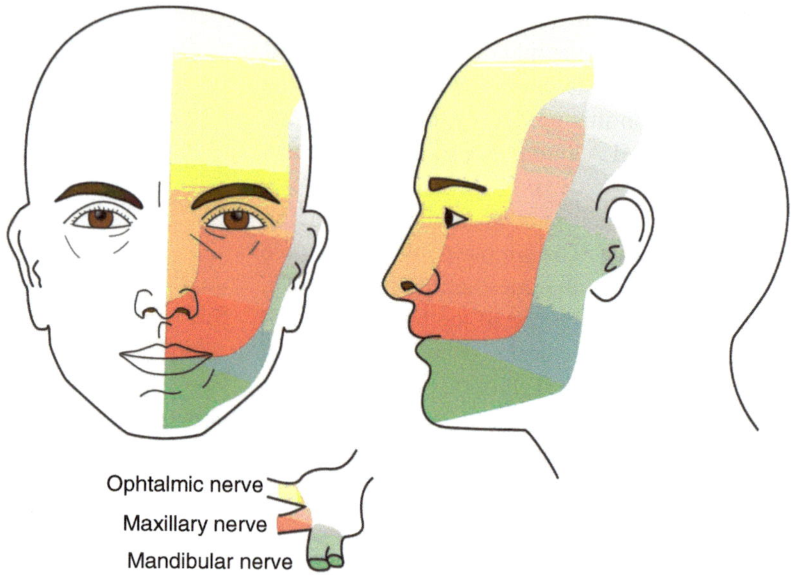

Fig. 5.1 Areas supplied by the main facial nerves (de Maio 2011)

> **Do's**
> - Do verify the type of preparation that will be used, 1 or 2 % with or without epinephrine before the injection.

> **Key Points**
> - The need of nerve blocks has tremendously decreased after the advent of fillers containing lidocaine.

5.6.1 The Supraorbital Nerve

5.6.1.1 Anatomy and Territory

The supraorbital nerve exits the skull through the supraorbital foramen, which lies along the supraorbital ridge in the midpupillary line. It supplies the forehead.

5.6.1.2 Technique

Inject 0.1–0.3 ml lidocaine right into the depression in the internal third of the eyebrows (supraorbital notch) with the needle pointed toward the forehead (Figs. 5.2 and 5.3).

5.6.2 The Supratrochlear Nerve

5.6.2.1 Anatomy and Territory

The supratrochlear nerve exits the skull along the medial corner of the orbit. It supplies the medial portion of the forehead.

5.6.2.2 Technique

Inject 0.1–0.3 ml lidocaine at the junction of the root of the nose and the upper rim of the orbit, just below the medial portion of the eyebrow (Fig. 5.4).

5.6.3 The Infraorbital Nerve

5.6.3.1 Anatomy and Territory

The infraorbital nerve exits the infraorbital foramen in the midpupillary line about 1 cm inferior to the infraorbital ridge. It supplies the lower eyelid, nasolabial fold, upper lip, and parts of the medial cheek and nose.

5.6.3.2 Technique

The infraorbital foramen can usually be palpated. There are two ways of blocking it: by a cutaneous and a mucosal approach. For cutaneous injections, the needle should be placed 1 cm below the

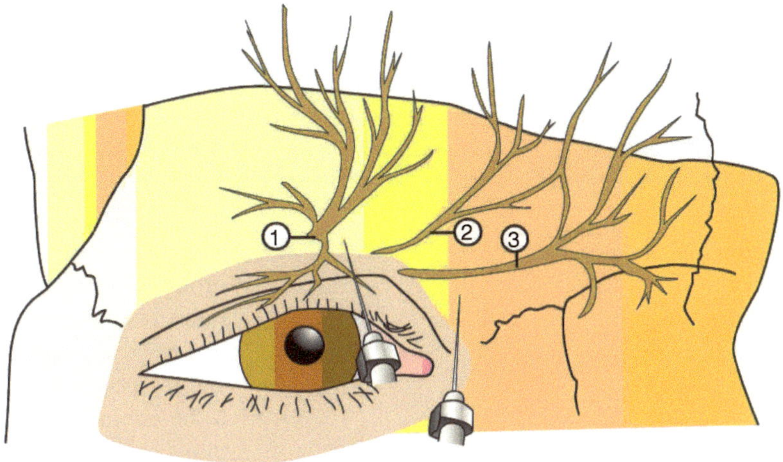

Fig. 5.2 Anatomy and blocking of the supraorbital nerve. (*1*) External branch of the frontal nerve and (*2*) and (*3*) internal branch of the frontal nerve (de Maio 2011)

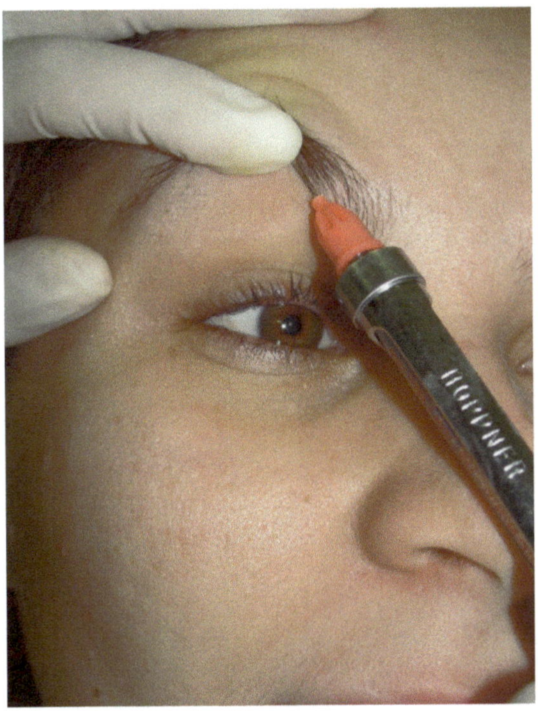

Fig. 5.3 Blocking of the supraorbital nerve

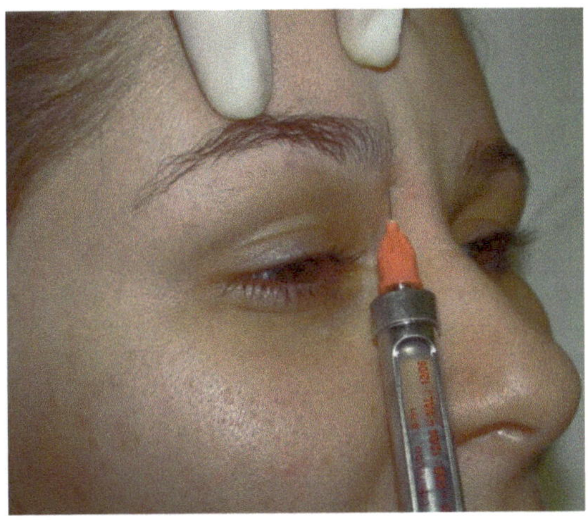

Fig. 5.4 Blocking of the supratrochlear nerve

inferior orbital rim in the midpupillary line and 0.1–0.3 ml lidocaine injected around but not into the canal. The needle should be advanced through the mucosa and then through the superior labial sulcus, aiming at the iris at the canine level. A total of 0.5–1 ml lidocaine should be injected using a retrograde technique. Control of the needle is undertaken externally with palpation (Figs. 5.5 and 5.6).

5.6.4 The Mental Nerve

5.6.4.1 Anatomy and Territory

The mental nerve exits the mental foramen approximately 2.5 cm away from the midline of the face in the midpupillary line. It supplies the lower lip and chin.

5.6.4.2 Technique

Inject 0.1–0.3 ml of lidocaine through the inferior labial sulcus, inserting the needle between the second and third inferior premolars aiming at the foramen mentalis (Fig. 5.7).

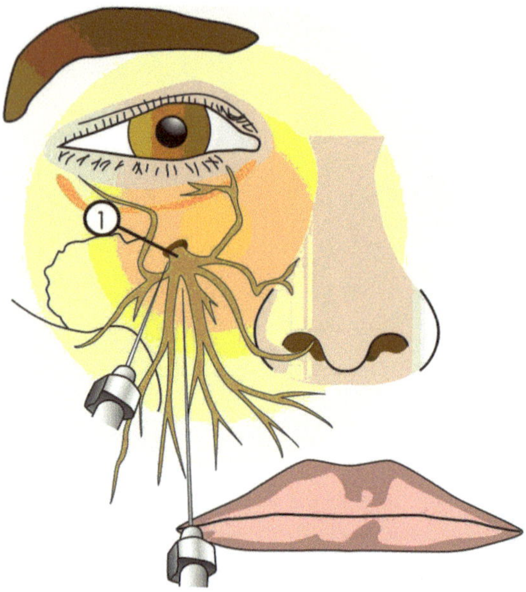

Fig. 5.5 Blocking of the infraorbital nerve (1) (de Maio 2011)

5.6.5 The Zygomaticofacial Nerve

5.6.5.1 Anatomy and Territory

The zygomatic nerve (temporomalar nerve, orbital nerve) is a branch of the maxillary nerve (a trigeminal nerve branch) that enters the orbit and helps to supply the skin over the zygomatic and temporal bones. The zygomatic nerve is not to be confused with the zygomatic branches of the facial nerve. The zygomatic nerve arises in the pterygopalatine fossa. It enters the orbit by the inferior orbital fissure and divides into two branches at the back of the cavity into two branches, the zygomaticotemporal nerve and zygomaticofacial nerve.

5.6.5.2 Technique

Inject 0.1–0.3 ml of lidocaine 1 cm below the lateral canthus and at level of the zygomaticofacial foramen in the zygomatic bone.

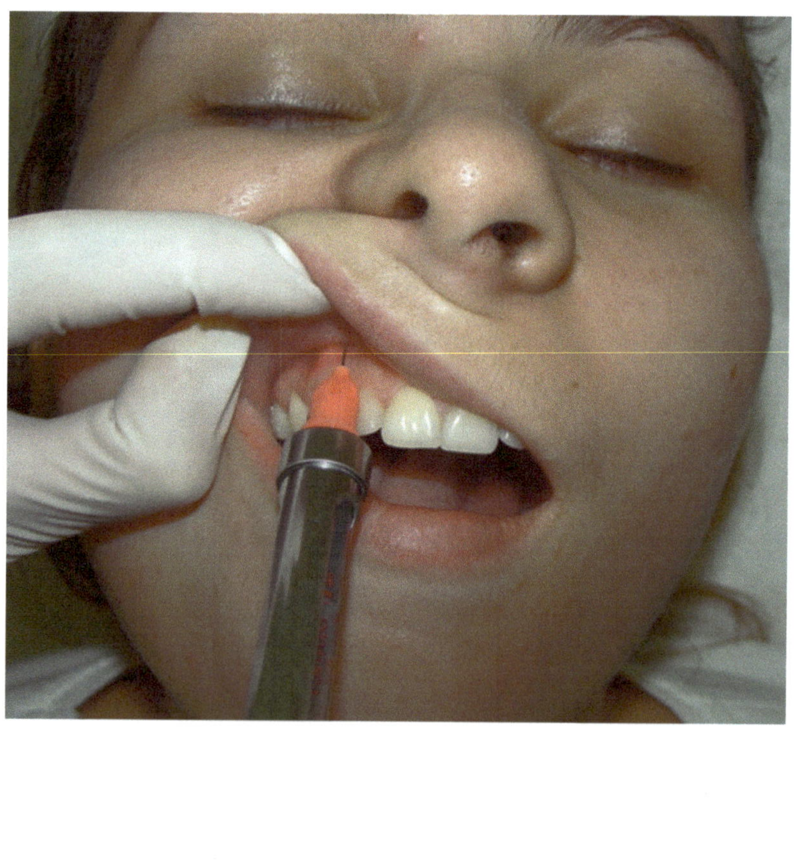

Fig. 5.6 The mucosal approach for infraorbital nerve blocking

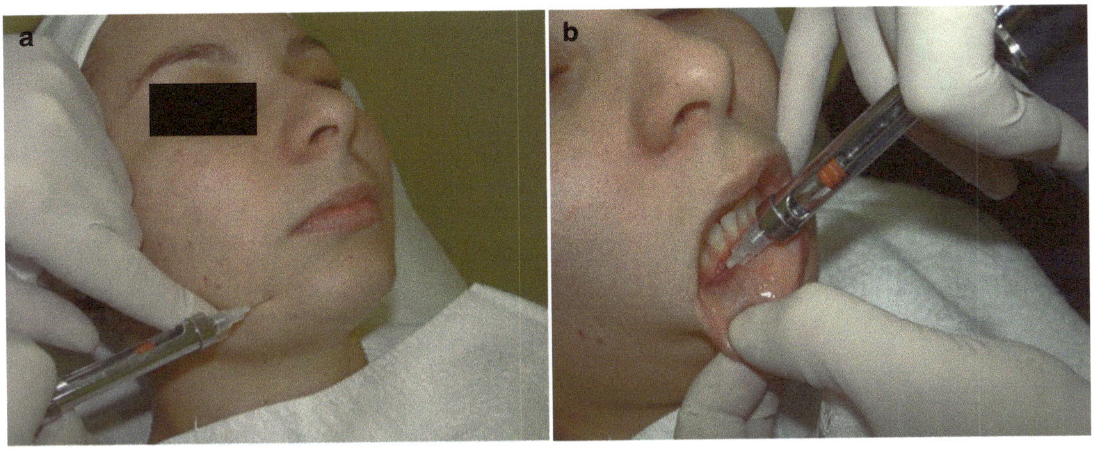

Fig. 5.7 (**a**) The mental nerve may be blocked either transcutaneously or through the mucosa (**b**)

5.7 Adverse Events

Adverse events can result from the anesthetic itself but are usually more common when epinephrine is used concomitantly. Short-term systemic reactions to epinephrine include tremor, tachycardia, restlessness, palpitations, headache, increased blood pressure, and chest pain (Grekin and Auletta 1988). Systemic reactions to local anesthetics can occur when toxic levels are reached. The use of larger volumes than recommended and inadvertent intravascular injection are the most common causes of toxicity.

Systemic toxicity of local anesthetics is characterized by central nervous and cardiovascular impairment. Signs and symptoms of toxicity depend on the velocity of injection and plasma concentration of the drug. The diagnosis of severe toxicity is mandatory: lip and tongue paresthesia, blurred vision, motor fasciculations, tinnitus, seizures, unconsciousness, coma, and respiratory and cardiovascular depression (Mather and Cousins 1979). Local anesthetics block sodium channels, causing myocardial depolarization and a reduction in nerve conduction velocity. Aesthetic treatment involving local anesthetics should therefore be carried out in conjunction with support measurements such as ventilation, oxygenation, and cardiovascular optimization.

Allergic reactions to anesthetics are rare but have been known to occur with ester preparations (Brown et al. 1981).

Key Points

- Short-term systemic reactions to local anesthetics containing epinephrine include tremor, tachycardia, restlessness, palpitations, headache, increased blood pressure, and chest pain.
- Real allergic reactions are very rare with local anesthetics.

5.8 Disadvantages of Local Anesthetics

The eutectic mixture of 2.5 % lidocaine and 2.5 % prilocaine may decrease the visibility of fine wrinkles, thus making it impractical for treatments involving very fine fillers such as some hyaluronic acid products. Nerve blocking might considerably change the shape of, for example, the nasolabial fold and the upper lip and may therefore encourage under- or overcorrection.

5.9 Tips, Tricks and Key Points

Never let the patients feel pain during aesthetic procedures. Any negative experience may mean that patients refuse to continue with facial improvement. Anesthesia should be seen as one of the most important steps during aesthetic treatment with fillers and volumizers.

Do's

- Do use products with lidocaine, or if the products (e.g., PLLA) do not contain a local anesthetic, add a local anesthetic to the solution/the filler. They reduce the patient's discomfort during the injection.
- Do perform nerve blocks if you are working with 21–18 gauge cannulas. It brings more comfort to the patient.

Don'ts

- Do not forget to slow down the speed of injection if you are working with products that contain lidocaine. It takes around 3–5 s to take effect.
- Do not get too hectic. If you are relaxed, the patient will be relaxed and therefore will experience less discomfort.

Key Points

- Products containing lidocaine have tremendously improved patients' comfort during the treatment, especially the most sensitive areas such as lips, perioral, and nose.

References

Arndt KA et al (1983) Minimizing the pain of local anesthesia. Plast Reconstr Surg 72(5):676–679

Brown DT et al (1981) Allergic reaction to an amide local anaesthetic. Br J Anaesth 53(4):435–437

Carvalho JCA, Mathias RS (1997) Chapter 22. Farmacologia Do's anestésicos locais. In: Manica JT et al (eds) Anestesiologia: Princípios e Técnicas, 2nd edn. Artes Médicas, Porto Alegre, pp 332–340

Cohen JL (2013) Pain management with a topical lidocaine and tetracaine 7 %/7 % cream with laser dermatologic procedures. J Drugs Dermatol 12(9):986–989

De Maio M (ed) (2011) Tratado De Medicina Estetica, 2nd edn. M. Ed. Roca, Sao Paulo

Grekin RC, Auletta MJ (1988) Local anesthesia in dermatologic surgery. J Am Acad Dermatol 19(4):599–614

Hallen B, Uppfeldt A (1982) Does lidocaine-prilocaine cream permit pain-free insertion of IV catheters in children? Anesthesiology 57(4):340–342

Laskin DM (1984) Diagnosis and treatment of complications associated with local anaesthesia. Int Dent J 34(4):232–237

Mather LE, Cousins MJ (1979) Local anaesthetics and their current clinical use. Drugs 18(3):185–205

McKay W et al (1987) Sodium bicarbonate attenuates pain on skin infiltration with lidocaine, with or without epinephrine. Anesth Analg 66(6):572–574

Snow J (1982) Manual of anesthesia. Little, Brown, Boston

The Most Common Indications 6

Mauricio de Maio and Berthold Rzany

Contents

6.1 **Forehead and Glabella** 70
6.1.1 Introduction 70
6.1.2 Anatomy 70
6.1.3 Patient Evaluation and Selection 71
6.1.4 Techniques 71
6.1.5 Tips, Tricks and Key Points 74

6.2 **Temples** 74
6.2.1 Introduction 74
6.2.2 Anatomy 74
6.2.3 Patient Evaluation and Selection 74
6.2.4 Technique 75
6.2.5 Complications 75
6.2.6 Tips, Tricks and Key Points 75

6.3 **Eyebrow** 76
6.3.1 Introduction 76
6.3.2 Anatomy 76
6.3.3 Patient Evaluation and Selection 77
6.3.4 Technique 78
6.3.5 Complications 79
6.3.6 Tips, Tricks and Key Points 79

6.4 **Epicanthal Fold and Sunken Upper Eyelid** 80
6.4.1 Epicanthal Fold 80
6.4.2 Sunken Upper Eyelid 80
6.4.3 Tips, Tricks and Key Points 81

6.5 **Infraorbital Hollow, Tear Trough, Cheekbones, and Cheek Reshaping** 83
6.5.1 Introduction 83
6.5.2 Anatomy 84
6.5.3 Patient Evaluation and Selection 85
6.5.4 Tear Trough and Infraorbital Area 85
6.5.5 Cheekbones 89
6.5.6 Cheek 92
6.5.7 Complications 96
6.5.8 Tips, Tricks and Key Points 96

6.6 **Nose Reshaping** 97
6.6.1 Introduction 97
6.6.2 Anatomy 98
6.6.3 Patient Evaluation and Selection 100
6.6.4 Technique 101
6.6.5 The Nasofrontal Angle 102
6.6.6 The Nasolabial Angle 102
6.6.7 The Tip and the Columella 102
6.6.8 Dorsum 103
6.6.9 Selection of Filler 105
6.6.10 Complications 105
6.6.11 Tips, Tricks and Key Points 106

6.7 **Nasolabial Folds** 106
6.7.1 Introduction 106
6.7.2 Anatomy/Structure 106
6.7.3 Patient Evaluation and Selection 108
6.7.4 Technique 108
6.7.5 Touch-Up 109
6.7.6 Complications 110
6.7.7 Tips, Tricks and Key Points 111

6.8 **The Earlobe** 112
6.8.1 Introduction 112
6.8.2 Anatomy/Structure 112
6.8.3 Patient Evaluation and Selection 112
6.8.4 Technique 113
6.8.5 Tips, Tricks and Key Points 114

6.9 **The Upper and Lower Lips** 114
6.9.1 Introduction 114
6.9.2 Anatomy 114
6.9.3 Patient Evaluation and Selection 116
6.9.4 Technique 117
6.9.5 Complications 120
6.9.6 Tips, Tricks and Key Points 120

6.10 **Marionette Lines** 123
6.10.1 Introduction 123
6.10.2 Anatomy 123
6.10.3 Patient Evaluation and Selection 123
6.10.4 Technique 123
6.10.5 Complications 123
6.10.6 Tips, Tricks and Key Points 124

M. de Maio, B. Rzany, *Injectable Fillers in Aesthetic Medicine*,
DOI 10.1007/978-3-642-45125-6_6, © Springer-Verlag Berlin Heidelberg 2014

6.11 **Jawline and Chin Reshaping** 125
6.11.1 Introduction 125
6.11.2 Anatomy 125
6.11.3 Patient Evaluation and Selection 126
6.11.4 Technique 127
6.11.5 Complications 128
6.11.6 Tips, Tricks and Key Points 129
6.12 **Other Facial Indications for Volumizers** 131
6.12.1 Introduction 131
6.12.2 Facial Advancement 131
6.12.3 Tips, Tricks and Key Points 132
References 132

In the following chapter, the indications will be discussed separately. However, one must be aware that treating one indication might influence the other indication, e.g., treating the temporal region may influence the position of the eyebrow and treating the cheek will influence the appearance of the tear trough and infraorbital hollow.

6.1 Forehead and Glabella

6.1.1 Introduction

The forehead and glabellar areas are characterized by extensive mimic movements of three main muscles: Mm. occipitofrontal, corrugator, and procerus. Horizontal forehead lines appear when the occipitofrontal muscle is activated. The vertical glabellar folds result from the continuous contraction of both corrugator muscles. The horizontal lines in the glabellar area arise from pronounced procerus muscle activity. With time, these lines become embedded into the skin and will not disappear after BoNT-A treatment. Therefore, the best possible overall effect may be gained using fillers (Fig. 6.1).

6.1.2 Anatomy

The aesthetic forehead unit comprises the upper one-third of the classical "facial thirds." It extends vertically from the supraorbital rim to the anterior hairline. The skin on the forehead is generally thicker than on the lower face, and five layers are encountered at this level: the skin, the subcutaneous tissue, the galea aponeurotica, a part of the submuscular aponeurotic system (SMAS), the loose subaponeurotic areolar layer, and the periosteum.

The fascia superficialis is known as the temporoparietal fascia in the temporal area and as the galea in the forehead. There is a fat pad called the galea fat pad in the glabella and above the eyebrows. The superficial fat is sparse in the forehead,

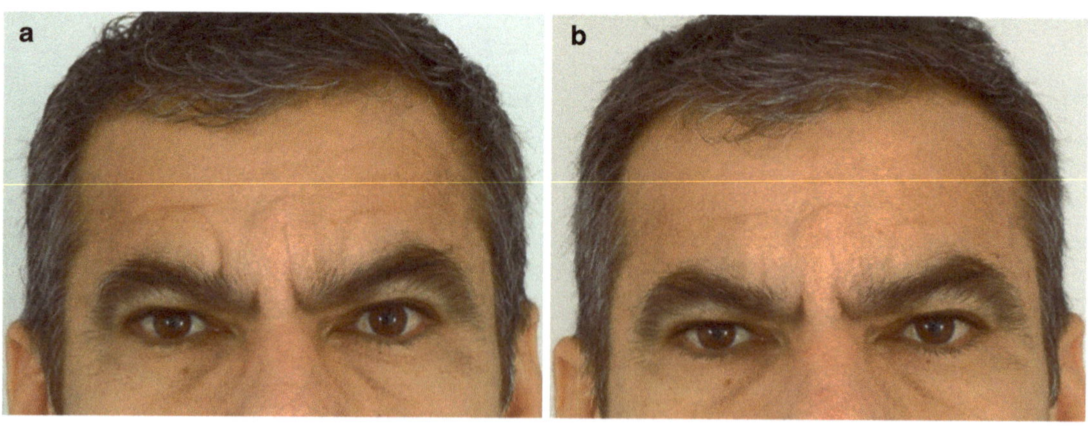

Fig. 6.1 (**a**) Analysis of the patient at rest: observe that due to overcontraction of the corrugators over time, the patient became hypertonic and is unable to relax these muscles anymore with the result of deep static wrinkles. BoNT-A alone would not be able to correct those lines or maintain a long-lasting result. (**b**) The patient was submitted to deep injection with HA with a 21G blunt cannula in both scar-like medial and lateral vertical wrinkles. No BoNT-A was injected and there is persistence of corrugators contraction

glabella, temporal, and orbital areas. It is dense due to fibrotic septa in the forehead region. Deep fat is dense in the temporal and periocular areas. At this level, the temporal extension of the deep fat pad of Bichat may be found. In the upper face, the SMAS denominated the galea aponeurotica, which envelops the frontalis, the occipitalis, and the procerus. The frontalis forms the frontal belly of the occipitofrontal muscle and is inserted into the galea aponeurotica. The galea connects the frontalis and the occipital muscles. In the central forehead, the frontalis muscle is paired and united by the superficial fascia. It raises the eyebrows and produces the forehead hyperkinetic lines. The frontalis antagonists are the corrugators, procerus, and orbicularis oculi.

The supraorbital artery is a terminal branch of the ophthalmic artery from the internal carotid artery. The superficial temporal artery is the terminal branch of the external carotid artery and divides into two major branches. The carotid veins accompany these arteries. The frontal branch of the facial nerve may be found within the temporoparietal fascia, from the midportion of the zygomatic arch up to its entrance to the frontalis muscle. It provides motor innervation to the frontalis, corrugator, and procerus muscles. It also innervates the cephalic portion of the orbicularis oculi (Pitanguy and Ramos 1966). The supratrochlear nerve exits the orbit between the periosteum and the orbital septum at the medial supraorbital rim. It runs along the caudal aspect and within the corrugator muscle and then superiorly on the inner surface of the frontalis fascia to supply sensation to the medial and central forehead. The supraorbital nerve exits between the medial and central thirds of the superior orbital rim and runs superiorly and laterally on the inner surface of the frontalis fascia and galea. It is responsible for sensation in the anterior lateral forehead and scalp.

6.1.3 Patient Evaluation and Selection

Patients should be critically appraised for possible pretreatment with BoNT-A; additional filler therapy in these areas often turns out to be unnecessary after pretreatment with BoNT-A. Persistent wrinkles after BoNT-A treatment as the residual wrinkles above the lateral eyebrows may benefit from the treatment with an injectable filler. Patients presenting deep forehead and glabellar folds will require a filler that can be injected more deeply (subcutaneous or intramuscular planes) to increase volume (Fig. 6.2). Patients presenting superficial forehead and glabellar folds or lines may benefit from a fine or very fine filler that must be injected more superficially (Fig. 6.3). Furthermore, for patients with advanced elastosis, repeated treatments with injectable fillers may rejuvenate the whole area. For deep and superficial forehead and glabellar folds, the appropriate fillers should be combined and the proper use of needles or cannulas should be considered.

6.1.4 Techniques

Anesthesia is not usually necessary. Most injectors use the retrograde tunnel technique (i.e., the filler is injected while withdrawing the needle), as it allows a faster application. However, the multiple injection site technique can also be used. This technique will help to blend the filler better into the surrounding area. Deep and superficial forehead and/or glabellar lines may require multilevel injections. The injection should not be too deep. An injection below the fascia may encourage migration of the filler (e.g., from the glabella to the perinasal area). To avoid an occlusion of the arteries, which have been reported for the glabella and forehead area, all injections should be done very carefully, if possible through a 30G or even blunt cannulas when deep planes are treated. Higher volumes should be avoided in this area. Usually 0.2–0.3 ml of an HA filler may be sufficient for the glabellar area (Bachmann et al. 2009). During treatment, avoid injecting into the direction of the upper eyelid if volume replacement at this level is not necessary.

Usually, volume requirement for the whole forehead is high especially when there is severe volume loss and depressions (Figs. 6.4 and 6.5).

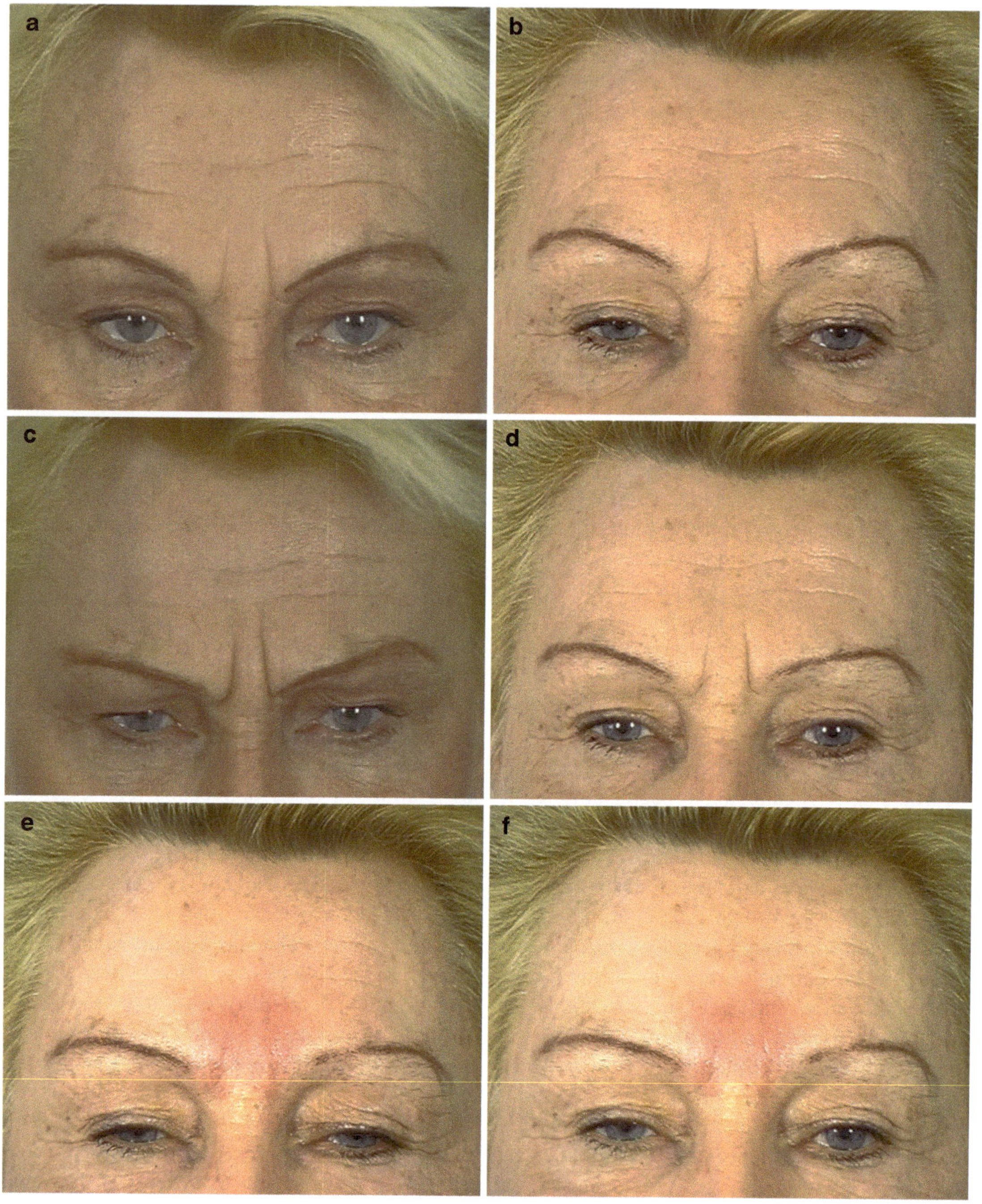

Fig. 6.2 (**a, b**) Before and 3 weeks after treatment with BoNT-A. Status: relaxed. (**c, d**) Before and 3 weeks after the treatment with BoNT-A. Status: at maximum frown. (**e, f**) Immediately after injection of hyaluronic acid relaxed and maximum frown. Please note: the erythema is not always necessarily present

Medium- to high-viscosity HA products are used with cannulas for forehead and glabella reshape to improve contour and volume loss. In elderly patients with severe dermal and subcutaneous atrophy, lower-viscosity HA products are preferred.

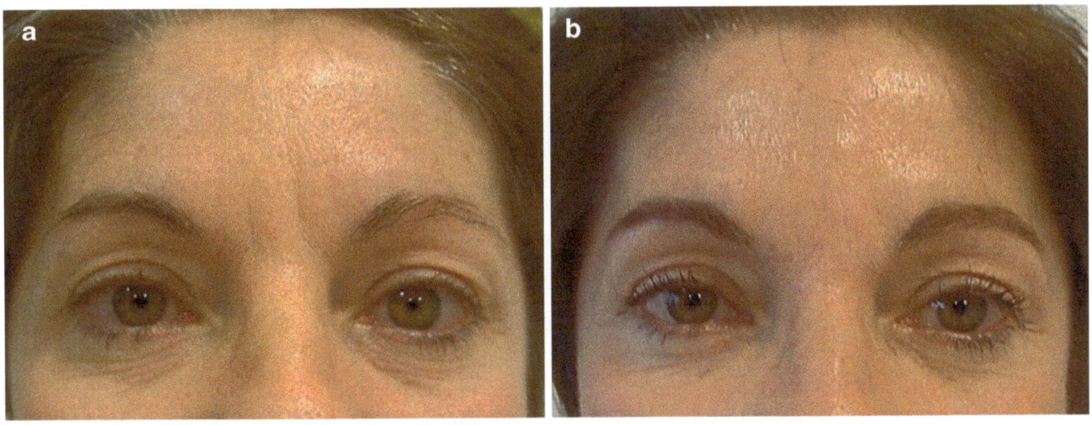

Fig. 6.3 (**a**) Superficial static lines over the glabella. (**b**) The patient was submitted to the injection of HA fine lines with a 30G cannula into the superficial dermis to avoid vascular occlusion. BoNT-A was not injected

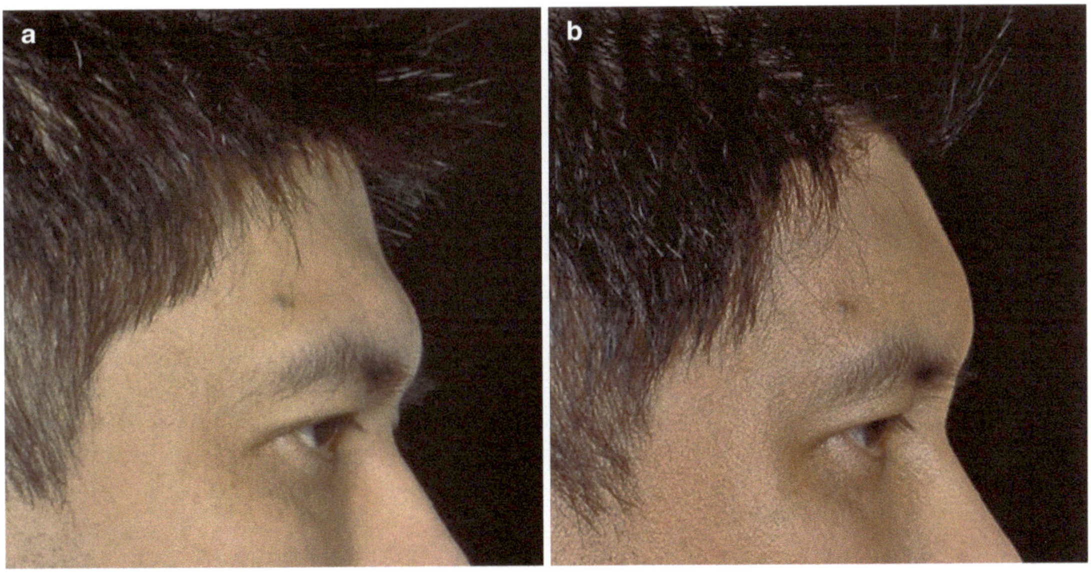

Fig. 6.4 (**a**) In Asians, due to structural aspect, concavity in the upper forehead and convexity at the glabella level may be found and is considered undesirable. (**b**) The patient was submitted to an injection of 4 ml Juvéderm Voluma with a single entry point in each eyebrow between the supratrochlear and supraorbital foramina. A 21G non-flexible blunt cannula was used. The after photo was taken after 8 months

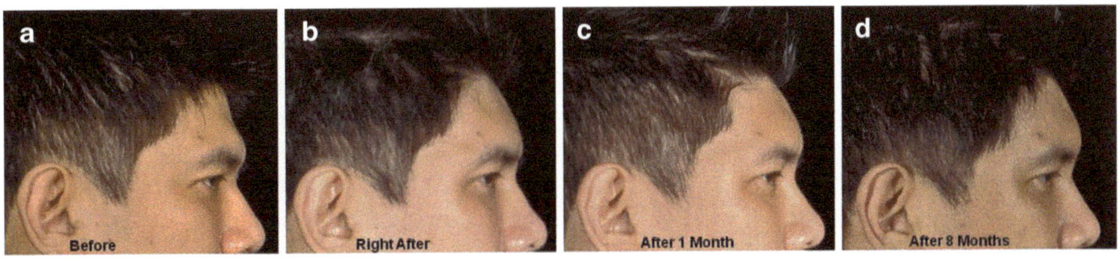

Fig. 6.5 (**a–d**) Before, immediately after, as well as 1 and 8 months after the forehead reshaping. Note: the consistency of the results over an 8-month period

6.1.5 Tips, Tricks and Key Points

Do's

- Before injecting a filler treating forehead and glabellar folds, it is recommendable to pretreat this area with BoNT-A. The combination of BoNT-A and an injectable filler usually leads to a better overall result. BoNT-A should be injected approximately 2 weeks before the filler, although both procedures can be performed at the same time in this area.
- Any remaining superficial lines above the eyebrow after treatment of the upper third with BoNT-A can easily be corrected with a biodegradable filler of low viscosity. Correction with small dosages of BoNT-A is also possible. However, this might carry a small risk of brow ptosis if a significant part of the M. frontalis is affected.

Don'ts

- Do not inject too much volume into the glabella and forehead area. In rare cases focal necrosis is reported after the treatment of the glabella and/or the forehead.

Key Points

- The glabella is a combination therapy area. BoNT-A therapy should go first.
- Do not inject too much volume into the glabella and forehead area. A little less may be preferable to decrease the risk of an unwanted arterial occlusion or extravascular compression.

6.2 Temples

6.2.1 Introduction

Thus far the temples are not frequently requested for treatment. However, when treating the whole face, this area should not be forgotten as it may impact the overall expression of the patient, e.g., the combination of full cheeks and hollow temples may not be aesthetically wanted. Furthermore, treatment of the temporal area may improve eyebrow positioning (see below) and thereby add further improvement to the upper face.

6.2.2 Anatomy

Lateral to the forehead region lies the temporal area. It is located above the zygomatic arch, limited by the temporal crest or linea temporalis (the junction of the frontal, temporal, and parietal bones) and laterally by the hairline. Below the skin and subcutaneous tissue, there are three fascial layers within the temporal region, comprising the superficial temporal fascia (or temporoparietal fascia), which is strongly attached to the subcutaneous tissue, and the superficial and deep layers of the deep temporal fascia attached to the bony floor. The trigeminal nerve supplies the sensory innervation of the temporal region. The temporal branch of the facial nerve passes posterior to the middle aspect of the zygomatic arch, where it lies quite superficially beneath the subcutaneous fat. The superficial temporal artery and vein are also found in the subcutaneous layer in the temporal area.

6.2.3 Patient Evaluation and Selection

Ideally, the temporal area should be slightly convex. With aging, it becomes straight, then concave. The concavity progresses from mild to moderate, then severe and very severe with a skeletonized appearance of zygomatic arch. The higher the volume loss, the higher volume replacement is required. A total amount of 0.5 ml of HA-based volumizer is enough for mild/moderate cases (Fig. 6.6) and an average of 1–2 ml per side in severe cases, and in very severe volume loss, a total of 4 ml of an HA-based volumizer may be required. A treatment of the temporal area may also have a beneficial effect on the lateral eyebrows. Some patients will

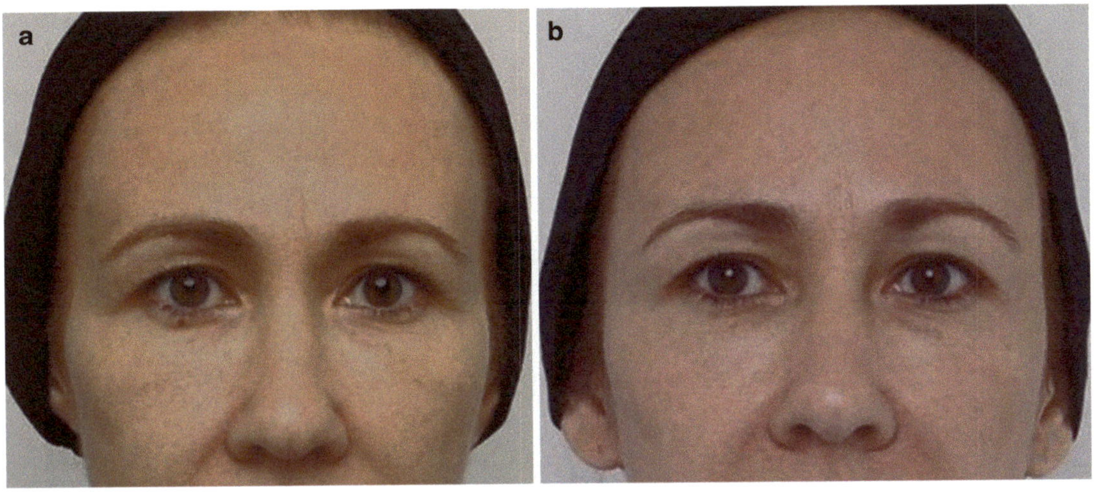

Fig. 6.6 (**a**) Volume loss and concave aspect at the temporal area down to the projection of the zygomatic arch before treatment. (**b**) After injection of 0.5 ml of Juvéderm Voluma per side, a convex aspect was obtained

present lateral eyebrow lifting only with injection into the temporal area.

6.2.4 Technique

Volume replacement at the temporal area may be carried out with needles or cannulas. Products may be placed deep down to the bone and/or subcutaneously. After marking the area of volume loss and identifying the superficial temporal artery (may be visible or may identifiable by its pulse) and the veins, the filler can be injected very safely by needle. The needle should be inserted perpendicular to the skin penetrating the epidermis, dermis, subcutaneous, superficial temporal fascia, temporal muscle, and deep temporal fascia up to the bone. The periosteum should not be scratched to avoid pain. After aspiration to rule out vascular injection, the filler/volumizer may be delivered safely. Advise the patient that (specifically with deep injections) a slight pressure at the temple level may be felt especially during mastication in the first post-treatment day. The disadvantage of this approach is more volume usage compared to the subcutaneous approach. The subcutaneous approach is the second possibility. As needles may lead to bruising and/or intravascular injections, cannulas are encouraged. However, specifically patients with severe subcutaneous atrophy may present irregularities of skin surface after subcutaneous filling with either needles or blunt cannulas.

6.2.5 Complications

With anatomical landmarks marked before, the injection itself is a very safe procedure performing deep temple volume replacement by needle. With the subcutaneous approach, bruising and surface irregularities may be found more commonly. As for the glabella and the nasolabial area also come cases of arterial occlusion have been reported for this area.

6.2.6 Tips, Tricks and Key Points

Most patients are not aware of volume loss at the temporal area. Therefore, the treating physician may suggest this area when designing the treatment plan.

Do's

- Remember that temporal volume replacement may be accompanied by lateral eyebrow elevation.
- The use of blunt microcannulas is encouraged using the subcutaneous approach for temporal elevation.

Don'ts

- Do not forget to assess and point out the volume loss in the temporal area in your patients. The sooner it is corrected, the lower the volume requirement will be.

Key Points

- Temple volume replacement has become more effective since the introduction of HA-based volumizers. We are able not only to correct the sunken aspect but also to lift the lateral aspect of the eyebrow. It is an important ally to BoNT-A treatments for the upper third.

6.3 Eyebrow

6.3.1 Introduction

One of the most important aspects of beauty concerns the position of the eyebrows. It has been established that "well-demarcated eyebrows should arch slightly at the junction of the medial two-thirds and lateral one-third of the face." Variations of color and texture of the hair contribute significantly to the overall perception of the image. However, it is the volume and mass at this level that determine the uniqueness of beauty. Eyebrow dimensions vary widely on an individual and ethnic basis. Eyebrow hair in the medial one-third is full and tends to sweep upward and laterally. In the middle one-third, hair direction is more horizontal and lateral; in the lateral one-third it points downward. It should be noted that normal eyebrow position differs from men to women, and this has to be taken into account when proper correction of undesired aspects of the eyebrows is considered.

The eyebrows not only frame the upward arc of the orbit but express emotions such as anger, frustration, and uncertainty. Any negative aspect concerning the eyebrow symmetry, position, and fullness influences the overall aesthetic balance of the face. Eyebrow position will change with age, as gravity and loss of soft-tissue support result in ptosis, thereby creating a tired and sad look. Eyebrow ptosis leads to lateral hooding of eyelids. The resulting skin excess influences the crow's feet lines. Hyperactivity of the frontalis muscle is an attempt to correct malposition of the eyebrow and results in transverse lines in the forehead.

Rejuvenation of the upper face may be accomplished using surgical and nonsurgical techniques. Nonsurgical techniques include ablative methods, BoNT-A, and fillers. The surgical approach includes the temporal lift, the endoscopic brow lift, and the coronal lift. Some of the surgical techniques targeting upper-third rejuvenation present certain limitations. Depending on the chosen technique, there may be no effect on glabellar and forehead lines or those in the middle and medium part of the eyebrow. Therefore, other methods, such as fillers and BoNT-A, are mandatory for a complete improvement.

6.3.2 Anatomy

The forehead and eyebrow positions are dependent on the frontal bone, the supraorbital rims, and the zygoma. The action of the frontalis, corrugator, and procerus muscles also influence their position. The underlying bone structure, rather than the soft tissues, can be responsible for aesthetic challenges. The contour of the orbital bone and its prominence, which can be targeted by fillers, is very important for the eyebrow position. The eyebrow is an important demarcation line dividing the upper and the mid-third of the face.

Understanding the eyebrow shape and its position with respect to the supraorbital rim is essential for promoting good results. The eyebrows should be 5–6 cm below the hairline. The medial portion of the eyebrow should lie on a perpendicular line that crosses the lateral portion of the ala nasi and rest around 1 cm above the inner canthus of the eye. The lateral eyebrow ends at an oblique line drawn from the alar base through the lateral canthus. The medial and lateral end of the eyebrow lies at the same horizontal

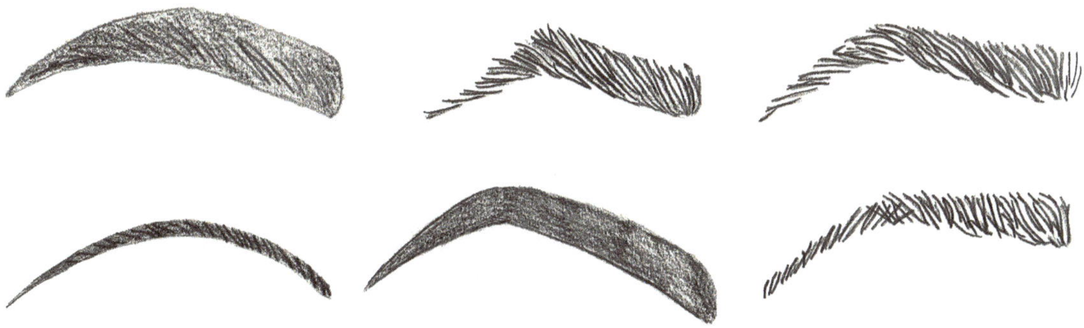

Fig. 6.7 Examples of different eyebrow shapes

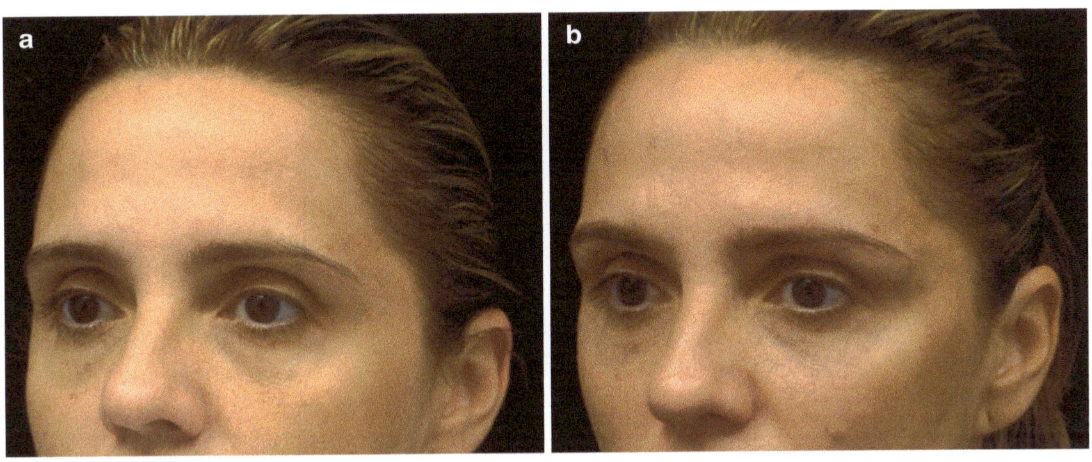

Fig. 6.8 (**a**, **b**) Patient before and after injection of 0.8 ml of Juvéderm Ultra Plus along the eyebrow per side and upper eyelid volume replacement with 0.8 ml of the same product per side both with a 21G blunt cannula. Note the projection of the upper lateral aspect of the orbit

level. In women, the eyebrow should lie above the supraorbital rim and in an arch shape with its highest point at the level of the lateral limbus of the eye at approximately the junction of the medial two-thirds and the lateral third of the eyebrow. In men, the arch must be smaller and must lie slightly lower at the supraorbital rim than in women. It also tends to be heavier in men than in women (Fig. 6.7).

6.3.3 Patient Evaluation and Selection

The initial consultation should include a physical evaluation and provision of education about the benefits that fillers may bring to brow reshaping. Patients should understand that it is not a surgical procedure. What fillers may promote is basically a mild volumetric augmentation of the lateral orbital roof and an elevation of the eyebrows in the range of millimeters (Fig. 6.8). Other aspects of the upper third such as hyperkinetic forehead and glabellar lines and the desire to have a major lifting of the eyebrows should be treated with BoNT-A or with selective endoscopic muscle transection. The patient should be evaluated for eyebrow position and mobility, eyelid function, and the presence of skin excess and eye bags. Pretreatment planning should include photographic documentation and a clear explanation of the final result.

Some clinical situations make treatment with fillers difficult or are contraindicated. Severe or

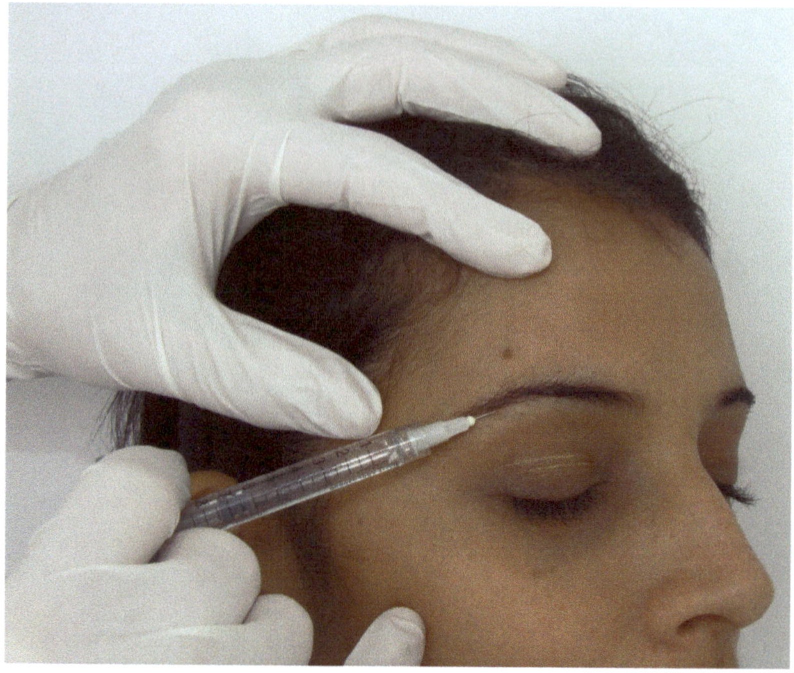

Fig. 6.9 In lateral eyebrow lifting, a small quantity of the product may be enough for the lateral upper part of the orbital roof

moderate ptosis of the eyebrows cannot be improved with fillers because of the inherent limitations of the procedure. The best results are those with symmetric mild ptosis of the eyebrows and thin skin. In these cases, the skin tends to have more mobility for both expansion and elevation. Mild upper eyelid skin excess can be improved in selected cases.

Eyebrow position is one of the common areas for asymmetry. It is quite difficult to find someone with eyebrows that are same shaped and positioned. Therefore, any asymmetry, which is quite common in middle-aged women, must be thoroughly documented before injection. Please note that most patients will present lateral eyebrow lifting only with injection at the temporal level.

6.3.4 Technique

Eyebrow elevation usually does not require local infiltration or nerve blocking prior to injection of the filler. Only topical or no anesthetic at all is usually required for this procedure. With the proper technique, this procedure may be considered quite painless.

After examining the patient, the requirement for medial, central, or lateral elevation must be evaluated. Before starting the injection, it is advisable to stretch up the eyebrow with the finger to verify the mobility of the medial, central, and lateral part of the eyebrow. When major expansion is desired, the entire eyebrow should be injected. In this case, the use of blunt cannula (21, 25, or 27 gauge) may minimize bruising.

If only lateral elevation is desired, a small quantity of the product (0.2 ml) is needed for the lateral part of the eyebrow and is usually performed with needles (Fig. 6.9). Mild differences in positions may be achieved by varying the quantity of the product injected.

Although the vast majority of fillers are designed for dermal injections, biodegradable products can be injected into all layers beneath the eyebrow for a better impression of the filler. The filler should be injected onto the periosteum, into the muscle, and subdermally, especially when volumizers are used to improve eyebrow contour and projection. The injection must be soft, and touching the periosteum (which would cause pain) should be avoided. While injecting, it is advisable to stretch the eyebrow and place the

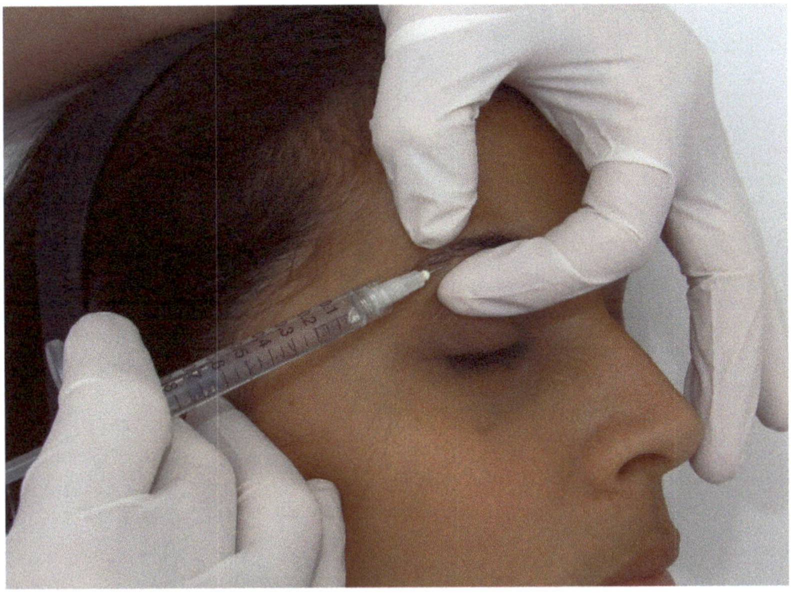

Fig. 6.10 Pinching the eyebrow with the fingers is helpful both to avoid migration of the product down to the upper eyelid. Furthermore, it might decrease pain

thumb on the upper eyelid to avoid migration of the product down this area (Fig. 6.10).

After injecting the entire eyebrow or into a specific area, it is advisable to compress the eyebrow for a few seconds to avoid bleeding and keep the product at the proper site. Bleeding is generally light and only minor edema usually occurs. Ice bags are put in place immediately after the procedure. Micro-tapes may be placed onto the site for 2 days to help maintain the eyebrow shape and to reduce edema and migration of the product down to the upper eyelid if we are treating restless patients. However, for the vast majority of patients, no tape is needed. Posttreatment pain is usually minimal and the use of any medication is rare. Patient's satisfaction is usually good if the limitations of the results have been understood. When fillers/volumizers are combined with BoNT-A treatment, the results tend to be longer lasting and more gratifying.

6.3.5 Complications

Bleeding at the injection site is rare and may cause local and upper eyelid ecchymosis. Proper delicate injection avoiding blood vessels may control bleeding. Immediate compression is advisable in these cases. Local pain and discomfort during injection is probably the result of touching the periosteum with the needle.

Edema after injection is quite common and should be explained to the patient beforehand. Surface irregularities result from irregular placement of the fillers. Asymmetry can be corrected with complementary injections of fillers.

The most feared complication is migration of the filler down to the upper eyelid. Using the proper technique and injecting only small quantities of the required product can avoid this. Other complications, such as those in association with surgical procedures (e.g., numbness, paresis, scars, alopecia, and nerve damage), do not occur in treatment with fillers.

6.3.6 Tips, Tricks and Key Points

Fillers injected into the eyebrow may be easily combined with BoNT-A in the upper part of the face. This will improve the eyebrow position, especially in its upper lateral part. Care should be taken to avoid migration down to the skin of the upper eyelid.

Do's

- Do remember that temporal volume replacement may lift the tail of the eyebrow in selected cases.

Key Points

- Eyebrow lifting is crucial for facial rejuvenation. When low positioning of eyebrows are associated with volume loss in the temporal area, the latter should be treated first to provide support for the lateral aspect of the eyebrow.

6.4 Epicanthal Fold and Sunken Upper Eyelid

The following two indications are advanced indications. The indication of the epicanthal fold applies almost exclusively to Asian patients. The sunken upper eyelid is an indication that applies for all ethnic groups.

6.4.1 Epicanthal Fold

Epicanthal fold, epicanthus, or simply eye fold are names for a skin fold of the upper eyelid covering the inner corner (medial canthus) of the eye. One of the primary facial features often closely associated with epicanthal folds is the nasal bridge. Indeed a lower-based nose bridge is more likely to cause epicanthal folds, and a higher-based nose bridge is less likely to do so. There are various factors influencing whether someone has epicanthal folds, including geographical ancestry, age, and certain medical conditions. Epicanthal folds are sometimes found as a congenital abnormality, e.g., in patients with Down's syndrome, the nasal bridge does not mature. Epicanthoplasty is the eye surgery to remove the epicanthal folds. It can be a challenging procedure because the epicanthal folds overlay the lacrimal canaliculi (tear drainage canals). Epicanthoplasty may leave visible postsurgical scar lines. A common corrective technique involves using a Z-plasty. The use of HA-based injectables with cannulas may be helpful to address epicanthal folds. This can be achieved by advancing the supraorbital ridge, the medial aspect of the orbit, and the nose. With this intervention the features can be improved without surgery. An office-based procedure with no time off may meet patients' expectations that are not inclined for surgical corrections (Figs. 6.11, 6.12, 6.13, 6.14, 6.15, and 6.16).

6.4.2 Sunken Upper Eyelid

When we are young the upper eyelid is full and there are only a few millimeters of the upper lid

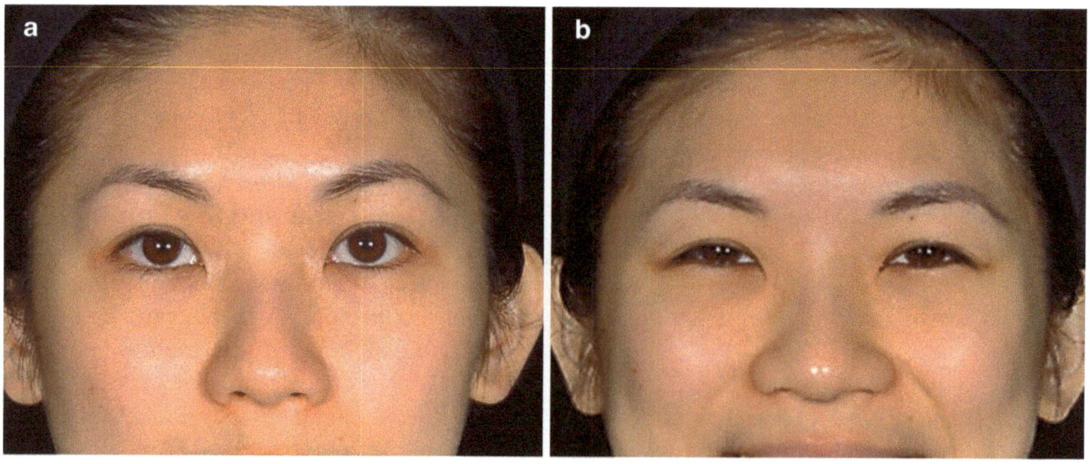

Fig. 6.11 (a) Epicanthal fold at rest. (b) Epicanthal fold on animation

showing. There is no shadow of the upper lid sulcus (see also Sect. 6.1). During aging the upper lid deflates, there is skin excess and folding where fullness was, and the shadow of the upper lid sulcus appears. The fold of the upper lid skin often droops and may reach the lash line and hide completely the upper lid. This status is an indication for aesthetic rejuvenation.

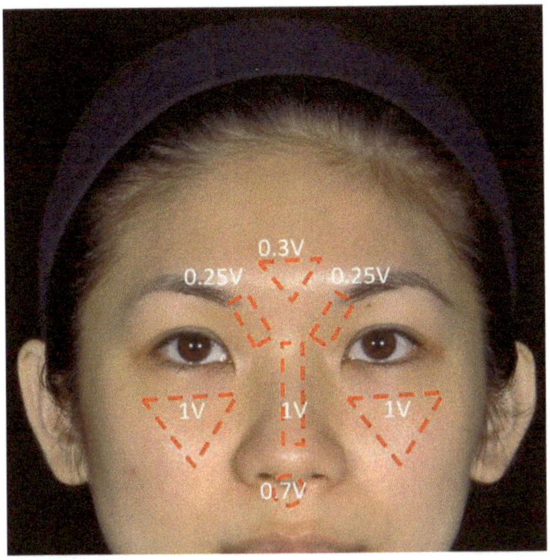

Fig. 6.12 Description of the areas and the quantity of Juvéderm Voluma injected with a 21G blunt cannula: glabella (0.3 ml), supramedial orbit (0.25 ml), nose (1.0 ml), anterior nasal spine (0.7 ml), and cheekbone (1.0 ml)

The treatment of the sunken upper eyelid with HA fillers should only be performed by experienced injectors that have already succeeded with the treatment of complex tear troughs. Persistent edema and mechanical impairment of the upper eyelid excursion may be found if inappropriate technique is performed. Serious risk of vascular injuries may happen if sharp needles are used. The use of blunt cannulas, gentle technique, and low volume is advisable to avoid complications. If proper technique is used, the result may be amazing and much better than fat grafting (Figs. 6.17 and 6.18).

6.4.3 Tips, Tricks and Key Points

These are tricky indications. Both of them should be restricted to advanced users.

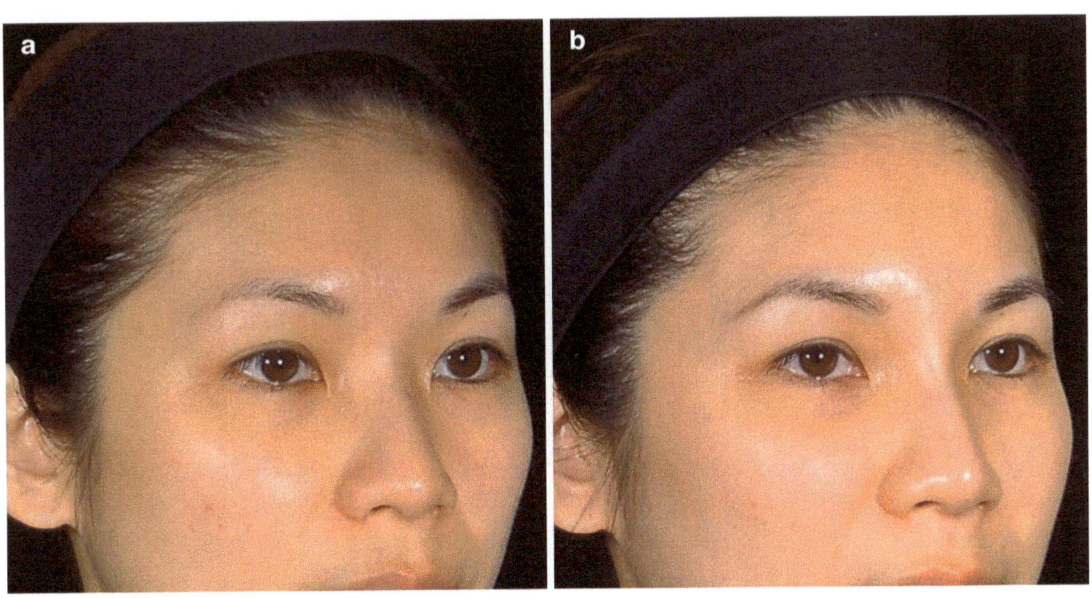

Fig. 6.13 (a) Sunken frontonasal angle and epicanthal fold. (b) After the augmentation of the glabella and nasal bridge, an improvement of the epicanthal fold can be seen

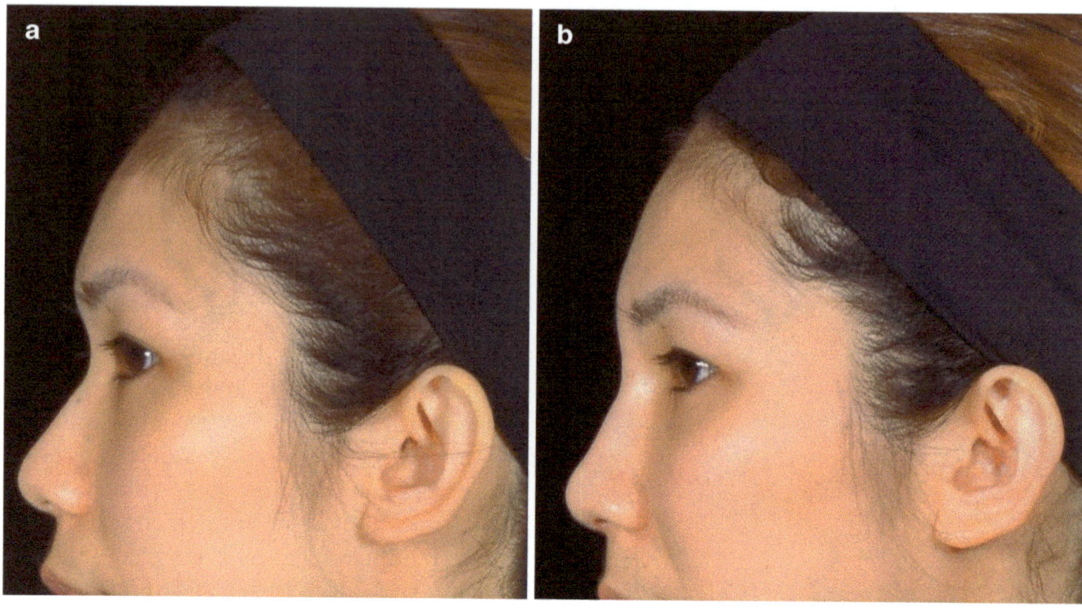

Fig. 6.14 (**a**, **b**) Profile view of the same patient: before and after augmentation

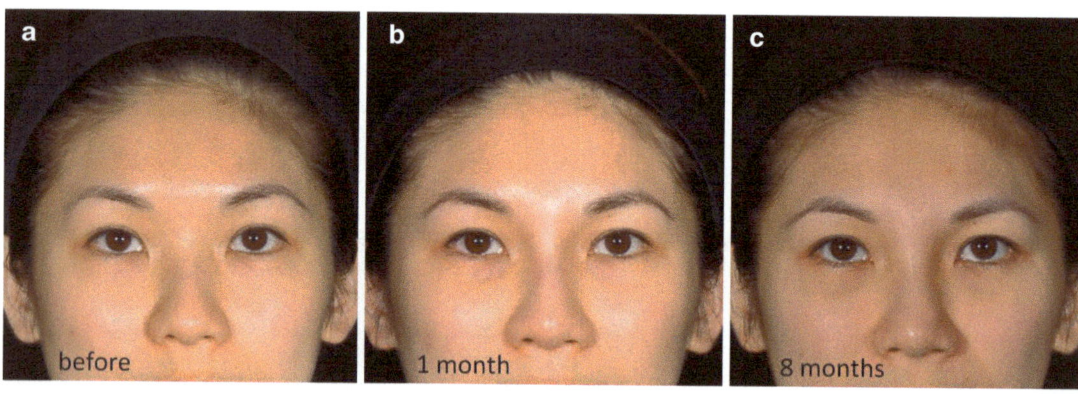

Fig. 6.15 (**a–c**) Frontal view of the same patient, before, 1 month, and 8 months after treatment

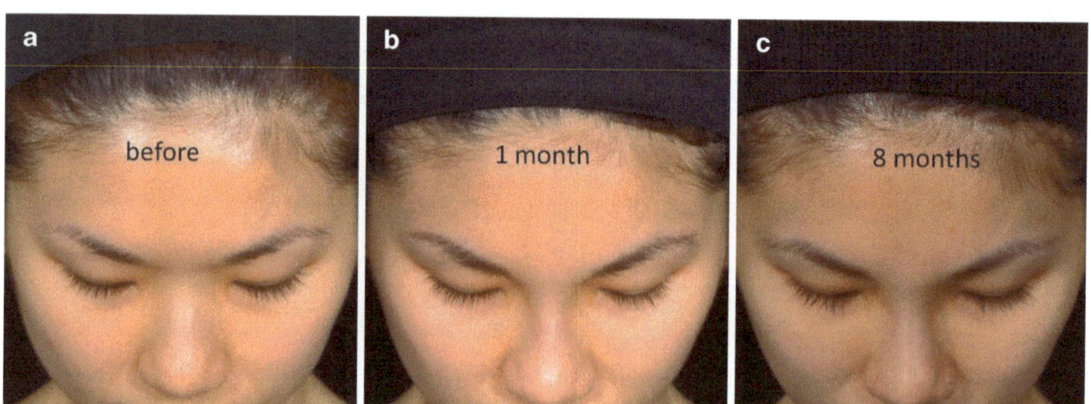

Fig. 6.16 (**a–c**) Observe the projection of the nose, the medial aspect of the upper part of the orbit, and the evolution of the epicanthal fold

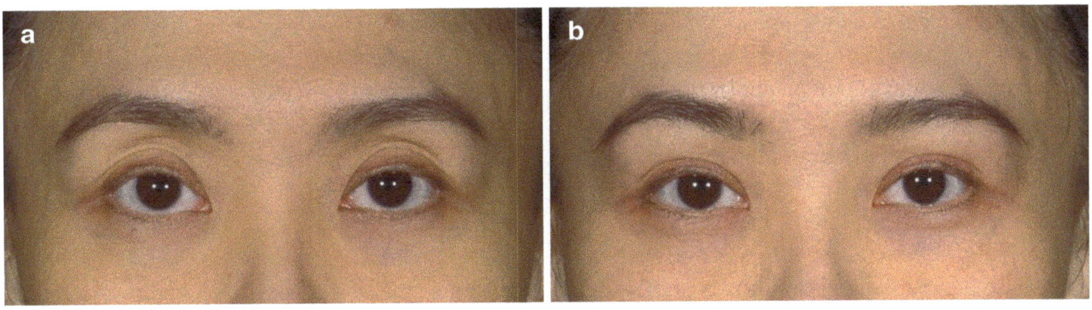

Fig. 6.17 (a) Frontal view: presence of sunken upper eyelid with excessive palpebral show. (b) The patient was submitted to an injection with a 21G cannula. A total amount of 0.45 ml of Juvéderm Ultra Plus was injected into the right side and 0.35 ml into the left side without any complications

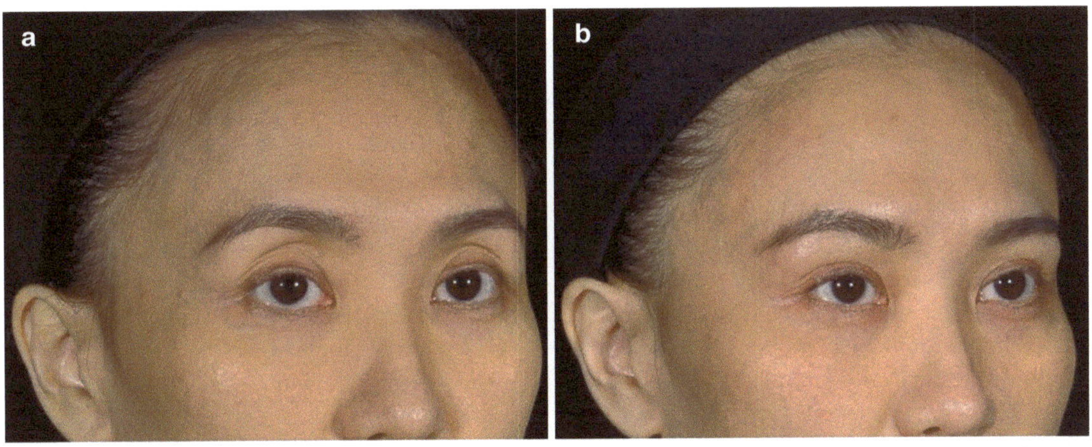

Fig. 6.18 (a) Oblique view: distracting appearance of the upper eyelid. That was patient's main complaint. (b) After the treatment, a more attractive look was achieved

> **Key Points**
> - We would recommend approaching these indications only after a specific training.
> - For the sunken upper eyelid, only HA fillers are recommended as in case of overcorrection or edema hyaluronidase might be easily used for correction.

6.5 Infraorbital Hollow, Tear Trough, Cheekbones, and Cheek Reshaping

6.5.1 Introduction

The midface specifically malar projection and full cheeks are important hallmarks of facial beauty and youthful appearance. Therefore, it is important to remember which signs mark a youthful appearance. In youth, the lower eyelid starts at the tarsal insertion and flows in a smooth convexity all the way down to the nasolabial fold and buccal region. The lid-cheek junction is smooth and short, and observing a youthful midface, there is no distinction between the lower eyelid and the cheek.

Volume loss in these areas is a very important landmark and so is the increase of shadows (Pessa 2000). In the lower eyelid, the loss of orbital volume may cause the infraorbital hollow and create a sharp distinction line or shadow that separates the lower eyelid from the cheek. The same loss of orbital volume may reveal the underlying orbital fat provoking eye bags (Lambros 2002). At the cheek level, the anterior view determines the volume loss creating the midface depression. Cheek ptosis with a depression parallel to the nasolabial fold and the face and the presence of the malar mound are important aging signs that are placed in the midface.

HA volumizers have dramatically changed the approach to the mid-third of the face. In the upper mid-cheek and upper lateral cheek area (cheekbone level), volume deficiencies are mostly corrected by the injection of volumizers at this level. Whenever a patient presents infraorbital hollow, tear trough, mid-cheek deficiency, and prominent nasolabial fold, always start by restoring volume at the cheekbone level which will usually lead to an improvement of the infraorbital hollow and the nasolabial fold.

6.5.2 Anatomy

The middle third of the face encompasses the area between the eyebrows and the base of the nose. The inferior third reaches from the nasal base to the menton. The ideal location of the cheekbone prominence is 10 mm lateral and 15 mm inferior to the lateral canthus. Deficits at this level are the result of maxillary elongation and are usually accompanied by a lack of midface projection. The cheek is framed superiorly by the malar complex and inferiorly by the mandible. The size and the shape of the cheeks are determined by the parotid gland, the musculature (mostly the m. masseter), and the buccal fat.

Any midface analysis must include the infraorbital, the tear-trough area, and the submalar triangle (Tobias and Binder 1994). Tear-trough deformities become visible in cases of infraorbital rim depression. The submalar triangle is an inverted triangular area of midfacial depression and is limited superiorly by the prominence of the zygomatic, medially by the nasolabial fold, and laterally by the body of the masseter muscle.

The SMAS comprises the superficial fascia and envelopes the majority of the midfacial musculature. The superficial fat to the SMAS is dense in the cheek, the nasolabial fold, and jowls. The superficial malar fat pad is divided into the cheek portion and the jowl portion. The deep fat is dense in the anterior and the middle cheek. The deep components of the malar fat pad may be encountered between the facial muscles. The buccal fat pad of Bichat is anterior to the masseter and lies deeper to the deep fascia at the buccal level.

The suborbicularis oculi fat (SOOF) is situated over the lower portion of the zygomatic body and beneath the muscles. It is separated from the periorbital fat by the thin orbital and the malar septum. The presence of malar bags may result from the ptosis of the SOOF.

In the cheek area, the buccinator muscle arises posteriorly from the pterygomandibular raphe. The buccinator muscle is localized deep to the buccal fat pad and extends anteriorly to attach the orbicularis oris. The masseter has a superficial and a deep part. The superficial part arises from the lower border of the anterior two-thirds of the zygomatic arch, and the deep part originates from the inner surface of the posterior third. It inserts the entire lateral ramus of the mandible. Its function is to elevate the mandible.

The malar prominence area has large musculocutaneous perforators. Just lateral to the nasolabial groove, there is a concentration of fatty tissue, the so-called malar fat pad. The facial nerve branches and the parotid duct are deep to the SMAS and superficial to the masseter and buccal fat pad. The zygomatical and buccal branches of the facial nerve become more superficial in the medial cheek (Hamra 1992). The infraorbital nerve is located deeply, along the bony midface. It is responsible for the sensitivity of the cheek and the lip.

As the aging process progresses, ptosis and pseudoherniation of the SOOF and the orbital fat pads occur. Malar bags result from the ptosis of the SOOF and occur below the level of the orbital rim. Loss of the midfacial cheek support causes accumulation of anterior and inferior cheek fat and loss of the lateral and superior cheek fat. This change of anatomy results in deep nasolabial folds, multiple folds in the cheek (while smiling), and a hollowness of the submalar area. The descendent vector will also produce a skeletonized appearance of the cheekbones.

6.5.3 Patient Evaluation and Selection

The use of fillers for reshaping the midface area must obey specific rules: the best results are obtained in patients with good midfacial fullness but insufficient malar projection and with minor malar and submalar deficiencies. It is also a good option for young patients with a good malar bone structure who complain of early onset of flatness in the midface.

Patients with extreme malar deformities and a severe submalar recess are not good candidates for fillers. Conventional malar implants must be considered. Patients with a deficient midface present a narrow nose with a shallow dorsum and a sunken and thin upper lip. The treatment of choice is usually maxillary advancement, and there is generally a 0.5:1 ratio of soft tissue to bony movement. Fillers and specifically the volumizers may also be helpful for complementing soft-tissue advancement.

Balancing the midface in selected cases may promote nice and natural results without the need of surgical procedures with their accompanying postoperative period with ecchymosis and edema.

The skin of the cheeks may show considerable elastosis. Patients with thin skin are in general also suitable for this procedure. Elastotic skin, however, may be difficult to treat. For the forehead area, for example, multiple sessions with a low-viscosity hyaluronic acid may be useful to increase its consistency. Alternatively (see Chap. 9) other interventions as fractionated lasers, peels might be used to improve the texture of the skin.

6.5.4 Tear Trough and Infraorbital Area

The term nasojugal groove was used to describe the concavity at the border of the eyelid and the cheek medially and was named as tear trough later (Flowers 1993; Loeb 1993). It refers to the medial one-third of the infraorbital hollow and may be the first early concavity at the lid-cheek junction in early aging. It is found at the inferior orbital rim down to the hemi-pupillary line. Depending on ethnicity, a trough may be seen in youth in many individuals, and it is its depth or true indentation that leads to a distracting appearance. The tear-trough deformity may be defined as the concavity at the junction of the thin eyelid skin above and the thicker and different nasal and cheek skin below, with attenuated subcutaneous tissue overlying the maxillary bone. The skin in the area of the concavity is indeed of different quality, texture, and color. Hyperpigmentation or full transparency may be found in the skin over the tear trough. Volume loss can be present laterally in more advanced aging, at or just below the orbital rim. At this level, the retaining ligaments are thicker and less distensible. In some individuals, the concavity in the groove is often associated with orbital fat herniation superiorly in the lower lid fat compartments, accentuating its appearance (Fig. 6.19). The orbicularis oculi muscle has a direct attachment to the inferior orbital rim from the anterior lacrimal crest to the medial limbus or approximately one-third of the orbital rim length. Laterally, bone attachment to the bone is given by the orbicularis retaining ligaments which may vary in length, then decreases laterally until these ligaments merge with the lateral orbital thickening in the lateral canthal region. The levator labii superioris

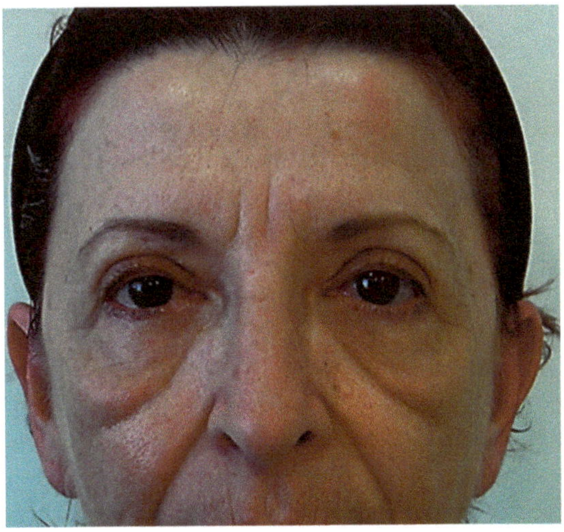

Fig. 6.19 Presence of prominent nasojugal fold, tear trough, and palpebro-malar sulcus. Observe the malar mound and the projection of the orbicularis oculi retaining ligament

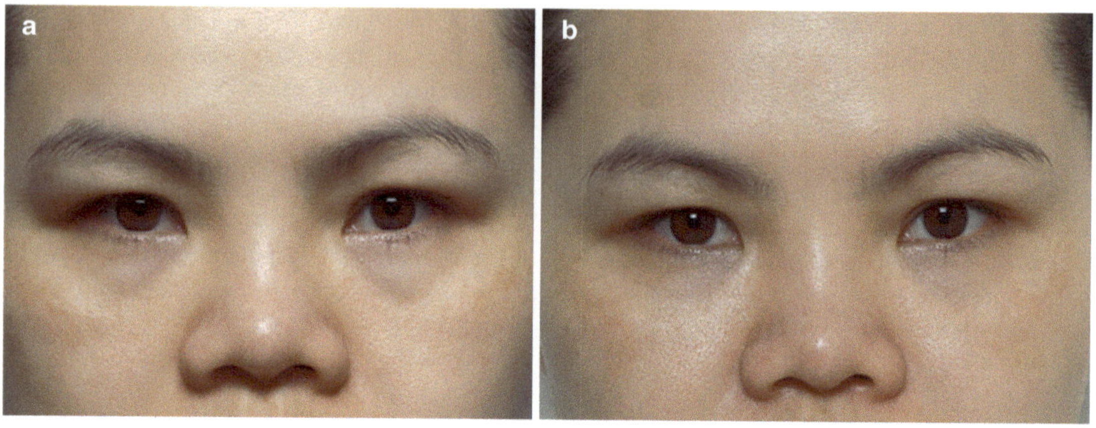

Fig. 6.20 (**a**) Presence of tired look with elongated lid-cheek junction. (**b**) After the injection of 0.5 ml of Juvéderm Voluma per side, the transition between the lower eyelid and cheeks was softened. A direct injection into the tear trough was not performed

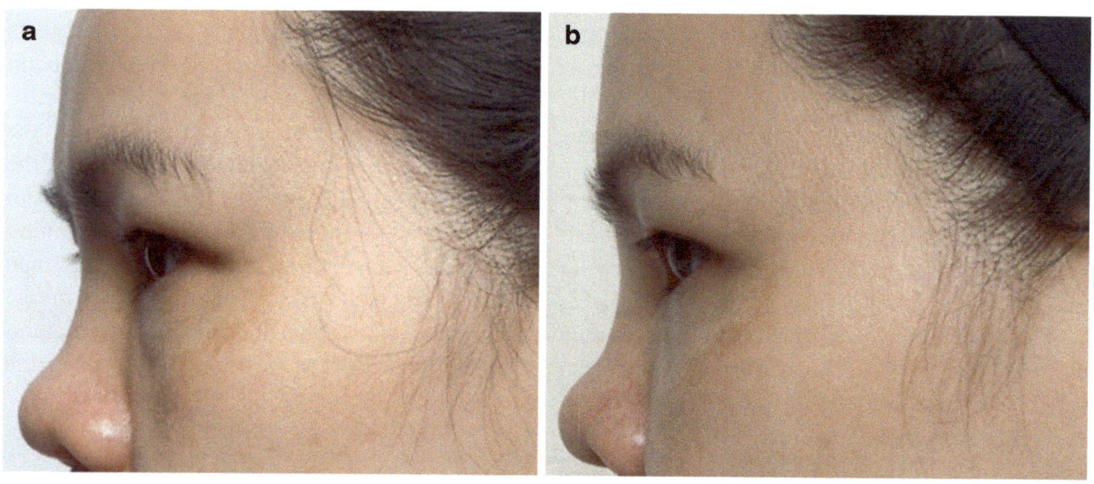

Fig. 6.21 (**a**) On the profile view, it is evident that the volume loss in the mid-cheek was the cause of the elongated lid-cheek junction and tired look. (**b**) After the treatment, there is no evidence of a noticeable transition line between both structures

originates just below the orbicularis oculi muscle attachment to the medial orbital rim (Muzaffar et al. 2002).

As there is scant subcutaneous tissue between the skin and the orbicularis muscle in this area, the tear-trough skin is attached direct to the orbital rim. The cause of the tear-trough deformity may include volume loss, orbital fat herniation, and skin laxity in different degrees of severity among patients.

Mild tear-trough deformities (e.g., infraorbital rim depression) are a good indication for fillers. The presence of fillers along the infraorbital rim may improve the suborbital groove. This is considered an advanced area for injectors, and complications are not rare, especially in the hands of inexperienced users who tend to use too much volume or inappropriate fillers. Minimizing adverse events is of utmost importance here.

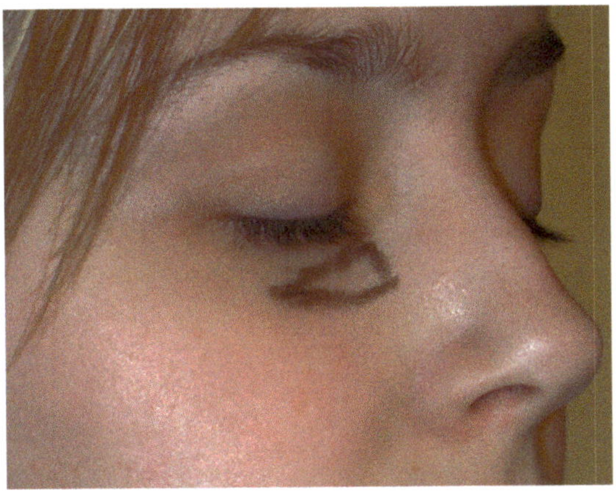

Fig. 6.22 Skin demarcation is very useful for treating the tear-trough deformity. After demarcation follows the injection. Care should be taken not to produce excessive ecchymosis

It is important to highlight that much of tear-trough deformities can be effectively treated only by mid-cheek volume replacement. Aging process provokes elongation of the lid-cheek junction, and shortening of the lower lid height can be also obtained only by volumizing the cheekbones (Figs. 6.20 and 6.21).

If a hydrophilic product such as HA is to be used at this level, undercorrection is advisable to avoid prolonged edema. Ideally, low-viscosity products are to be injected at the tear-trough level due to the thin aspect of the skin. However, other products as low-viscosity HA preparations may be injected in this area too – provided they are injected deeply.

Treatment in the infraorbital area starts with the marking (Fig. 6.22). The patient should be in upward position and should bend the head forward with "chin down, eyes up." This position enables more accurate distinction of the elongated lid-cheek junction and accentuates the tear-trough deformity and volume loss along the infraorbital and cheekbones areas. The inferior orbital rim is usually higher, so any intraorbit injection is avoided if the upper limit of this marked line is respected. Usually only topical anesthetics and/or ice packs are used. Infraorbital and zygomatic facial nerves block might be needed if working with larger cannulas and with HA products without lidocaine.

Volume replacement in the infraorbital and cheekbone areas can be performed with either needles or blunt cannulas. Deep injections touching the bone at the infraorbital foramen level must be avoided to high risks of complications. Both bolus and retrograde techniques can be performed at the cheekbone level. The accurate choice will depend on the degree of volume loss and bone projection. Flat bone and universal volume loss at this level is better treated with retrograde or small bolus injection to avoid irregularities. High volume concentrated in a single point could lead to difficulty in molding the product and higher risk for unwanted effects.

In general, volume replacement in the infraorbital and cheekbone areas may solve totally or partially problems at the lid-cheek junction especially when it is not a real tear-trough deformity. If direct injection into the tear trough is needed, the volume requirement will be lower and so will the risk of adverse events such as Tyndall effect or prolonged edema after HA injection. It is important to avoid injecting a large continuous column of filler along the tear trough because a "sausage" appearance can result. Multiple entry points with either micro bolus (0.01–0.02 ml per point) or retrograde product delivery along or preferably below the inferior orbital rim may be considered for needles or cannulas. Low volume is desirable for both injection types. Gentle massage with finger or cotton buds is advisable (Figs. 6.23, 6.24, 6.25, 6.26, and 6.27).

The advantages of cannulas at this level include fewer entry sites and more safety if correction above the orbital rim of sunken and/or skeletonized eyes either genetic or post-blepharoplasty is needed.

The duration of results has been longer than expected in the infraorbital and tear-trough areas. For most patients, results can be expected for 1 or even 2 years in younger patients.

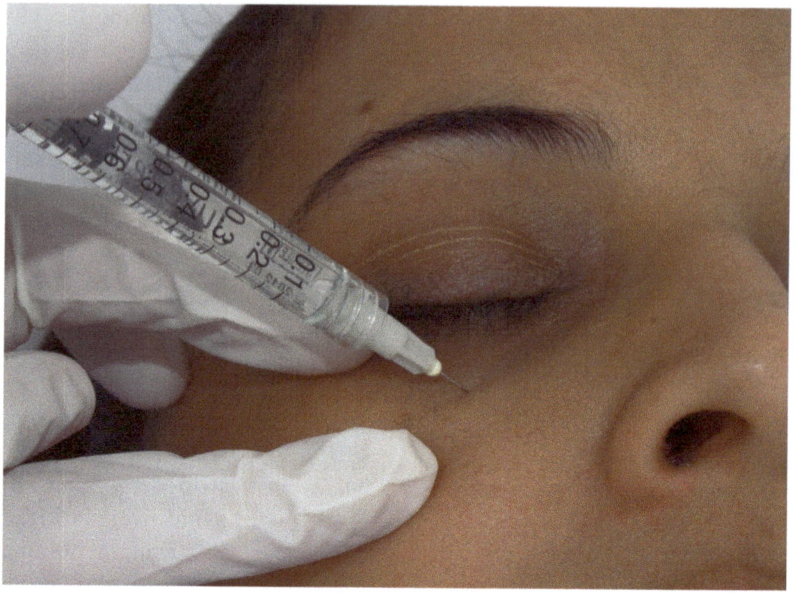

Fig. 6.23 Careful injection into the tear trough may expand the skin and decrease the deformity

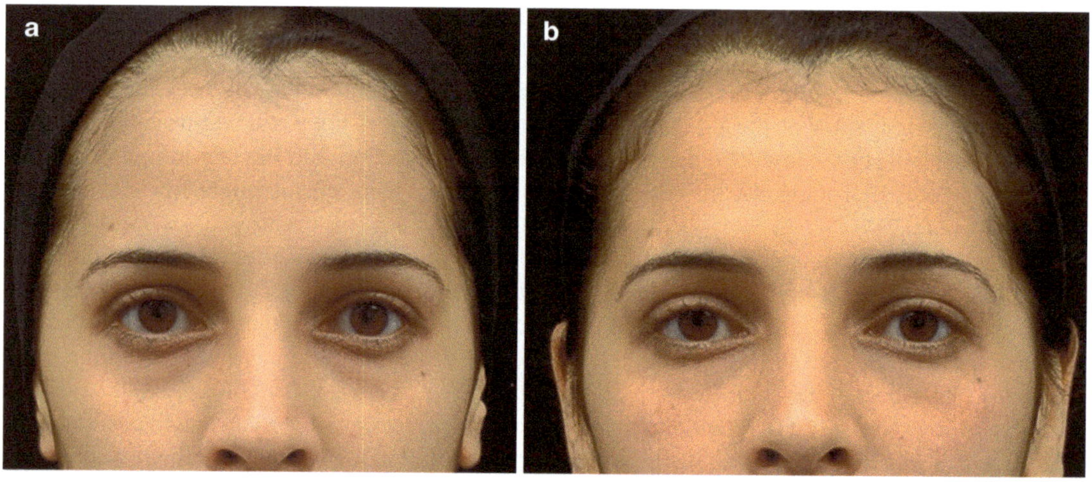

Fig. 6.24 (**a**) This patient presented eye bags in the lower eyelid. She was searching a nonsurgical solution. (**b**) She was submitted to the injection of 1 ml of Juvéderm Volbella per side in a single entry point with a 25G microcannula. The product was delivered along the periosteum of the inferior orbital rim and under the m. orbicularis oris. Note that the eye bags have completely disappeared. No late edema was found

Key Points

- It is important to differentiate the real tear-trough deformity from elongated lid-cheek junction, eye bags, and skin excess. Inaccurate diagnosis might lead to unwanted effects or even complications.

Do's

- When correcting the infraorbital area, undercorrection is advisable. The use of cannulas in this area might reduce the risk of postinjection hematoma.

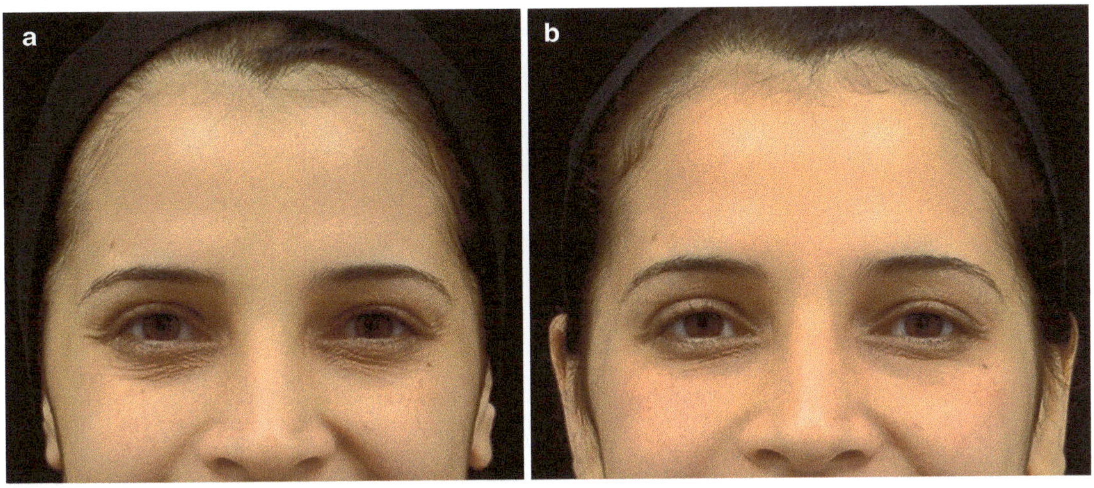

Fig. 6.25 (**a**, **b**) The same patient before and after treatment smiling. Please note the reduction in the number of suborbicular wrinkles

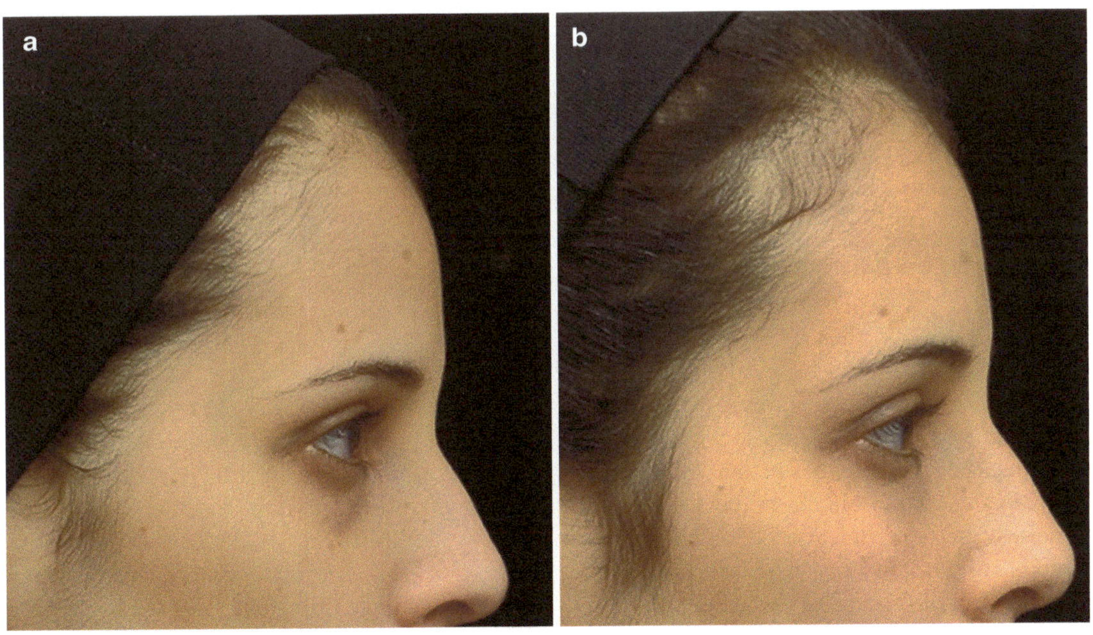

Fig. 6.26 (**a**, **b**) Profile analysis of the same patient before and after treatment. Observe shortening of the lid-cheek junction and improvement of dark circles through tissue expansion with the HA

Don'ts

- Do not use high-viscosity HAs for this indication.

6.5.5 Cheekbones

There has been a huge change in cosmetic practice since the introduction of volumizers in the market. Before that when assessing the midface,

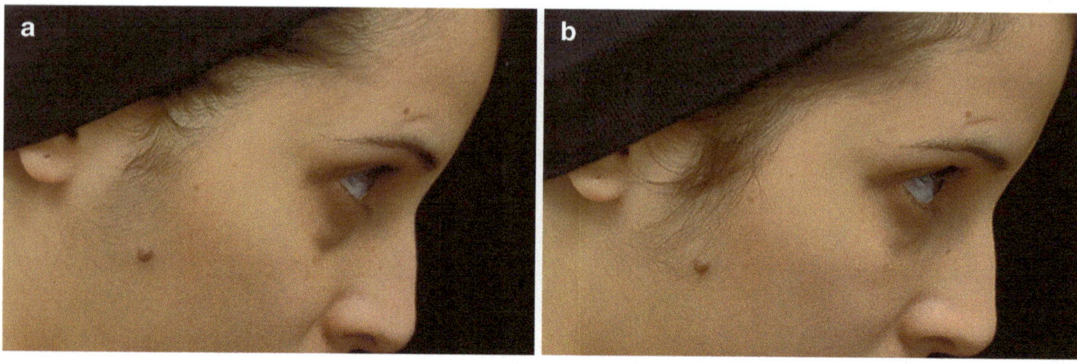

Fig. 6.27 (**a**, **b**) Profile analysis of the same patient leaning forward with "chin down and eyes up." In this position the protrusion of the eye bags makes it easier to understand the importance of lower eyelid by the injected HA

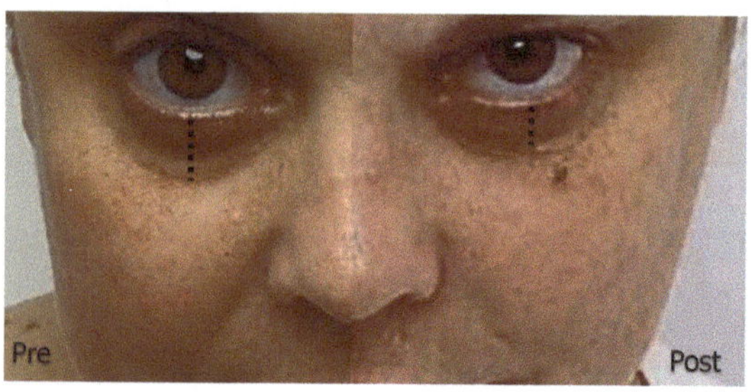

Fig. 6.28 Split photograph: patient is leaning forward. Note before treatment the elongation of the lid-cheek junction, ptosis of cheek, and the prominent nasolabial fold (*right side*). After volume replacement with 2 ml of the Juvéderm Voluma (*left sided*), there is improvement of the mid-third of the face (right and left is based on the patients perspective)

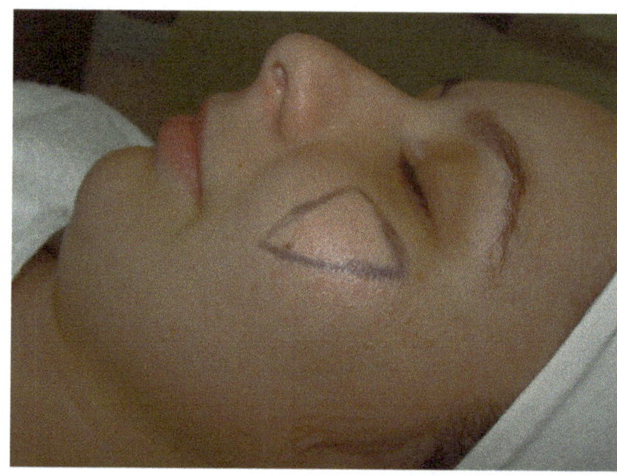

Fig. 6.29 A small *triangle* is demarcated at this level. Both the frame and the internal area should be filled

both injectors and patients would focus on the nasolabial fold and sometimes in the tear-trough area, but cheekbones were in the "blind spot." The introduction of volumizers did show us how important the replacement of volume loss in the cheekbones is. Not only have we noticed the WOW effect in our patients but an additional improvement in the nasolabial fold and tear trough.

There are different approaches to volume replacement in the cheekbones. It is important to mark the lid-cheek junction and the volume loss in the mid and lateral aspects of the cheekbones. I usually perform the marking with the patients with "eyes up and chin down." This position enables a more accurate definition of the areas to be treated as well as a very efficient way to verify the immediate response (Fig. 6.28).

Either no anesthetic or only topical anesthesia is usually required for this procedure especially when the product contains lidocaine. Nerve blocks may be necessary if cannulas are to be used especially 18 and 21 G. Outlining the entire area with, e.g., an eyeliner before injection may promote accurate filling and easy removal of the marking (Figs. 6.29 and 6.30).

Depending on the HA volumizer preparation, injections should be deep down to the bone. However, for some volumizers as Juvéderm Voluma injections may be performed in the superficial and deep fat malar compartment. This enables a better lifting effect with less quantity of product. The multilayer approach is recommended when the deficiency also results from lack of good bone projection. There are different approaches that may lead to the same result.

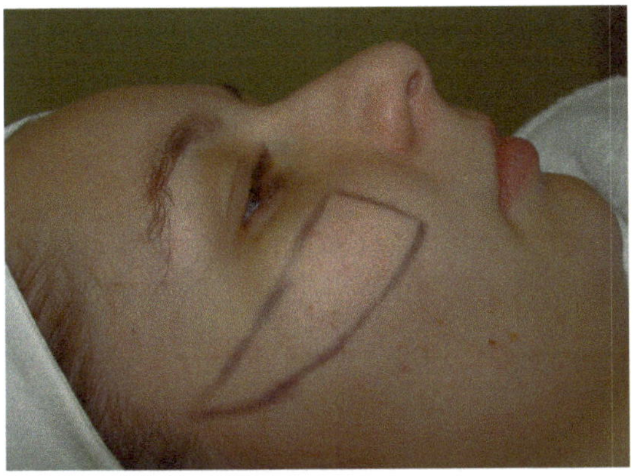

Fig. 6.30 When major projection is desired, the zygomatic arch level is also filled

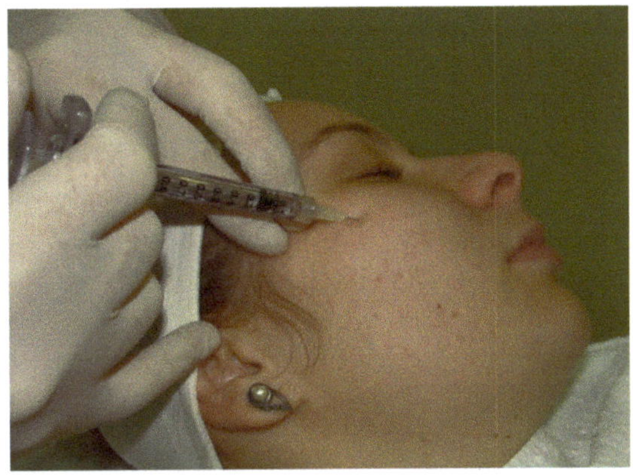

Fig. 6.31 Injection is performed after an injection plan of the area to be treated has been drawn. At this level, the malar prominence is enhanced

Bolus or small bolus, retrograde/anterograde techniques are possible at this level. Massage is very important to smooth out any irregularity.

Both cannulas and needles can be used for cheekbone volume replacement, and care should be taken to avoid deep direct injection into the infraorbital foramen. It is also noticeable that more volume is used when the treatment is delivered with cannulas. Maybe it is due to the fact that more superficial product placement is obtained with needles.

During the injection, the fan technique is undertaken from each edge of the drawing in order to promote a crossing of micro-tunnels. M multilayer injections are conducted. The deep reticular dermis will be filled by starting more superficially with the needle almost parallel to the skin. Opening the angle of the needle to 30–45° will allow it to reach the subcutaneous and the muscular layers (Fig. 6.31). After filling all layers, a soft massage is conducted and a final analysis of the obtained projection is undertaken. Finally, if needed, the needle must be inserted at a 90° angle almost touching the periosteum on the most prominent parts of the malar bone for major projections. Drapes are may be applied to reduce edema but are usually not necessary and for correct maintenance of the position of the filler. After the edema has subsided, the final result may be evaluated (Fig. 6.32). The filling of the cheekbones should be subtle and increase slightly the midface width (Fig. 6.33).

The amount of product will vary according to the degree of volume loss: mild deficiencies may require 0.5 ml, moderate deficiencies may be improved with 1.0 ml per side (Fig. 6.34), severe deficiencies may need a minimum of 2.0 ml per side, and very severe may require up to 4.0 ml when submalar deficiency is also present. Volume restoration in the mid-cheek may also be helpful to promote facial advancement (Figs. 6.35 and 6.36).

A frequent challenge that can be seen is the over-injection at the cheekbone level, what is considered not aesthetically appealing. Patients and injectors need to be aware about balance and proportion in this area. A simple rule to be followed includes the following: treatment should stop if at rest we still believe that a little more product is required, and then the patient will be good on animation. If full cheekbones are slightly big at rest, the result may be catastrophic on animation!

Key Points

- The injection of volumizers in the cheekbone area has changed the understanding of treatment sequence. Patients presenting elongated lid-cheek junction, volume loss in the cheekbones, and prominent nasolabial fold sometimes might only need treatment at the cheekbone area, and improvement of the tear trough and nasolabial fold will not be necessary.
- Overtreatment of the cheekbone area is not recommended.

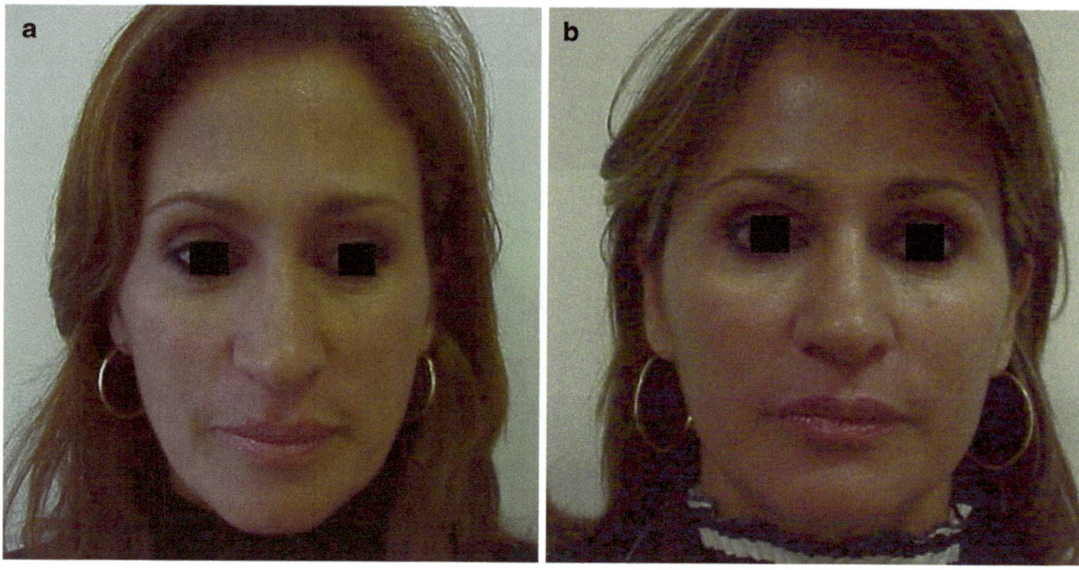

Fig. 6.32 (**a, b**) Before and after injection of the cheekbone area. After treatment, with the improvement of the mid-third of the face, a more youthful appearance is evident

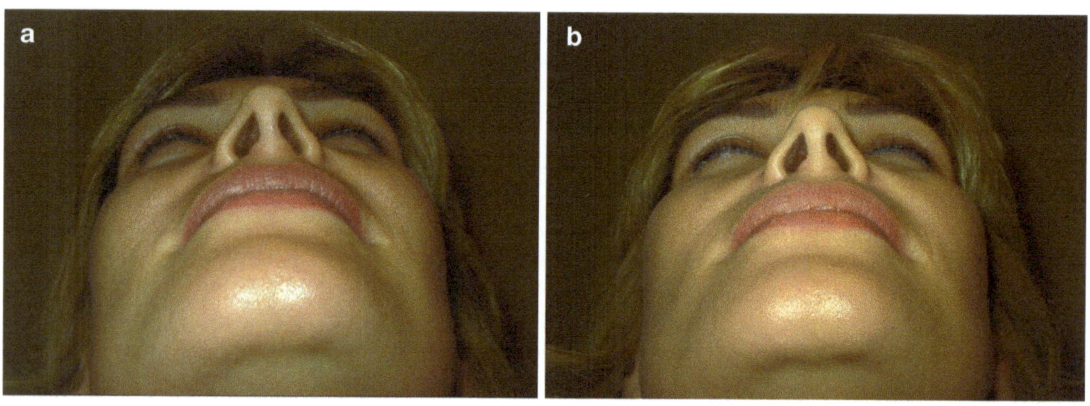

Fig. 6.33 (**a, b**) The filling of the cheekbones must be subtle and increase slightly the midface width

Do's

- Do not forget to get a three-dimensional view of your patient. What looks good from the front might not look good from the sides.

Don'ts

- Do not create bean-shaped cushion-like depots in the cheekbone area. It rarely looks good.

6.5.6 Cheek

Cheek augmentation follows the same initial steps as that of the cheekbones. Topical anesthesia is usually sufficient for this area if the treatment is with needles and the product containing lidocaine. Visual analysis is important to establish the markings, which should be done with the patient in an upright position and leaning forward (eyes up and chin down). When the patient is leaning forward, we may mark the NO GO areas (Fig. 6.37). These are the areas that if injected may worsen by causing bulging areas

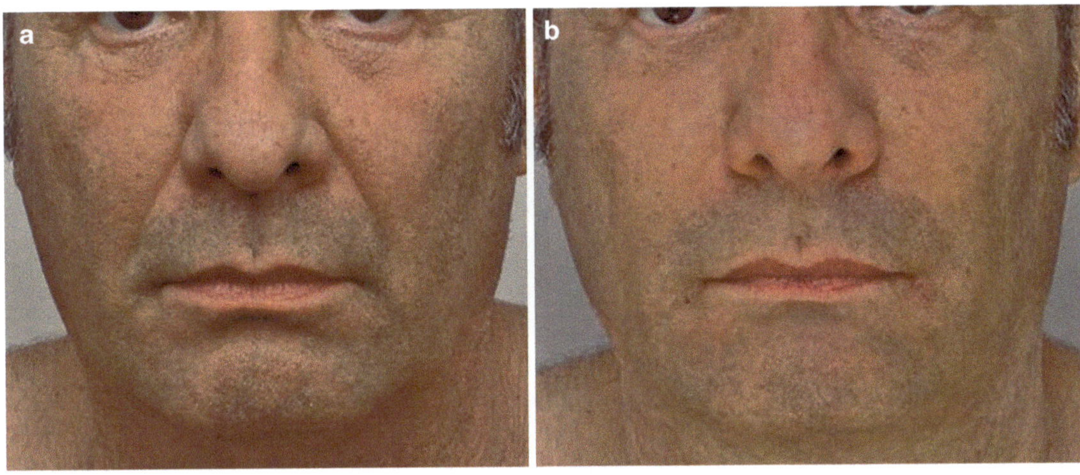

Fig. 6.34 (**a**, **b**) A male patient with elongated lid-cheek junction, volume loss in the mid-cheek, and prominent nasolabial fold before and after 2 ml of Juvéderm Voluma into the cheekbones and nasolabial fold

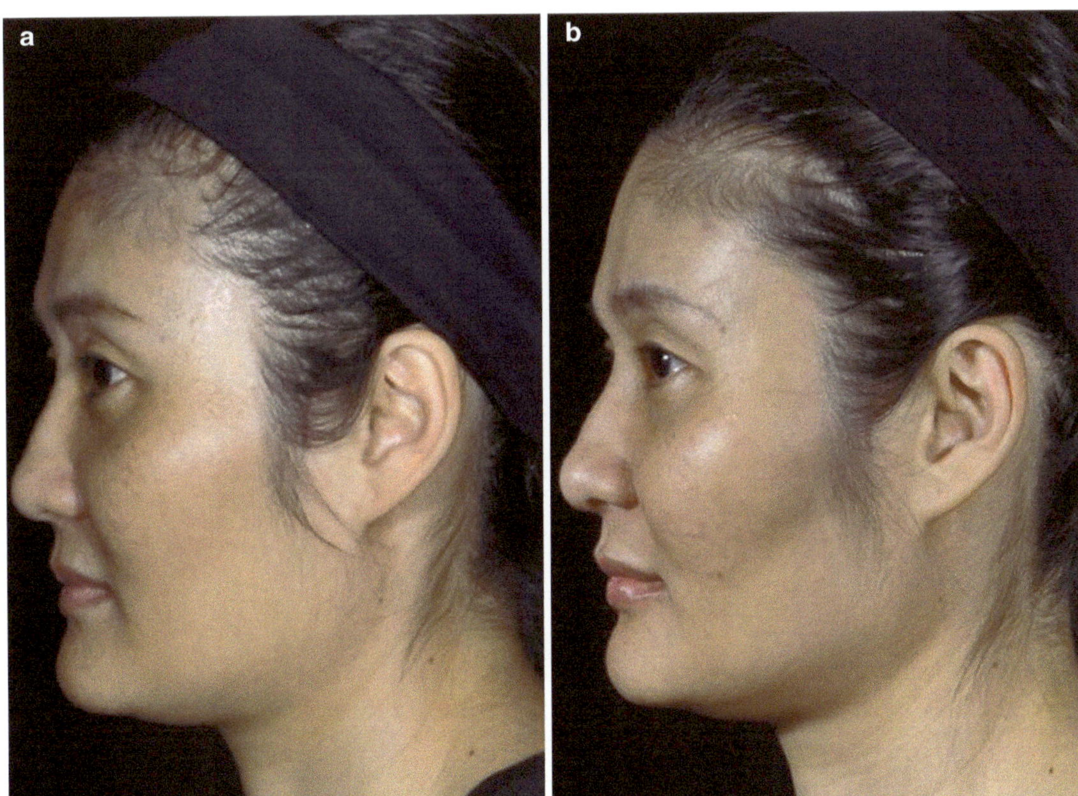

Fig. 6.35 (**a**, **b**) Asian patient with volume loss in the mid-cheek and retruded upper maxilla before and after 2 ml of Juvéderm Voluma per side for the mid-cheek and canine fossa and 1 ml Juvéderm Ultra Plus injected into the lips. The injections in the midface were done with a 21 G blunt cannula

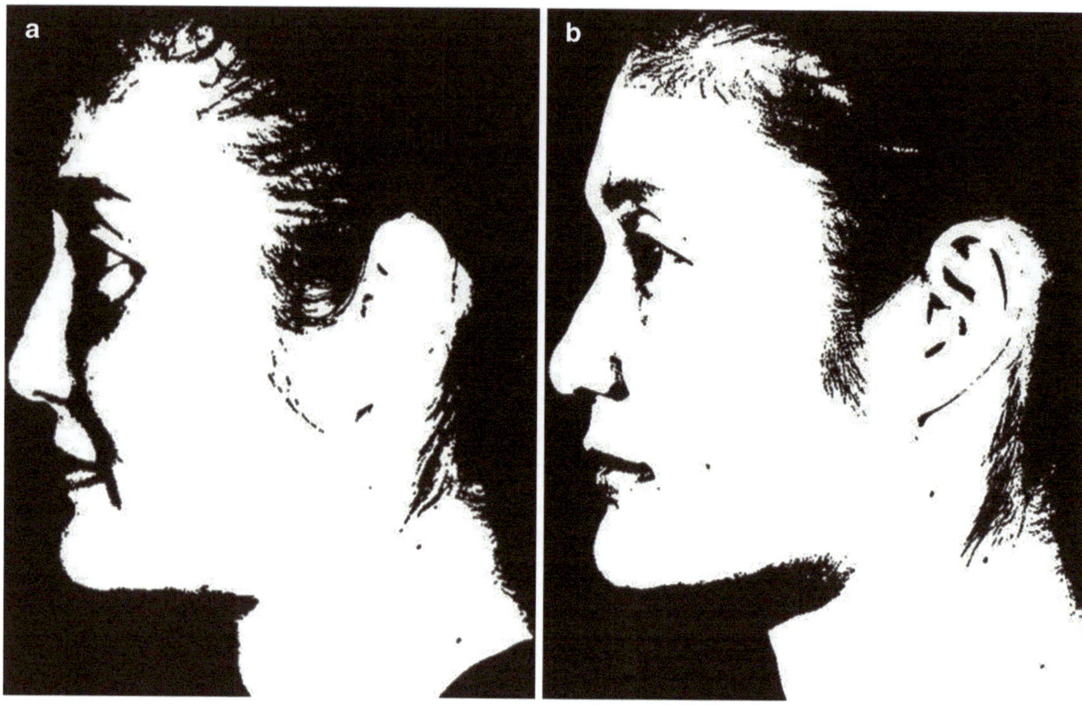

Fig. 6.36 (**a, b**) Same Asian patient as before in negative photo analysis. Observe that after advancement of the mid-third of the face with injectable fillers, less concavity is obtained and consequently less shadow is noticed. The negative photo analysis is an alternative way of reviewing improvements in volume restoration. Shadow vs light analysis after volumizing cheekbones

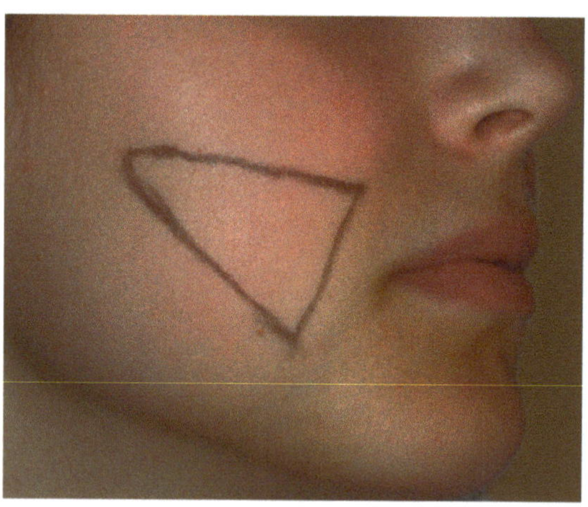

Fig. 6.37 Skin demarcation for injection: it is helpful to delimitate the area that be injected

both at rest and on animation. Pinching the skin at this level may also indicate the area where the skin and underlying tissues are atrophic. A triangle is usually drawn to limit the area to be treated (Fig. 6.38). Retrograde injections are

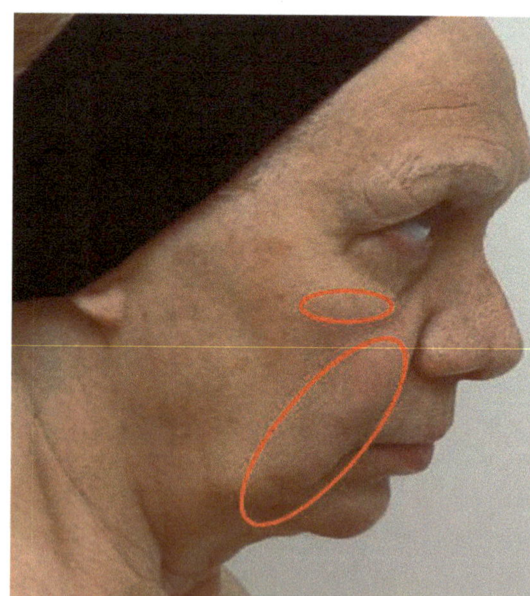

Fig. 6.38 When the patient is leaning forward, the NO GO areas should be marked to avoid any inadvertent injection into areas of laxity such as the malar mound and jowls

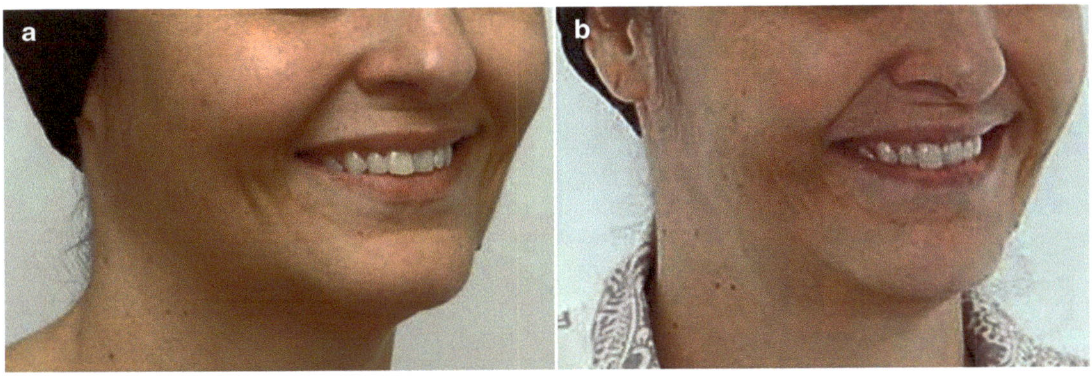

Fig. 6.39 (**a, b**) Cheek lines before and after injection of 1 ml of Juvéderm Voluma per side. The injections were done with a 21G cannula. By this a deep support at the M. buccinator was provided and resolution of the lines obtained. Please note that direct injection with needles usually does not lead to prolonged correction

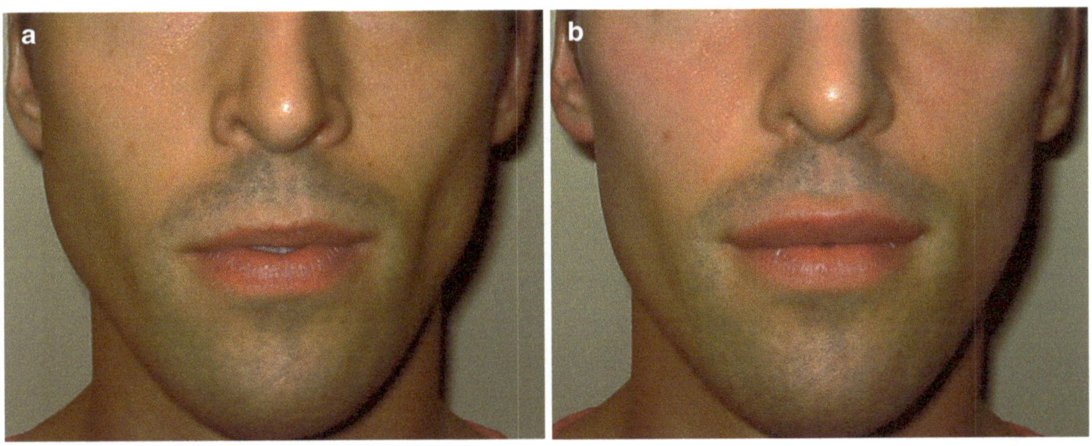

Fig. 6.40 (**a, b**) Both the left cheek and the upper lip were filled. Symmetry and balance were obtained after the filling procedure

undertaken beneath the lines. Placing the thumb against the cheek intraorally may be helpful during the injection, especially when the internal part is treated. Immediately after the fan technique, a smooth massage with both the thumb and the index finger will make the surface more uniform and make any small untreated areas evident. Both cannulas and needles may be used in this area. The treatment of accordion lines is better handled with blunt cannulas (Fig. 6.39). In some cases only one specific area needs to be filled to promote facial balance and correct asymmetries (Fig. 6.40). In other situations, cheek volume replacement may contribute to fight gravity (Fig. 6.41) Besides HAs PLLA is the product for cheek rejuvenation. As here the results are based on gradual collagen stimulation, the desired effect will show only after several sessions over several months. PLLA should be diluted with 9 ml (see Sect. 1.3.4) to avoid unnecessary adverse effects. For cheek augmentation, PLLA should be injected deeply approximately 0.3 ml per 1 cm^2 following the cheekbone. In the lower cheek area, subcutaneous injections of approximately 0.1 ml/ cm^2 are recommended (European Expert Recommendations for Sculptra, unpublished data).

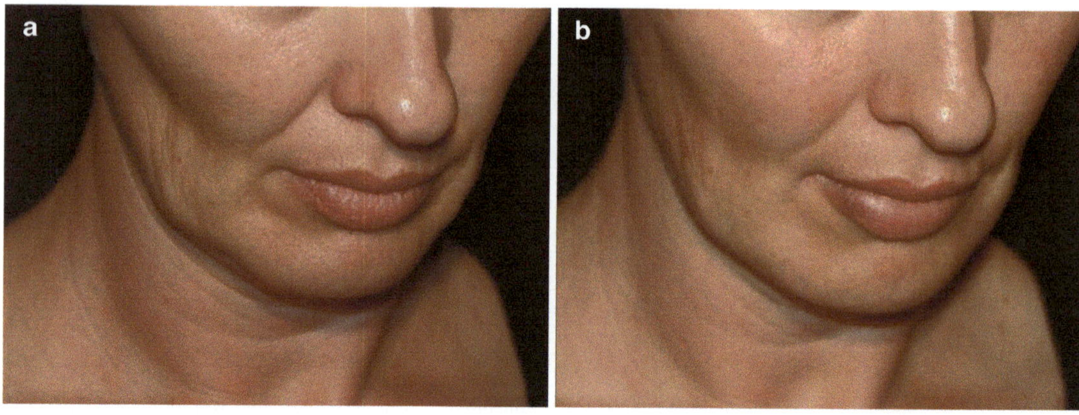

Fig. 6.41 (**a**, **b**) Before and after treatment of the volume loss and sagginess of the cheeks with 2 ml of Juvéderm Voluma per side by a 21G cannula. Besides correcting the volume loss, observe the improvement of sagginess

Key Points

- For severe volume loss at the cheek level, it is better to inject HAs with blunt cannulas as several tissue layers should be injected. Inadvertent vascular and nerve injury is reduced. Extensive bruising is not uncommon when needles are used.
- In severe volume loss treatment might also be done in steps. When volume replacement is distributed in several steps, the outcome might be more natural.
- Besides HAs this is an area for PLLA treatment.

6.5.7 Complications

The most common adverse events for cheekbones and cheeks include edema, bruising, visible nodules, and overcorrection. The infraorbital hollow/tear-trough area is more prone to adverse events compared to the cheekbone area and cheeks.

Some of the complications that are found in the tear trough result from the presence of highly hydrophilic products such as some preparations of HA when the injector inadvertently injects too superficially or promotes full correction of the deformity to please the patient. As a suggestion in this case, undercorrection is advisable for it may reduce Tyndall effect and prolonged edema.

6.5.8 Tips, Tricks and Key Points

The most important advice for this area is a careful approach that follows the patient's anatomy. As for the lips, a three-dimensional view is recommended. For example, results should always be seen not only from the front but also from both sides.

Do's

- Do start the treatment of tear-trough deformity by volumizing the mid-cheek. We may not need direct injection there.
- Do ask your patient to be with "eyes up and chin down" before marking the tear-trough and cheekbone volume loss. Use also this position to evaluate immediate results.

Don'ts

- Do not over-treat the tear-trough area with HAs. It is likely to produce Tyndall effect and prolonged edema.
- Do not use PLLA for tear-trough rejuvenation. PLLA is a good product for cheekbone and cheek augmentation.
- Do not over-inject cheekbones. If they are already slightly big at rest, they will be catastrophic on animation.

- Do not aim for round faces when reconstructing cheeks (specifically in male patients). Most patients will naturally present some concavity here.

Key Points
- Whenever a patient presents infraorbital hollow, mid-cheek deficiency, and prominent nasolabial fold, start always by restoring volume at the cheekbone level, and improvement in both the infraorbital hollow and nasolabial fold is obtained.

- The best results for cheekbone reshape are obtained in patients with good midface fullness but insufficient malar projection and with minor malar and submalar deficiencies.

FAQs
- For cheekbone volume replacement, which one should we choose: needles or cannulas?

  Both tools can be used in this area. A simple rule is asking yourself: Is it possible to solve this problem with a needle? If yes, needles might be very helpful. The reasons include less pain, lower quantity of product, and more lifting effect due to more superficial product delivery. However, if the patient presents very severe lipoatrophy, which means the skin is adhered to the bone and multiple layering and more products are required, there is an option for cannulas.
- When should be HAs used and when PLLA?

  If an immediate effect is desired, HAs are the first choice. When gradual rejuvenation is desired, the choice can be PLLA, however, never in the tear-trough area.

6.6 Nose Reshaping

6.6.1 Introduction

The surgical approach to the nose may be seen as a quite invasive procedure, especially when surgery is based on fracturing the nasal bone. Reshaping the nose with injectable fillers, however, is a minimally invasive technique with a quick recovery time that has revolutionized cosmetic practice. Reshaping the dorsum and lifting the tip of the nose can be effectively achieved with injectables, what was only possible with surgery before. It is known that distracting noses are usually corrected during adolescence for those who are bothered with their nose appearance. However, the vast majority of people get into adulthood with distracting noses that tend to worsen during aging process. It is very much unlike that senior and adult patients go to operating room to have their nose fixed with surgery even when they are unhappy with it. That is the reason why injectables have become a powerful tool for nose reshape and will be a more frequent solution than surgery to improve the distracting or aging nose.

The knowledge of anatomy and gold standards of the nose are important tools for those who are willing to start working in this facial region. Not only because it is an important area but also due to serious complications as tip necrosis that may happen in the hand of inexperienced injectors. Due to the risk that this area presents, it is highly advisable that appropriate training is performed.

Reshaping the nose with injectables is a method from which there is quick recovery time with no need for general anesthesia or sedation and does not result in ecchymosis. It definitely may produce similar final results as surgery, but they are not as long lasting if biodegradable fillers are used. Lately, the use of newer volumizing HA products has filled the duration gap, and longer results for more than 2 years can be expected for this indication (Fig. 6.42).

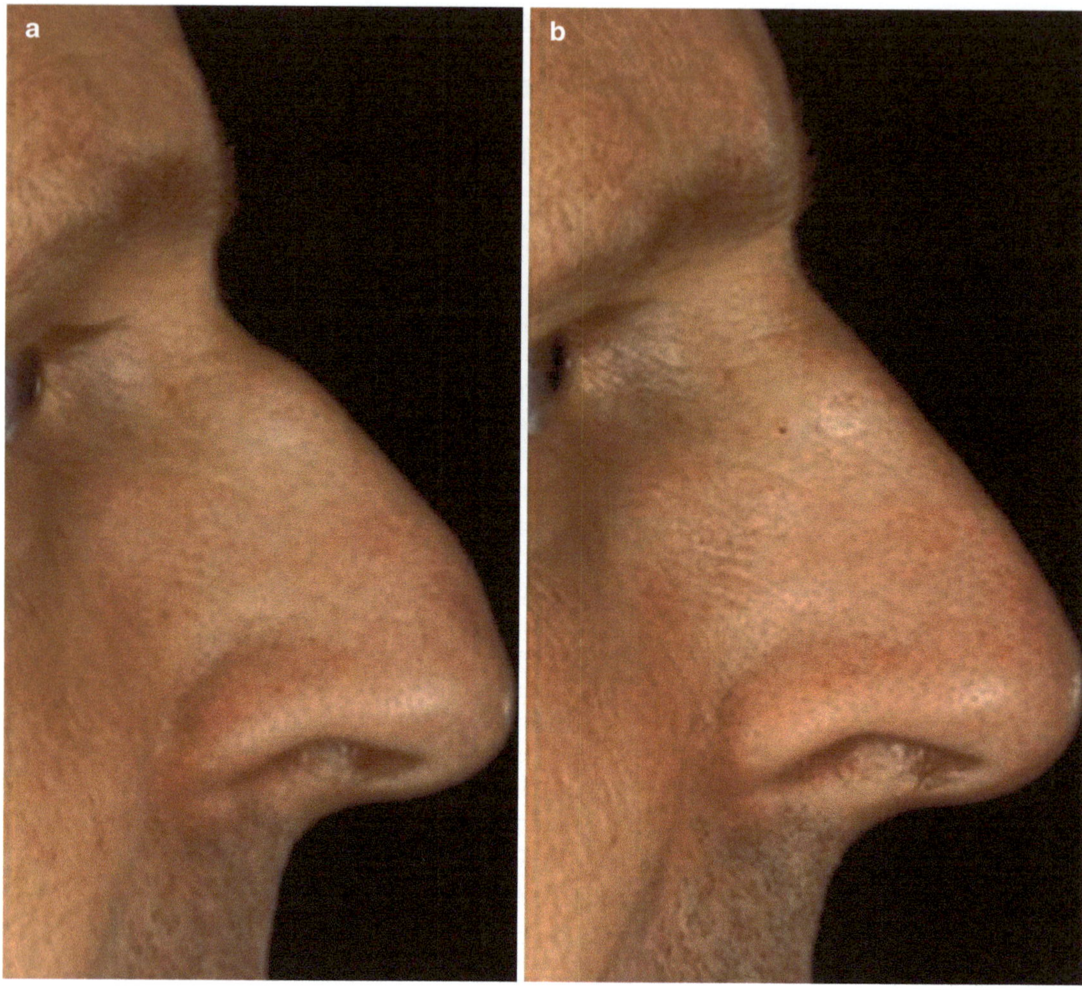

Fig. 6.42 (**a**) At rest, there is an evident nose hump and caudal rotation of the nose tip. This patient considered his nose to be distracting but he was not open for surgery. (**b**) He accepted the nonsurgical approach with HA fillers. Injections into the frontonasal angle, supratip, and tip areas were carried out. A total amount of 1 ml of HA-containing lidocaine was injected

6.6.2 Anatomy

The nose consists of a framework of skin, cartilage, and bone that is supported by connective tissue and ligaments that hold them all together. The skin is thicker and adherent in the lower third of the nose and is thinner and more mobile in the upper two-thirds. The blood supply to the external nose is based on the facial artery. The superior labial and the angular artery are the main branches that respectively form the columellar branches and the lateral nasal branch. Both of them supply the tip of the nose. The dorsal nasal and the external nasal arteries are branches of the ophthalmic artery. The lateral nasal vessels are 2–3 mm above the alar groove and together with the columellar artery arise deep at the nasal base and end at the tip in the subdermal plexus (Rohrich et al. 1995; Fig. 6.43).

The skeletal component of the nose consists of bone and cartilage. The nasal bones are paired and the frontal process of the maxilla is found laterally. The dorsum of the nose is where the lateral surfaces of the upper two-thirds join the midline. The upper lateral cartilages are continuous with the nasal bones. The lower lateral

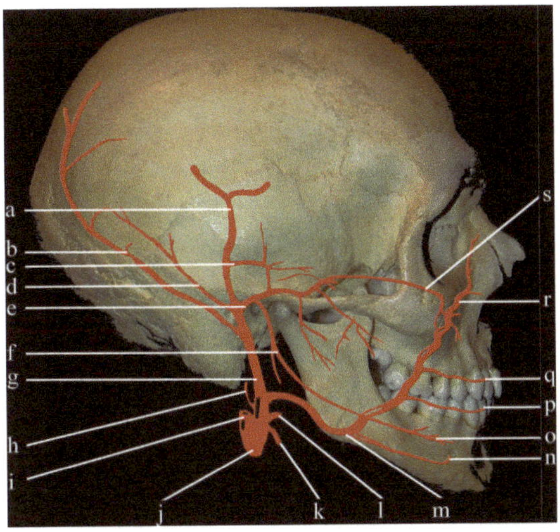

Fig. 6.43 The nose blood supply: *a* superficial temporal artery, *b* occipital a., *c* transverse facial a., *d* posterior auricular a., *e* maxillary a., *f* inferior alveolar a., *g* external carotid a., *h* ascending pharyngeal a., *i* internal carotid a., *j* common carotid a., *k* superior thyroid a., *l* lingual a., *m* facial a., *n* submental a., *o* mental a., *p* inferior labial a., *q* superior labial a., *r* angular a., and *s* infraorbital a

cartilaginous vault is comprised of the medial, middle, and lateral crura. The anatomic dome is the junction of the medial and lateral crura. Depending upon the intrinsic relationship of these structures, the tip of the nose can be normal, bulbous, or boxy. Tip support is basically a combination of skin, ligaments, and cartilage.

The depressor septi nasi is the most important muscle that acts on the tip and lip complex. It shortens the upper lip and drops the tip when smiling. Surgical resection or blocking with BoNT-A may be necessary to enhance the result of fillers. However, this is not the rule (Figs. 6.44 and 6.45).

When reshaping the nose with fillers, the angles with the lips and the forehead are quite important. The former is the nasolabial angle and should be between 90° and 100° in men and between 100° and 110° in women. The latter is the nasofrontal angle, which is between the forehead and the nasal dorsum (Fig. 6.46).

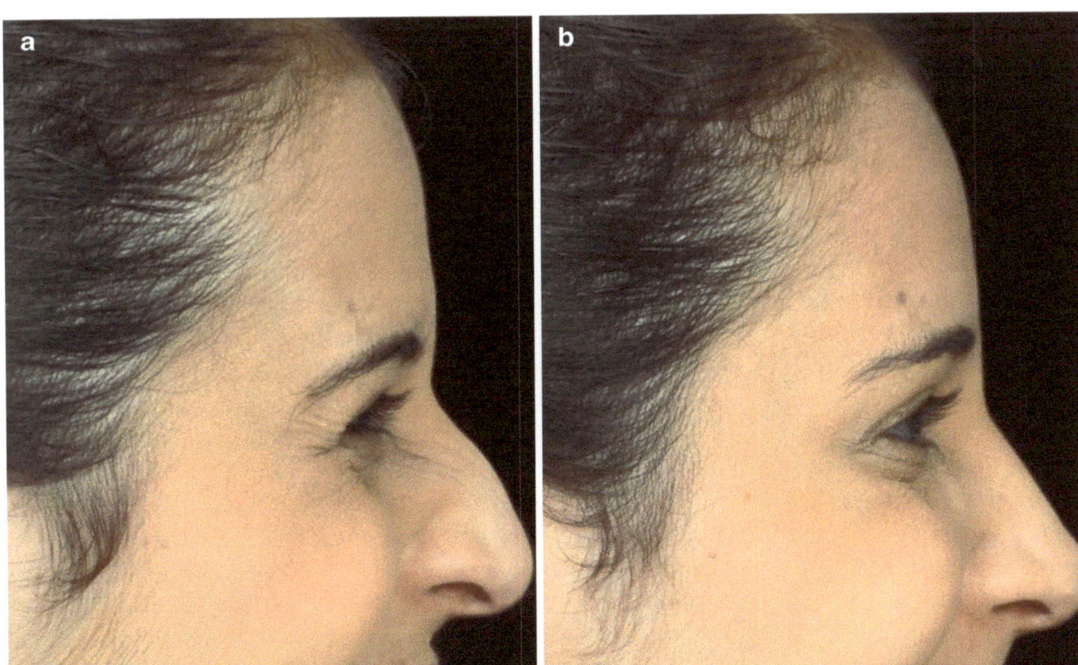

Fig. 6.44 (**a**) During animation, a downward rotation of the nose tip can be noticed. Note the presence of an evident nose hump. (**b**) After the injection of 1 ml of Juvéderm Voluma into the nasal dorsum and into the nasolabial angle, straightening of nasal dorsum is observed

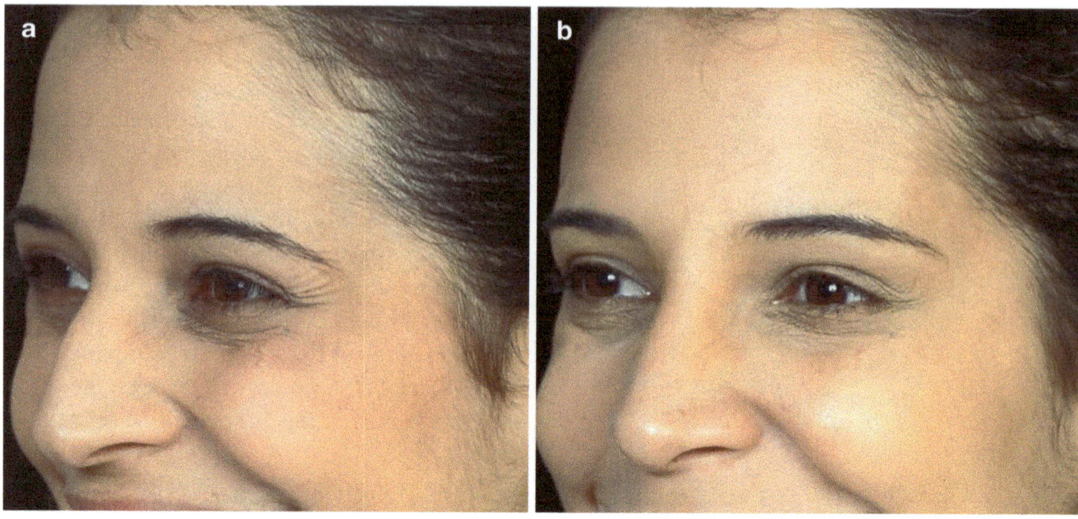

Fig. 6.45 (**a**, **b**) Nose reshape with 1 ml of Juvéderm Voluma. Note the straightening of the nose dorsum

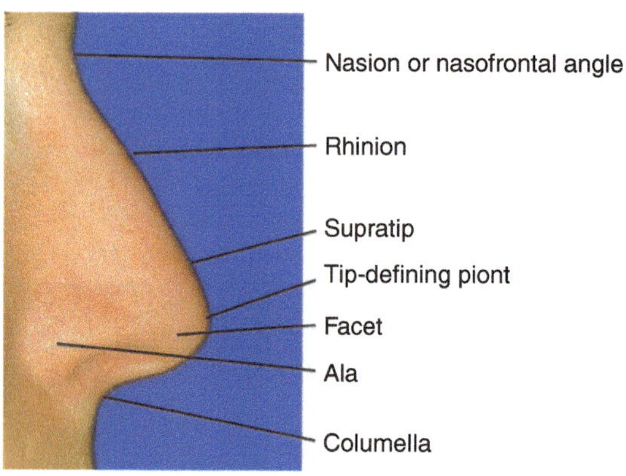

Fig. 6.46 Anatomy of the nose

6.6.3 Patient Evaluation and Selection

Patient selection is of utmost importance for nose reshaping with fillers. Both thin and thick skin is suitable for fillers. Patients with thinner skin usually require less product. In these patients in particular, however, any mistake (too much material either absolutely or relatively) can be evidenced during and after treatment. Biodegradable substances, although temporary, are thus the best to start with. The vast range of products available nowadays enables the right choice for each case. Small molecules can provide a subtle result and are the first choice for beginners in patients with thin skin. Thicker skins do not expand as easily as the thinner ones and usually require more product or larger molecules.

Another aspect to be analyzed should be the presence of deviations. Deviations can be evidenced with an imaginary line from the midglabellar area to the middle of the chin, crossing the nasal tip and the Cupid's bow. The width of the alar base should be the same as the intercanthal distance. The columella should be only slightly visible on the frontal view. If the columella is too small, filling may produce a nicer aspect of the nose. The ratio between the columella and the nasal lobule should be 2:1. If the nostrils are flat, increasing the height of the columella may be desirable. On the basal view, the nose should be like an equilateral triangle (Farkas et al. 1986).

When analyzing the profile, some important aspects must be evaluated: the nasofrontal angle, the nasolabial angle, and confirmation of the presence of a supratip break. The nasofrontal angle should be gentle and a concave curve. It is the connection between the brow and the nasal dorsum. Lack of tip projection is found in short noses. An imaginary vertical line adjacent to the projection of the upper lip should divide the distance between the nasal base and the apex of the nasal tip. If less than 50 % of the tip is anterior to this line, augmentation should be conducted.

The nasal dorsum should be evaluated after treating the tip projection. Ideally, the dorsum

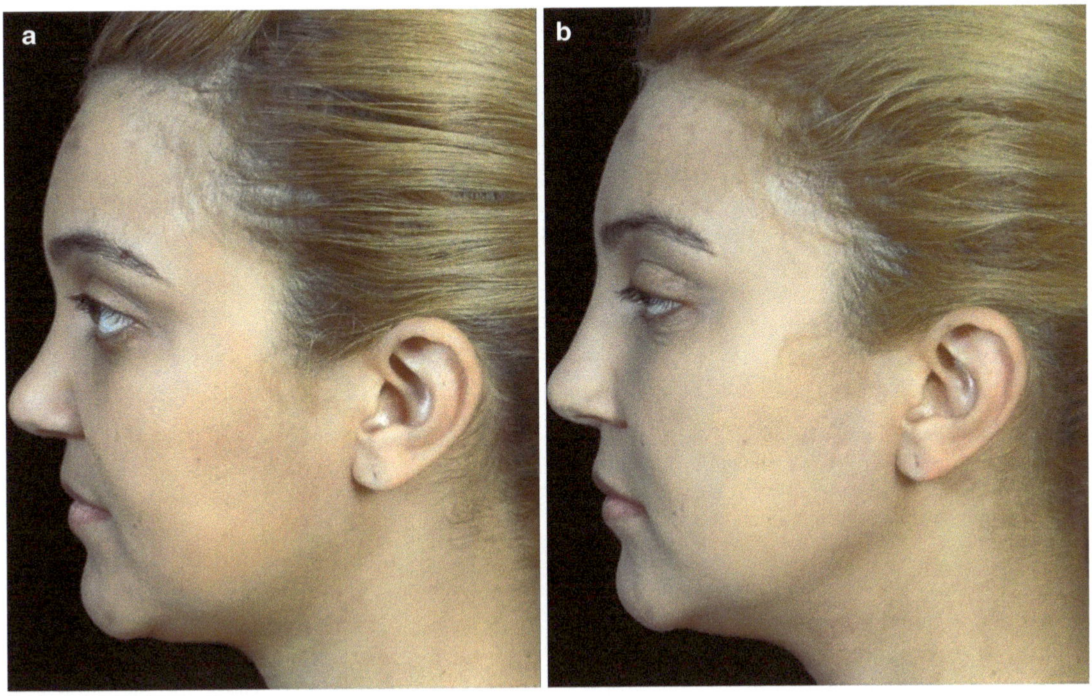

Fig. 6.47 (**a**) This female patient presents a low nasal dorsum and an excessive concave frontonasal angle giving the impression of a frontal fossa. This pattern may be found in infants and Afro-descendants. (**b**) Nose reshape was done with 1 ml Juvéderm Voluma using a 25G blunt cannula through correction of the saddle appearance of the nose and the retruded columella

should lay 2 mm posterior to a parallel line from the nasofrontal angle to the nasal tip in women and a little less in men. The best cases to be treated with fillers are those too far posterior to this line; in these cases the whole dorsum should be augmented. If the dorsum is on the line or projects over it, filling the tip and the nasofrontal angle should be the choice.

Nose reshaping with injectables can enhance dorsum projection, correct nose hump, lift the nose tip, and improve the retruded columella (Fig. 6.47).

6.6.4 Technique

As the nose is quite a sensitive area, topical anesthesia might not be sufficient. Therefore, a block of the fibers of the ophthalmic and maxillary nerve branches is recommended. Usually blocking the supratrochlear and infraorbital branches will suffice especially when cannulas are to be used. Lately, HA preparations containing lidocaine have brought enough comfort for patients during the injection, and the use of nerve blocks is unnecessary when working with needles.

Tissue expansion is easier on the bone dorsum and more difficult in the lower third. Care should be taken with the vessels that pass within the subcutaneous tissue above the muscles. The injection of any substance into patients with oily skin and large pores may be followed by extrusion and loss of the product, so injections should always be below the subdermis and the bevel down. When contrasting thin with thick nasal skin, the latter will require larger polymers and quantities of products. Any mistake will become quite evident in patients with thinner skin. For safety reasons beginners are advised to start with biodegradable products. As mentioned previously, HA preparations are lasting longer and the use of permanent fillers tend to decrease.

The use of cannulas for nose reshape is the best alternative to treat very low and flat noses

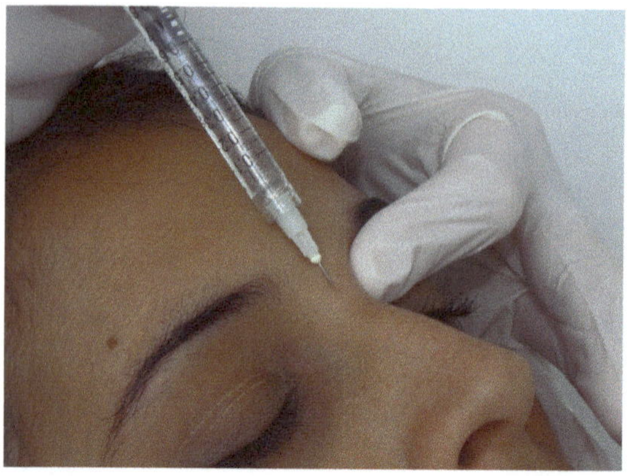

Fig. 6.48 Treatment of the nasofrontal angle must be undertaken closely to the periosteum, injecting into the muscular and subdermal layers. This filling will make the bone dorsum more even and straighter

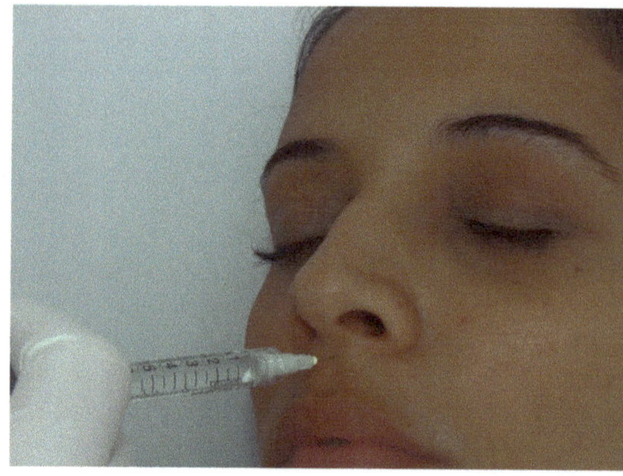

Fig. 6.49 The nasolabial angle filling enables the lifting of the tip of the nose. For women, this angle must be 100° or 110°. It produces a delicate appearance of the nose

such as those found in Asian patients. One of the challenges to enhance nose projection in those patients is to maintain the height of dorsum projection. By creating a single connective tissue tunnel with a cannula, lateral displacement is avoided and projection is maintained.

6.6.5 The Nasofrontal Angle

The best patients to fill are those whose nasofrontal angle is too deep. When the dorsum is excessive, filling the nasofrontal angle and reducing its concavity may straighten the dorsum and the nose may look smaller (Fig. 6.48). If too much product is injected into this area, the nasofrontal angle may become too shallow, producing an undesirable effect. This area is not painful and patients do tolerate the injection without any anesthetic at all. Nose deviation may occur especially if the injection is performed by the side of the patient instead of the cranial approach. Usually 0.1–0.2 ml is needed at this level.

6.6.6 The Nasolabial Angle

The opening of the nasolabial angle is obtained with the filling of the anterior nasal spine (Fig. 6.49). Injecting deeper adjacent to the nasal spine will expand the inferior part of the membranous septum. If necessary, the columella base can also be injected, especially if widening of the medial crura is desired. More volume is needed here especially if the columella is retruded or underdeveloped such as in Asian patients. A total of 0.5 ml may be required. Elongation of the upper lip may occur and should be avoided. Longer upper lip is distracting in the vast majority of patients. However, patients with excessive short upper lip and gummy smile may benefit from it.

6.6.7 The Tip and the Columella

6.6.7.1 Columella Height

The medial crura should be expanded if the nostrils are flat. It should be teardrop shaped. A retracted columella can also be filled. Depending on the degree of retraction, soft-tissue expansion should be handled in more than one session. Expansion is undertaken with an injection into the membranous septum. Injecting into the footplates of the medial crura may increase tip projection (Fig. 6.50). Before injecting, it is advisable to pinch the columella to check how expandable it is.

6.6.7.2 Supratip Deformation

Care should be taken not to erase the supratip break. Filling into this point may cause supratip deformation and consequent dropping of the nasal

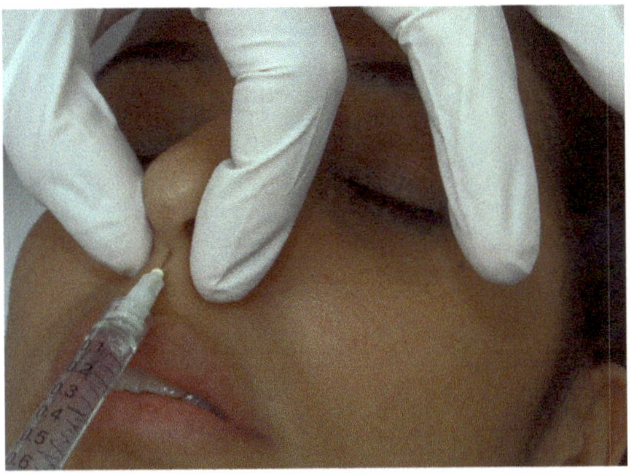

Fig. 6.50 When injecting into the columella basis, care should be taken not to wide this area too much. So, the thumb and index finger must be in a position to avoid it

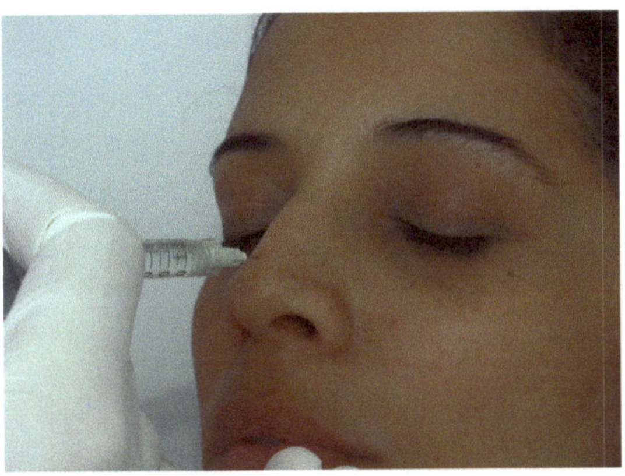

Fig. 6.51 Injecting into the cartilaginous dorsum must be carefully performed to avoid a supratip deformation and a falling of the tip

tip (Fig. 6.51). To enhance the supratip break, there must be a difference in height between the domes and the septal angle; a tiny injection into the tip of the dome may produce this effect.

6.6.7.3 Tip Projection

To evaluate whether the filling of the tip was correctly performed, the final tip projection must equal the width of the alar base. An increase in tip rotation is conducted in patients with a reduced nasolabial angle. Increasing the nasal tip projection may be undertaken by direct injection into the domes (Fig. 6.52). When treating the tip, it must be established whether the patient needs augmentation of the domes and/or the middle crura. When only the domes need augmentation, injections must only be made into the upper portion of the tip. If the whole tip must be treated, upper and lower injections must be undertaken. This is a nice solution for patients with thin skin who present surface irregularities on the tip.

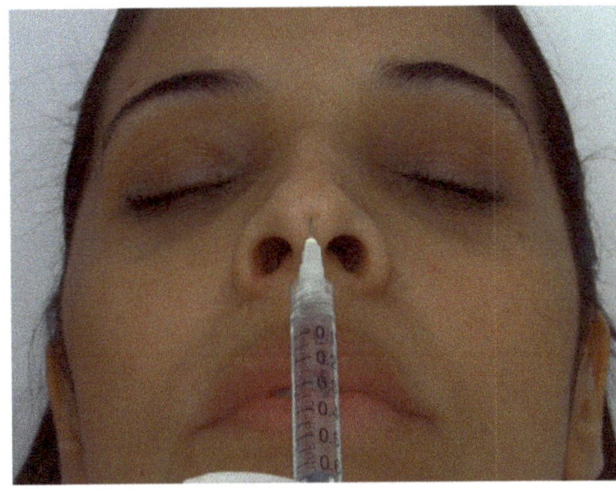

Fig. 6.52 The tip filling: a direct injection into the tip of the nose promotes both lifting and projection increase. Too much of the injected product may provoke a boxy deformation

Care must be taken not to inject too much product as this may produce widening of the middle crura and a boxy tip aspect, which is undesirable. During the injection, pinching the tip may be helpful to avoid excessive filling. A delicate caudal injection into the tip may produce an increase in tip projection and a nice upward tip rotation. When a major increase in tip projection is necessary, filling into the soft tissue of the premaxilla is advisable.

Injection into the tip should be carried out with caution. The use of biodegradable products is recommended.

6.6.8 Dorsum

When the tip of the nose is adequate but the nasofrontal angle and dorsum are low, fillers are very suitable for nose reshaping (Fig. 6.53). The tip height helps to give an idea of the quantity of product to be injected. Injections should start with the nasofrontal angle to reduce its concavity up to the point where it equals the tip height. The dorsal

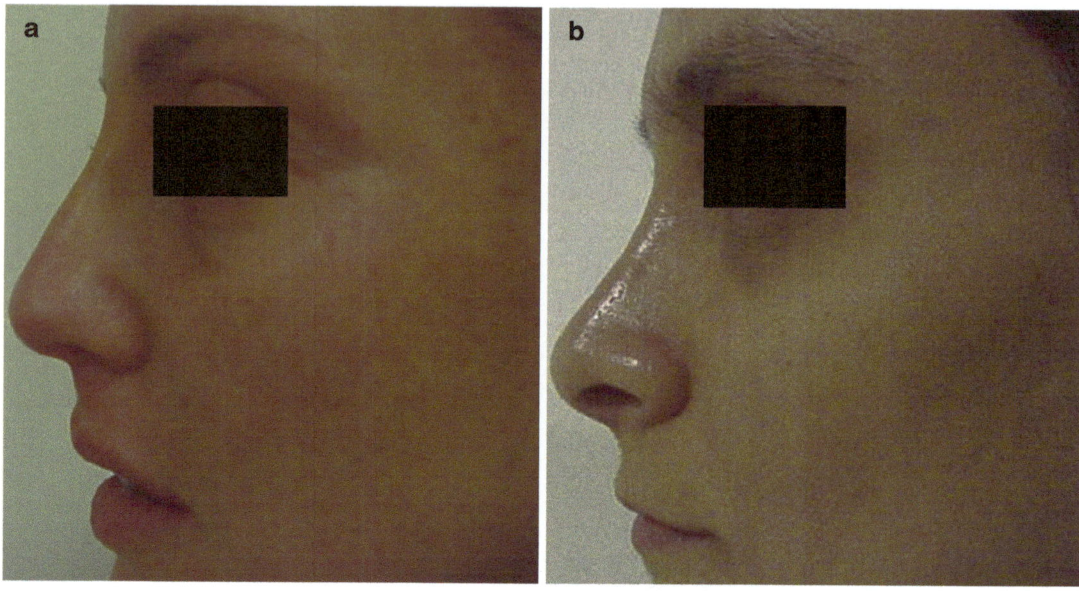

Fig. 6.53 (**a**, **b**) Saddle deformity after rhinoplasty before and after treatment with a filler. Fillers may be an important ally to prepare patients for surgery or may even be the only treatment

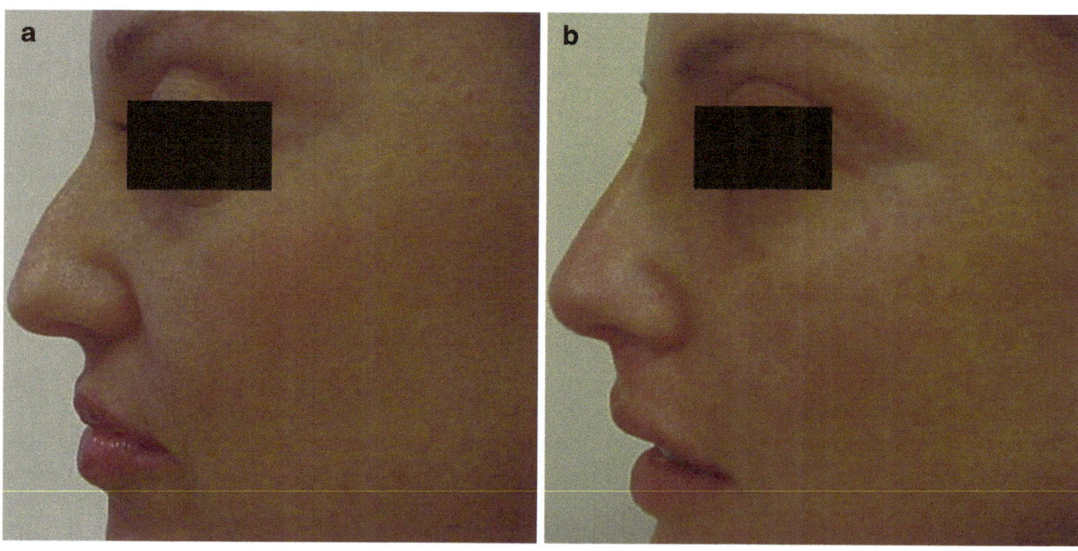

Fig. 6.54 (**a**, **b**) This typical surgical nose was only treated with fillers. After a 5-min procedure, the patient could leave the office with no postoperative period, no ecchymosis, and no bandages

augmentation should almost reach the imaginary line between these two points. Injections should be carried out with a retrograde technique. Any irregularity should be treated with a slight massage.

In the past, the dorsal hump was treated mainly by surgery. However, a very good alternative is to use injectables (Fig. 6.54). After treating the tip, injections must be made into the nasofrontal angle, onto the bone and cartilaginous dorsum, and into the nasolabial angle. Care should be taken not to produce a supratip deformation.

6.6.9 Selection of Filler

If it is the first time that the nose has been injected, it is preferable to get experience with biodegradable products. Only experienced physicians should handle nonbiodegradable products. Even some experienced physicians only use biodegradable products to avoid complications. Hyaluronic acid enables a good start; although the results did not last long in the past, new HA preparations such as Juvéderm Voluma or comparable HA products have increased dramatically the performance and duration of nose reshape. Due to its hydrophilic properties and pseudoplasticity, it can be easily molded (Fig. 6.55).

Nonbiodegradable products are a good choice for longer-lasting results, but care should be taken with blood vessels. Accidental injection into the nasal blood vessels, especially into the columella base, may result in tip necrosis, which may lead to a catastrophic result. PMMA preparations are examples of products that usually produce longer-lasting results but tend to be used each time less as longer-lasting HA preparations are coming into the market

6.6.10 Complications

The most frightening complication associated with nasal reshaping is necrosis and blindness. It is rare and occurs mainly with nonbiodegradable products. Blood vessel impairment with biodegradable materials is much less common, and if an HA filler is inadvertently injected into a blood vessel, a massage should be promptly undertaken to break up the polymers and hyaluronidase should be immediately used.

Excessive filling of the cartilaginous dorsum may lead to supratip deformation and irregularities. The nasofrontal angle and the nasolabial angle rarely produce deformities if properly injected, but nose deviation may result though. Care should be taken not to produce a widening of the nose at these areas. If too much product is injected into the tip of the nose, a boxy deformation may occur.

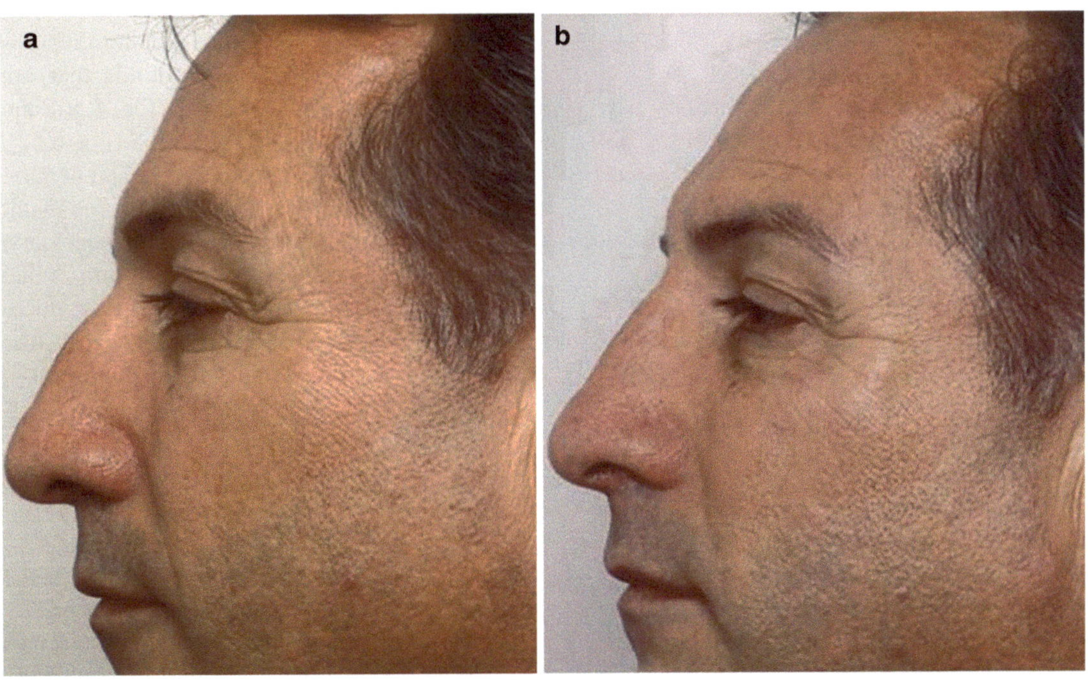

Fig. 6.55 (a, b) Presence of nasal hump and a droop of nasal tip. The treatment was carried out with 1.0 ml of Juvéderm Voluma. A straightening of the nasal dorsum and correction of the tip were obtained

6.6.11 Tips, Tricks and Key Points

Nasal filling should be undertaken with care and knowledge of the anatomy. Some of the results are comparable to those achieved with surgery. This is a good option for patients who are not willing or are unable to submit to surgical procedures.

Do's

- Do educate your patients with nasal deficits about the benefits of nose reshape with injectables.
- Please remember that nasal injections will not change the physiology of the nose. In case of a distorted nasal septum, surgery is the option.

Don'ts

- Do not inject noses if you are not properly trained.

Key Points

- Nose reshaping with injectables have filled a gap to the treatment of the distracting or the aging nose when we had only surgical solutions in the past.
- To have good results and avoid adverse events, extreme care in technique and proper antisepsis is of utmost importance.

FAQs

- What are the benefits and limits of nose reshape with injectables?

  Nose reshape with injectables may have limited results in the correction of a bulbous tip, but it definitely can enhance dorsum projection, correct nose humps, lift the nose tip, and improve the retruded columella.
- Needles or cannulas for nose reshape?

  It depends on the case. Needles are useful to correct dorsal humps and lift the tip of the nose by injecting into the nasolabial angle but may be limited in very flat and low noses where cannulas are the best option.

6.7 Nasolabial Folds

6.7.1 Introduction

Nasolabial folds are still the major indication for injectable fillers. Furthermore, they are the best investigated filler indications as the FDA requests this indication for fillers entering the US market. Based on these studies we have for the investigated products good data to answer simple questions as the following: (1) How much filler do I need to inject on average? (2) How long will the filler last? After one injection? After repeated injections? And what is the safety of this procedure?

There is no such thing as *the* nasolabial fold. There are deep nasolabial folds and more superficial ones; there are nasolabial folds that are induced by strong facial mimics (Fig. 6.56) and those induced by ptosis of the SMAS (Fig. 6.57). Each of these folds requires special attention with regard to the injection technique, the material to be used, and the amount of filler necessary. Last but not least, a word of caution: this is like the glabella, an area where an inadvertent injection in an artery (a. nasalis) might lead to the occlusion of the vessel with subsequent necrosis, e.g., of the ala nasi (see Sect. 8.5.3).

6.7.2 Anatomy/Structure

Nasolabial folds – the small triangle between the ala, the nose, and the cheek – can be deepened by contracting the levator labii superioris alaeque nasi and the levator labii superioris muscles. Both muscles are activated when patients wrinkle their nose. Strong muscular tonus might lead to very deep wrinkles at quite an early age (Fig. 6.58). The depth

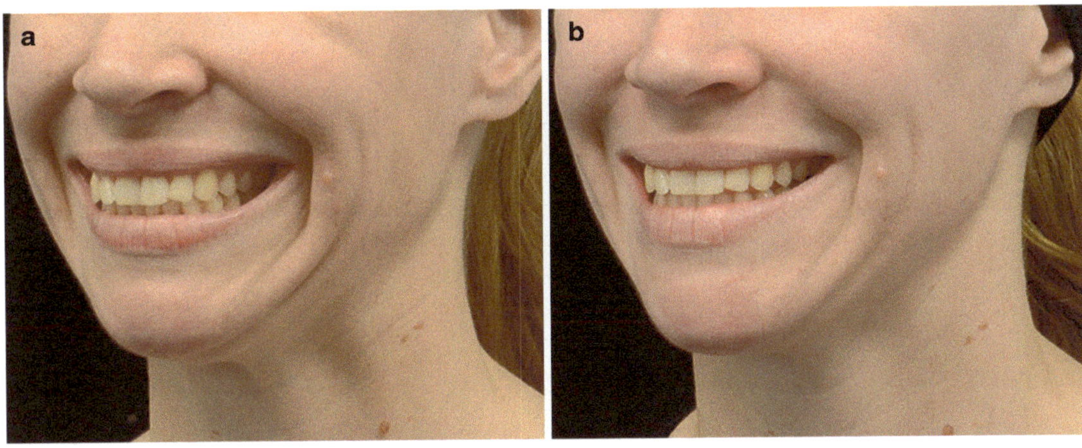

Fig. 6.56 (**a**, **b**) Nasolabial fold on animation before and after correction with Juvéderm Volift (0.4 ml in the NLF and 0.1 ml in the marionette line per side)

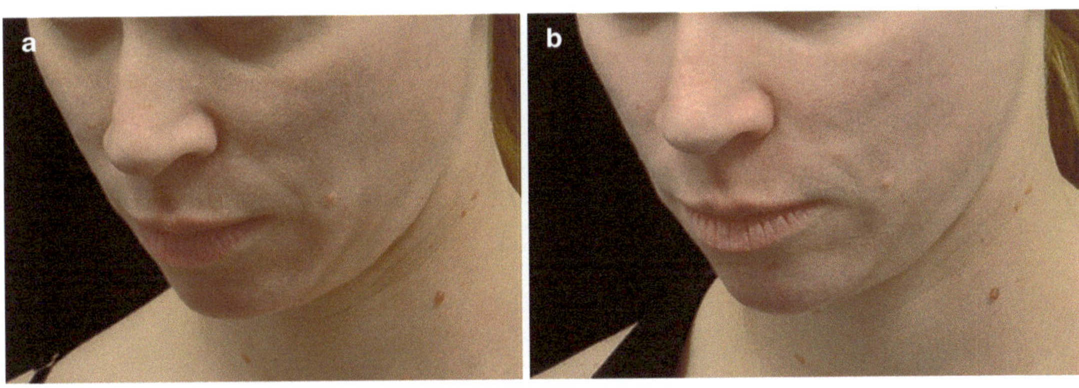

Fig. 6.57 (**a**) Before treatment, patient is leaning forward to show and analyze the degree of skin laxity at the nasolabial fold and cheek. (**b**) After treatment of the nasolabial folds and marionette lines, mechanical support was provided and less sagginess resulted

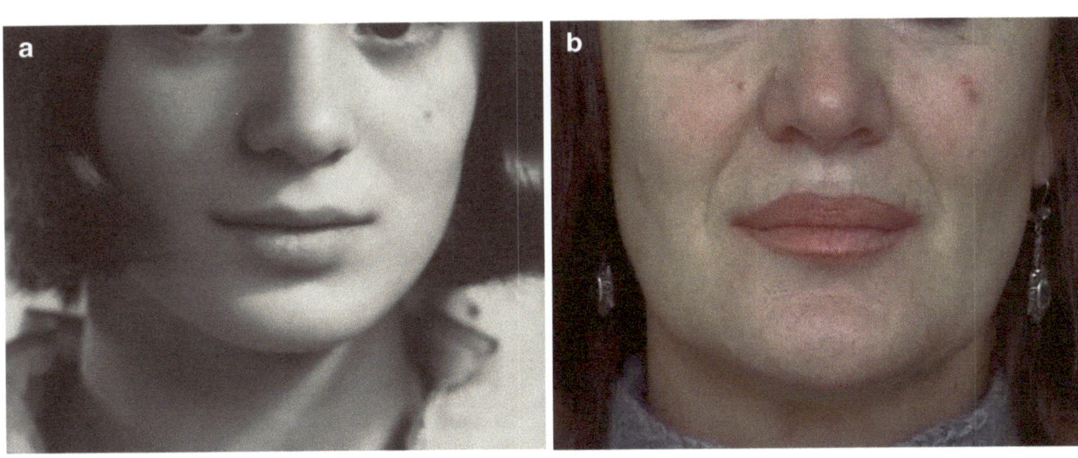

Fig. 6.58 The same patient in her twenties (**a**) and her forties (**b**). Please note the deepening of the nasolabial folds

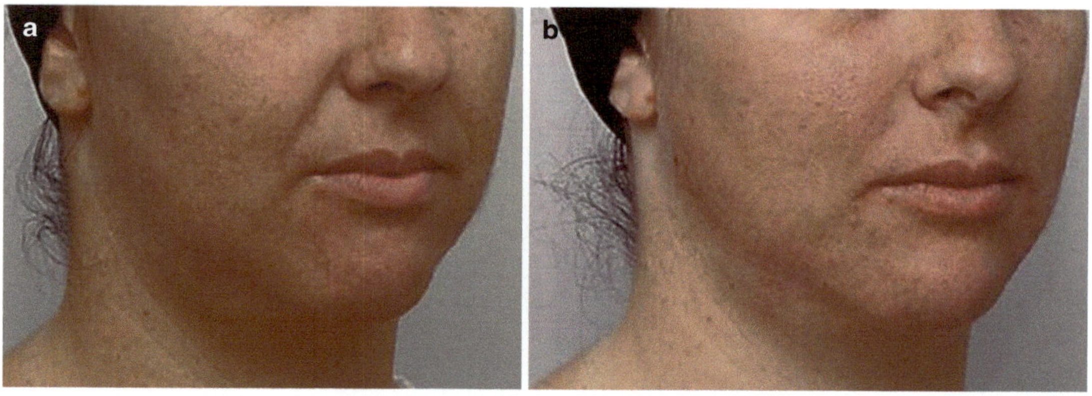

Fig. 6.59 (**a**, **b**) Before and after treatment or the nasolabial fold with 1 ml of Juvéderm Voluma per side. The lips were treated with 0.6 ml of Juvéderm Ultra Plus

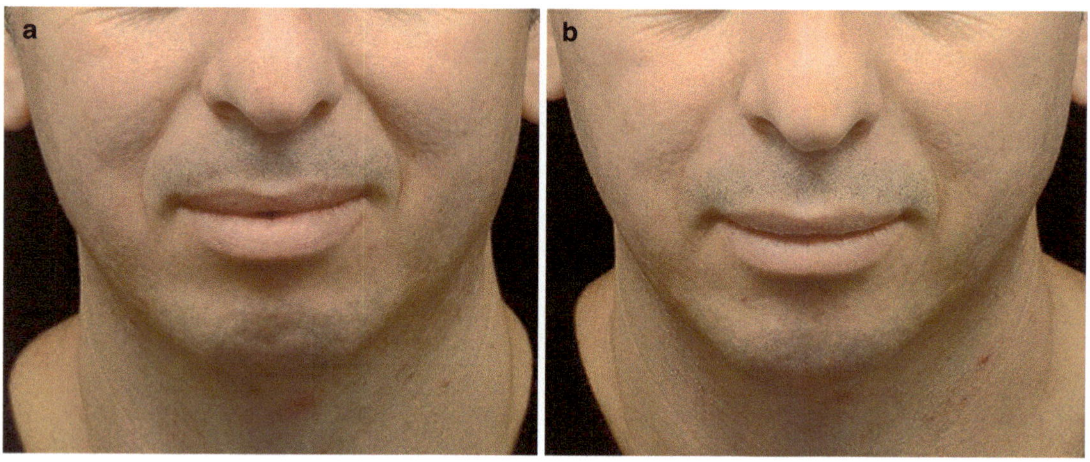

Fig. 6.60 (**a**, **b**) Before and after treatment of the nasolabial fold of a male patient. A total of 1 ml of Juvéderm Volift was injected by side. Note the softening and natural aspects of the folds

of the nasolabial folds at rest in contrast correlates well with the degree of cutaneous elastosis and the tonus of the SMAS. Therefore, nasolabial folds are one of the signature folds to be affected by aging.

6.7.3 Patient Evaluation and Selection

The nasolabial folds must be analyzed prior to filler injection. If there is an active contraction of the levator labii superioris alaeque nasi and the levator labii superioris muscles, fillers may be accompanied by a pretreatment with BoNT-A of these muscles. In addition, the amount of filler required should be realistically estimated. In older patients with very deep folds, for example, it might be necessary to inject up to 2 ml per site. The best results are obtained in patients with either no or mild saggy skin over the nasolabial fold (Figs. 6.59 and 6.60). With the introduction of HA volumizers in the market, nasolabial folds are often treated in a second step, e.g., after volume replacement in the cheekbones (Fig. 6.61).

6.7.4 Technique

Stretching the skin between two fingers prior to injection helps to visualize the fold and to ensure that the material is injected where it should be (Figs. 6.62 and 6.63). To avoid an increase in the

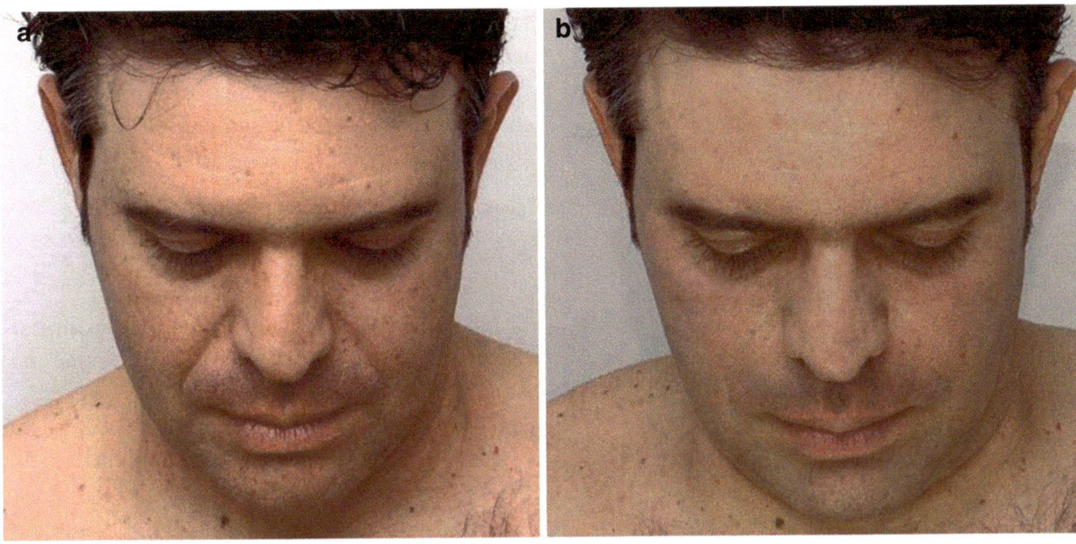

Fig. 6.61 (**a**) This male patient is leaning forward. A worsening of the nasolabial fold is seen. (**b**) To be sure the correction of the nasolabial fold will be long lasting, observe if the correction is still maintained with the patient leaning forward, after treatment. If the nasolabial fold is not fully corrected under this position of stress, short-lasting result may be expected. A total of 4 ml of Juvéderm Voluma was injected into the cheekbones and NLF. With this a duration of the result should last over 18 months

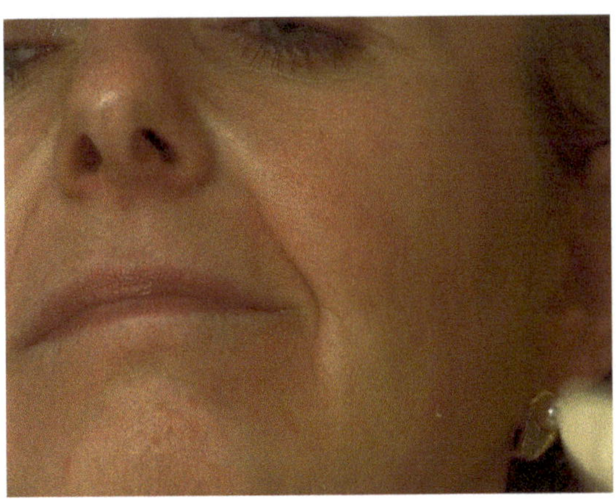

Fig 6.62 Native nasolabial fold

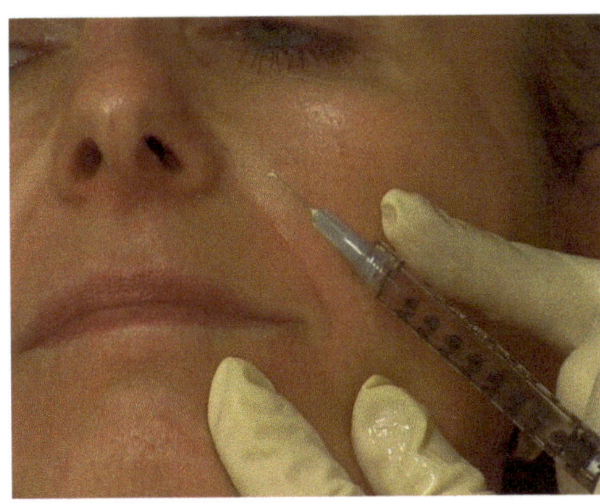

Fig. 6.63 Stretching of the skin of the nasolabial fold prior to injection

visibility of the fold, especially in patients with SMAS-related deep folds, the injections should be performed slightly more medially (Fig. 6.64).

Nasolabial folds are quite easy and fast to treat with the retrograde injection technique. Cannulas and sharp needles might be used. The multiple injection site technique can be applied, too. This technique will help to blend the filler better in the surrounding area. Deep nasolabial folds and folds in patients with elastotic skin might require a multilevel approach, e.g., applying the filler or different fillers on different levels of the skin.

6.7.5 Touch-Up

When using a biodegradable filler for deep nasolabial folds, a touch-up will prolong the durability of the effect. The touch-up can be early

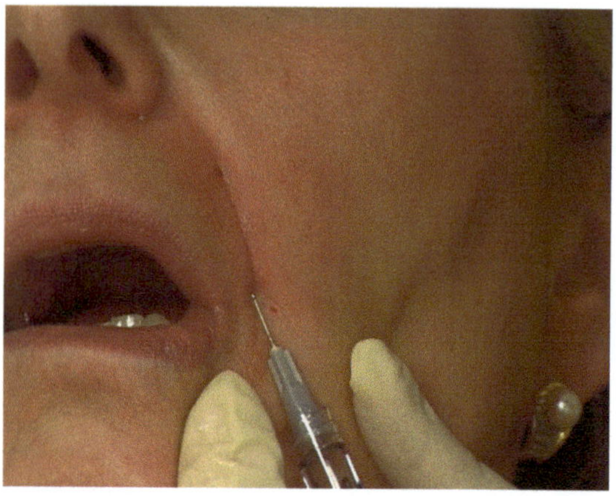

Fig. 6.64 Medial injection with an HA in a patient to avoid an unwanted increase of the cheek ptosis

approximately 3–4 weeks after the initial treatment (when the result after the initial treatment is not sufficient) or late 4.5–9 months after the treatment (when a prolonged durability is intended) (Narins et al. 2008; Figs. 6.65 and 6.66).

6.7.6 Complications

There are some general pitfalls that are attributable to an inappropriate injection technique that should be avoided:

1. The sausage: the sausage constitutes the remains of a filler that was too superficially

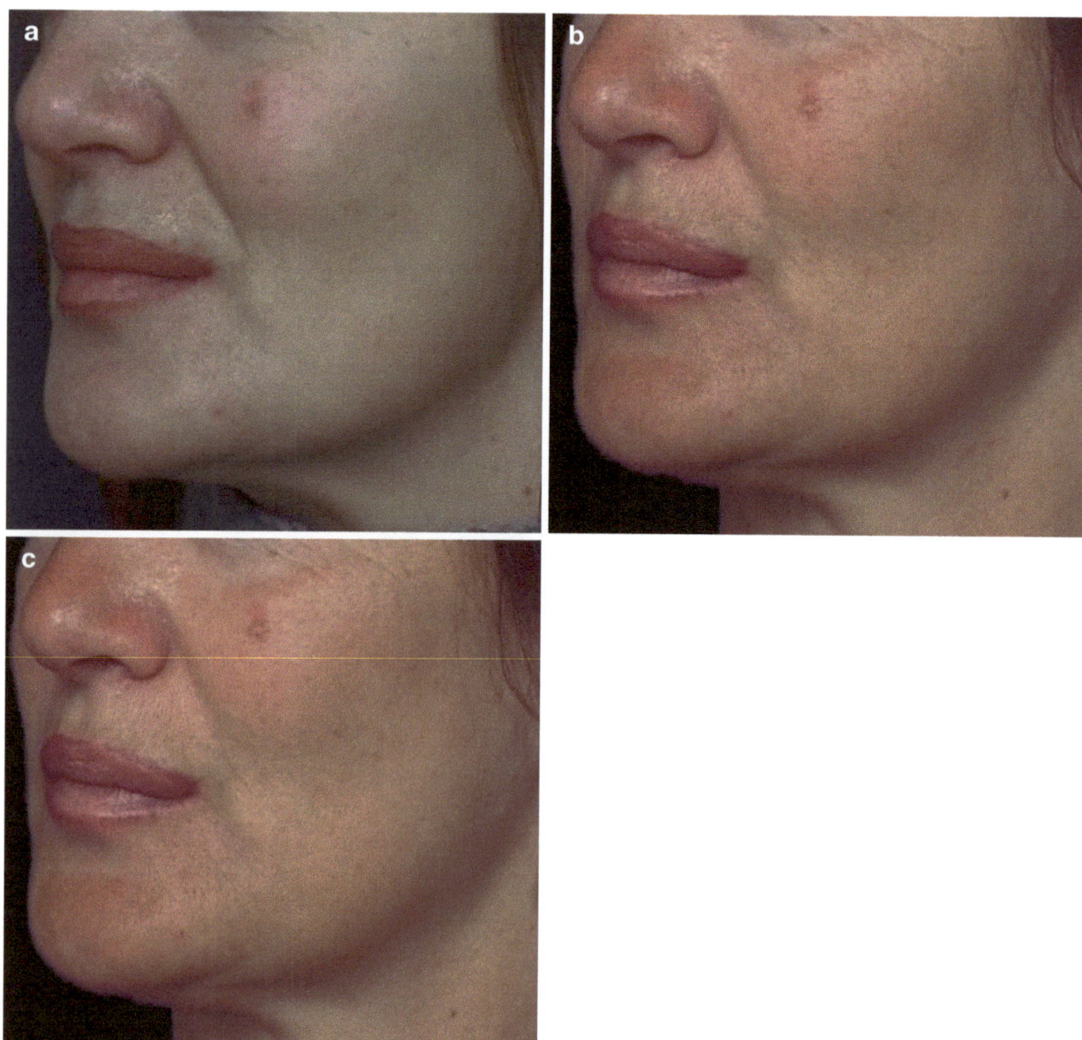

Fig. 6.65 (a–c) Deep nasolabial folds treated with PLLA prior to and immediately after treatment and 5 months later

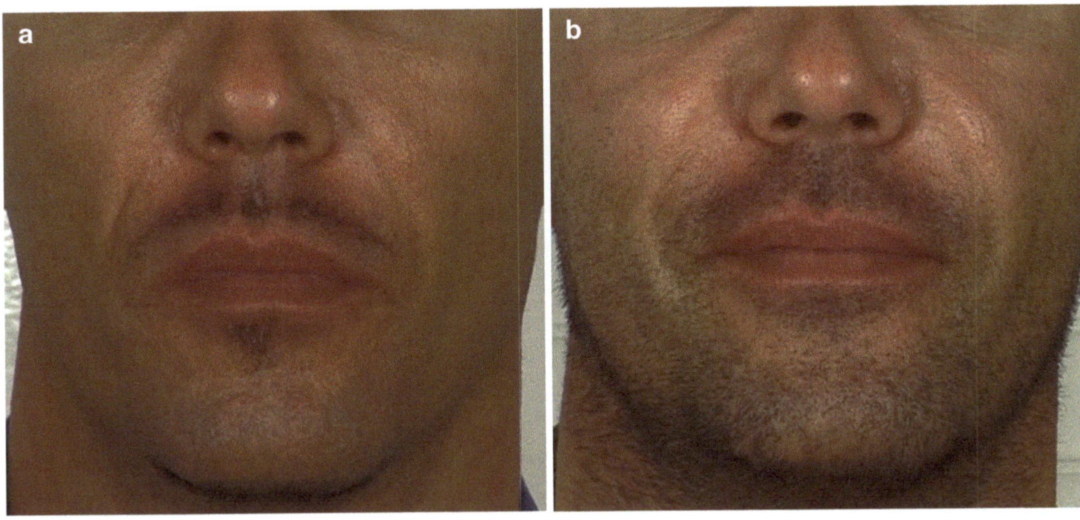

Fig. 6.66 (**a**, **b**) Superficial nasolabial lines in a patient successfully pretreated with PLLA for deep nasolabial folds before and 3 months after the superficial injection of a total of 1.4 ml of a low viscosity hyaluronic acid

injected (n.b. the sausage can be found in other areas as the infraorbital area, too).

2. The lump: injecting large amounts of a filler will result in filler depots that might be palpable for several weeks.
3. The increased fold: in a patient with SMAS-related ptosis of the cheek, an injection made too laterally will lead to an increase in the depth of the fold.
4. A necrosis of the ala nasi: thankfully this is a rare complication. If severe pain during injection is reported and a whitish discoloration develops, the injection has to be immediately stopped, and if an hyaluronic acid is injected, hyaluronidase should be injected immediately (see also Chap. 8).

6.7.7 Tips, Tricks and Key Points

Do's

- Have the patient comfortably sit up either during the whole procedure or at the end to make sure that you evaluate the nasolabial folds at maximum gravity.
- In patients with moderate to extreme nasolabial folds, consider a planned touch-up after 4.5–9 months to increase the durability of the injections.

Don'ts

- Do not inject too laterally in patients with saggy skin. If you inject too laterally, the fold might be become more visible.
- Do not inject if not enough. If you inject just one syringe in a patient who in fact needs two or three syringes per side, the patient will not be happy because the visible changes are not as the patient would have liked them.
- If the patient has strong marionette lines too, please do not forget to treat them in the same session. Otherwise the patient might look quite weird.

Key Points

- Despite all the talk on the overall volumization of the face, the correction of the nasolabial fold is still a major individual indication. One reason for that is that patient might more easily afford one or two syringes instead of three or more.
- If you start to work with injectable fillers, start with this indication. The treatment is straightforward and the results predictable.
- Always inject enough but do not overcorrect.

6.8 The Earlobe

6.8.1 Introduction

Earlobes have been ornamented with jewelry for thousands of years, traditionally by piercing of the earlobe. In some cultures, ornaments are placed to stretch and enlarge the earlobes. Tearing of the earlobe from the weight of heavy earrings, or from traumatic pull of an earring (e.g., by snagging on a sweater), is fairly common. Patients with loose or atrophic earlobes can benefit from injectables (Fig. 6.67).

6.8.2 Anatomy/Structure

The earlobes are composed of 2 portions – an attached upper part and an unattached lower part. There is significant variability in the shape and contour of the earlobes. Ideally, the earlobe should comprise about 20 % of the length of the ear. The average length of the lobe itself is about 18 mm. Most people are born with unattached earlobes. About 30 % of people have attached earlobes, which represents a recessive gene (Figs. 6.68 and 6.69).

6.8.3 Patient Evaluation and Selection

As we age, the unattached portions of the earlobes increase in size. The earlobes also "deflate" by losing some of the fat under the skin. This results an increase in wrinkles and creases. Just like elsewhere on the face, the earlobe skin is susceptible to sun damage. Sun exposure also contributes to wrinkling of the earlobe as well as discoloration.

Atrophic earlobes that present wrinkles and creases can effectively be improved with injectables that will plump them back up, resulting in more youthful appearance. Torn or stretched ear piercing holes are to be repaired by surgery. However, orifice narrowing may also be improved with injectables. Patients who received a face lift and present deformities in the earlobe may also benefit from injectables.

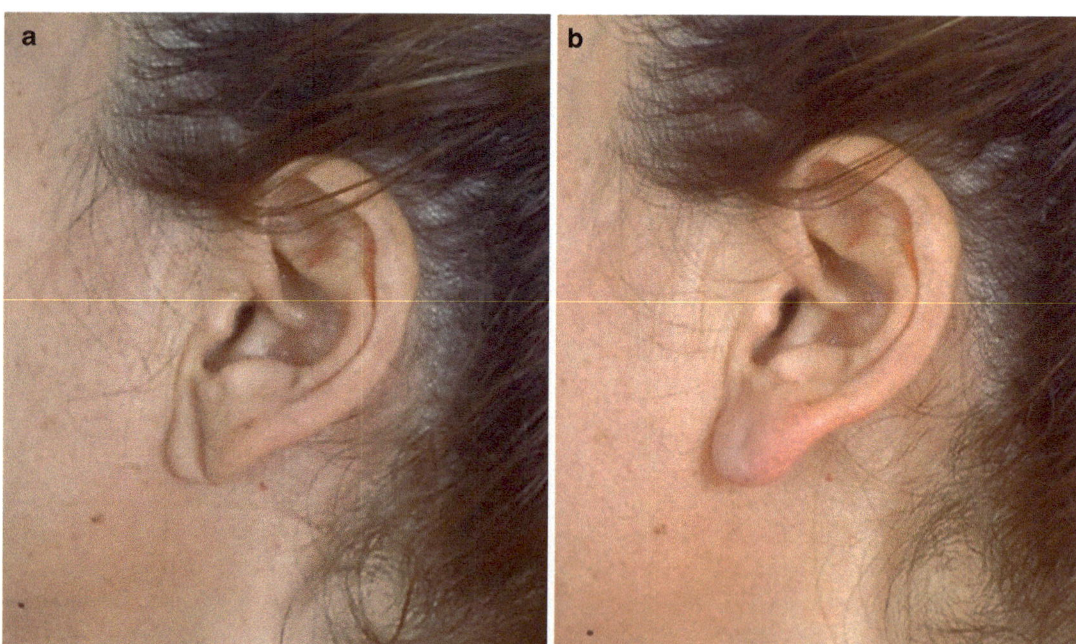

Fig. 6.67 (**a**, **b**) Before treatment, there is a deflation of the earlobe and presence of a vertical wrinkle. After injection of 0.5 ml of Juvéderm Ultra Plus per side, volume restoration is achieved

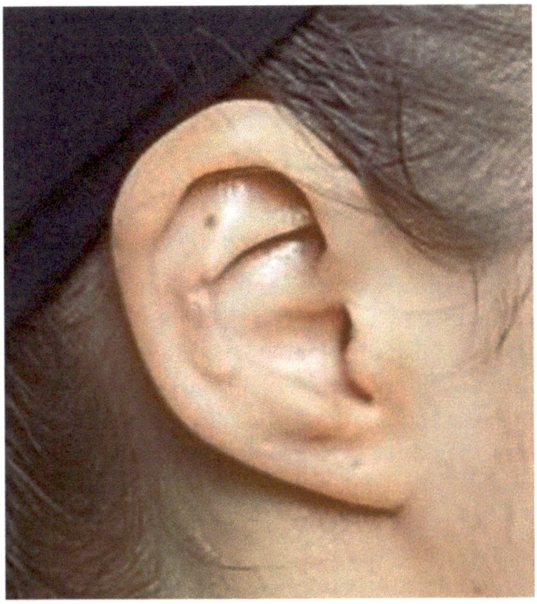

Fig. 6.68 A typical attached earlobe

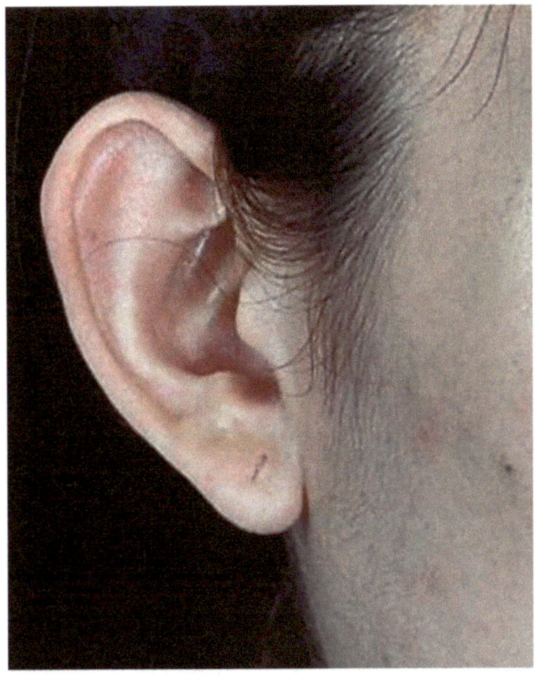

Fig. 6.69 The unattached earlobe

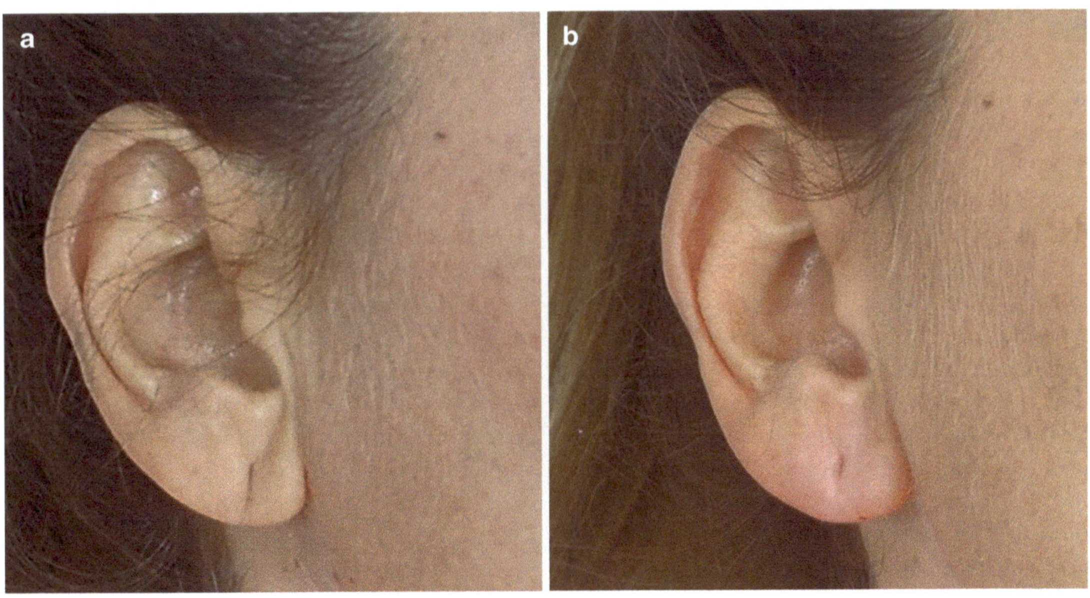

Fig. 6.70 (**a, b**) Before treatment, it seems that it is a ripped earlobe with an enlarged orifice. Usually, this patient would be submitted to surgical correction for improvement. Right after the injection of 0.5 ml of Juvéderm Ultra Plus per side, the torn aspect is resolved

6.8.4 Technique

The skin is stretched and then the filler is injected in the subdermal tissue. Usually 0.2–0.5 ml of the filler should be sufficient. If narrowing of the orifice is needed, HA may be injected around to constrict it (Fig. 6.70). Usually no anesthesia is required.

6.8.5 Tips, Tricks and Key Points

Do's
- Stretch the skin while injecting.

Don'ts
- Do not overdue it – the patient does not want a big lump as an earlobe.

Key Points
- This is usually an indication of which the patient is not aware. You might point this out in case you have a patient with loose earlobes while treating another indication.

6.9 The Upper and Lower Lips

6.9.1 Introduction

The lips are very important for social interaction. A wide spectrum of emotions is represented by the lips, from happiness to sadness and sorrow. It also plays an important role in the expression of sensuality and sexuality. When the sphincter mechanism is intact, normal lip function promotes a competent oral seal for liquids and solids, especially the lower lip. The free movable nature of the vermillion and cutaneous skin makes this area quite suitable for distortion. The use of BoNT-A, although sometimes quite helpful, may lead to asymmetries and temporary loss of function (see Sect. 9.4). Fillers, on the other hand, are highly suitable for both lip augmentation and improvement of perioral wrinkles.

Nevertheless, one has to be aware that the variety of lip shape, occlusion, and muscle activity at this area make the treatment of the lips a challenge. Lack of understanding of the lip anatomy and muscular activity patterns may lead to undesirable results that even for lay persons are detectable. Together with the eyes, the perioral area is under direct attention and any inadvertent injection will lead to distraction.

6.9.2 Anatomy

The lips cover more than the area of the red part of the mouth. They also include the skin adjacent to the red part of the mouth. It must be considered as an anatomic unit with extensions superior to the nose and inferior to the chin. Perfect lip structure includes a visible white or transition line between the mucosa and skin, a "V"-shaped Cupid's bow, fulfilled medial tubercle and vermillion, and ascendant line in the oral commissures. The ratio between the upper and lower lips, at golden proportions, is 1:1.618.

A very important topographic landmark is the philtrum. The midpoint of the upper cutaneous lip is highlighted by the two vertically oriented ridges of the philtrum. The Cupid's bow is the concavity at the base of the philtrum (Fig. 6.71). It is also very important to take into account the surroundings of the lips, which are the labiomental and nasolabial lines. If too deep, these lines may give an older appearance which will prevail even after a sufficient augmentation by a filler.

The skin of the upper lip is very thin and lacks subcutaneous fat. The lack of additional support at this level and excess of muscular movement may lead to the breakdown of the perioral area, producing wrinkling (Fig. 6.72).

The major muscle of the lips is the orbicularis oris muscle. It has circumferential fibers that are responsible for the sphincter function of the mouth. There are circumoral muscles, which are intimately associated with the orbicularis oris. These muscles elevate, depress, and retract the lips, producing complex movements during normal function. The levators lie from medial to lateral: the labii superioris alaeque nasi levator, the labii superioris levator, the zygomatic minor and major, the levator anguli oris, and the risorius muscles. The depressors include the depressor anguli oris, the depressor labii inferioris, the mentalis muscles, and the platysma.

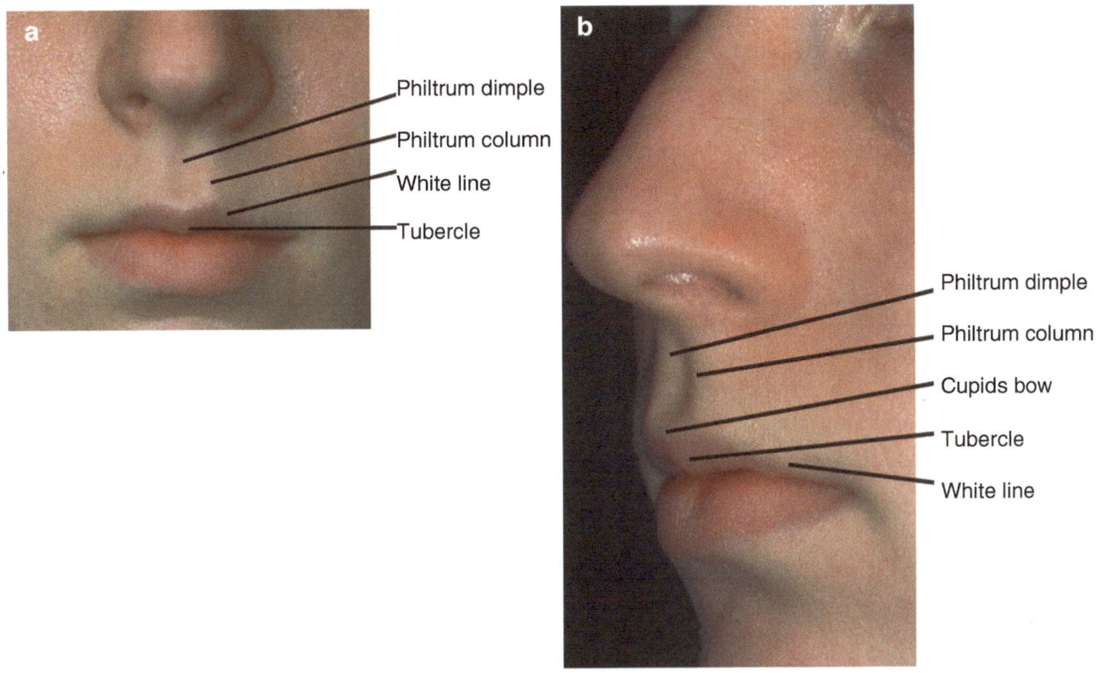

Fig. 6.71 (**a**, **b**) Frontal and lateral view on landmarks of the upper lip

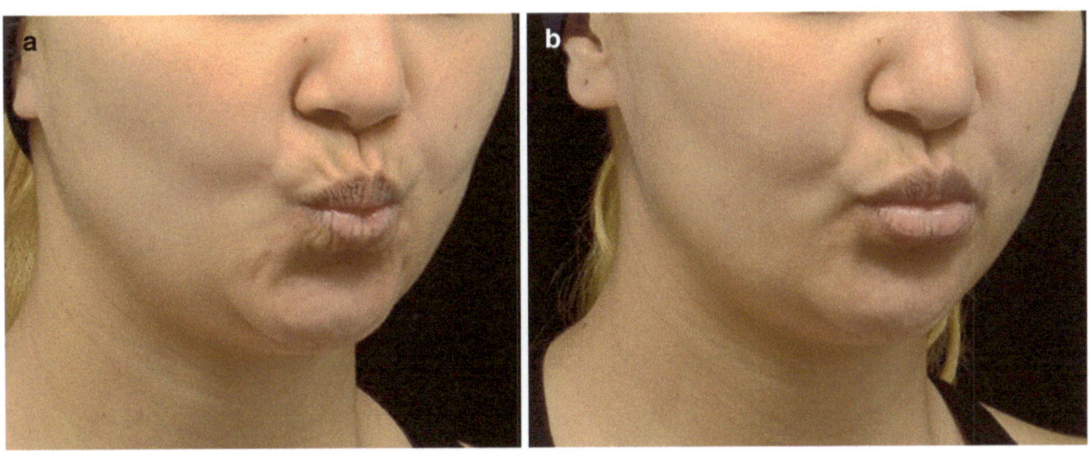

Fig. 6.72 (**a**, **b**) At the age of 28 this patient already presents excessive perioral wrinkling on animation. If left untreated, these dynamic rhytides are likely to become static as well. After the injection of 1 ml of Juvéderm Volbella into the vermillion, less wrinkling is observed and a younger condition is provided

The upper and lower lips are supplied respectively by the superior and inferior labial arteries within the submucosa. Both of these are branches of the facial artery.

Sensory innervation of the upper lip is provided by the infraorbital nerve. The lower lip is innervated by the mental nerve. The motor innervation of the orbicularis oris is provided by the buccal branches of the facial nerve. The muscles that act around the mouth are either innervated by the buccal or the marginal mandibular branches of the facial nerve.

6.9.3 Patient Evaluation and Selection

The best results and most natural results are found in young patients who desire lip augmentation and present with preserved lip landmarks (Fig. 6.73). Sometimes even in younger female patients, the mouth may present with perioral radial grooves and a decrease in the volume of the lips that tend to worsen with aging process (Fig. 6.74). Lip reshaping will require not only augmentation but also improvement of the radial grooves (Figs. 6.75 and 6.76). The patient's expectations should be established to avoid unrealistic results.

The physical examination is of utmost importance in lip reshaping. Both the upper and lower dental arcades promote an important role in lip augmentation. Sometimes, advancement of upper maxilla is necessary to promote balance of the perioral area (Figs. 6.77 and 6.78). If the teeth (central and lateral incisors) are inclined backward, lip projection is extremely difficult and mucosal approach should be used to compensate it (Fig. 6.79). Muscular activity in patients with very thin lips should also be evaluated. During the smile, there may be excessive inversion of the vermillion, especially in patients with gummy smile. Fillers may not produce the desired effect in this case.

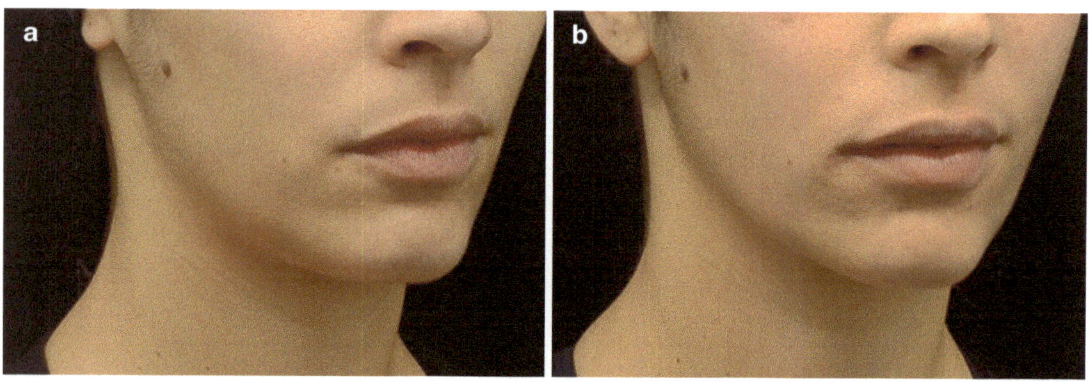

Fig. 6.73 (**a**, **b**) Analysis of the young lip before and right after treatment with 1 ml of Juvéderm Volbella injected into the upper and lower vermillion through small boluses and massages. Note the absence of edema, bruising, or unnatural appearance of the lips

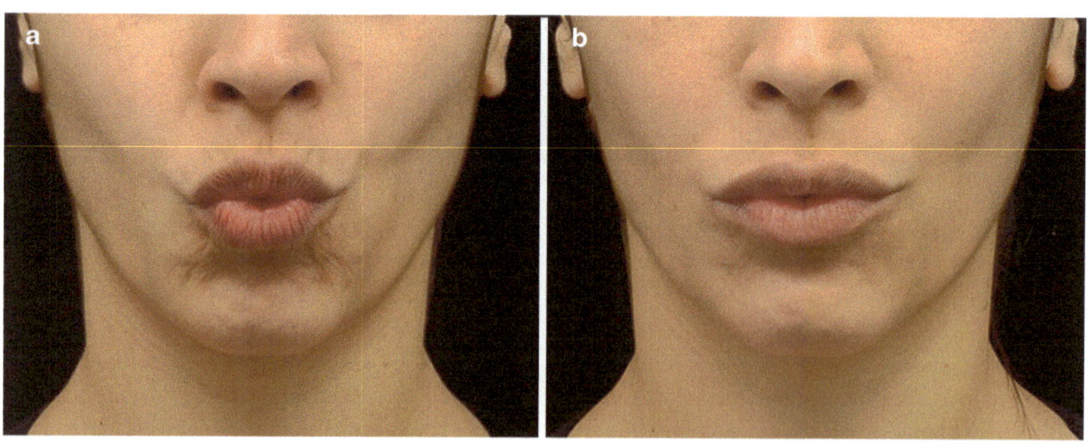

Fig. 6.74 (**a**, **b**) The same patient 20 days after treatment. Despite her young age (32 years old), she presents perioral wrinkling on animation. After the treatment of the vermillion, better structure and less wrinkling were observed. The presence of the product avoids excessive puckering of the lips

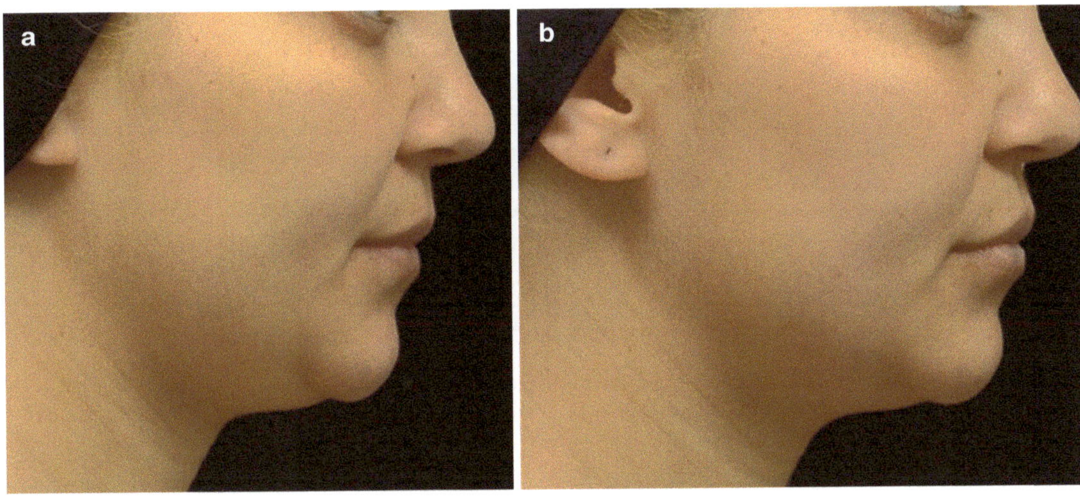

Fig. 6.75 (**a**, **b**) Profile analysis of photos before and right after the patient has been treated with 1 ml of Juvéderm Volbella injected into the upper and lower vermillion through small boluses and massage. Note the adequate and pleasant projection of both the upper and lower lips

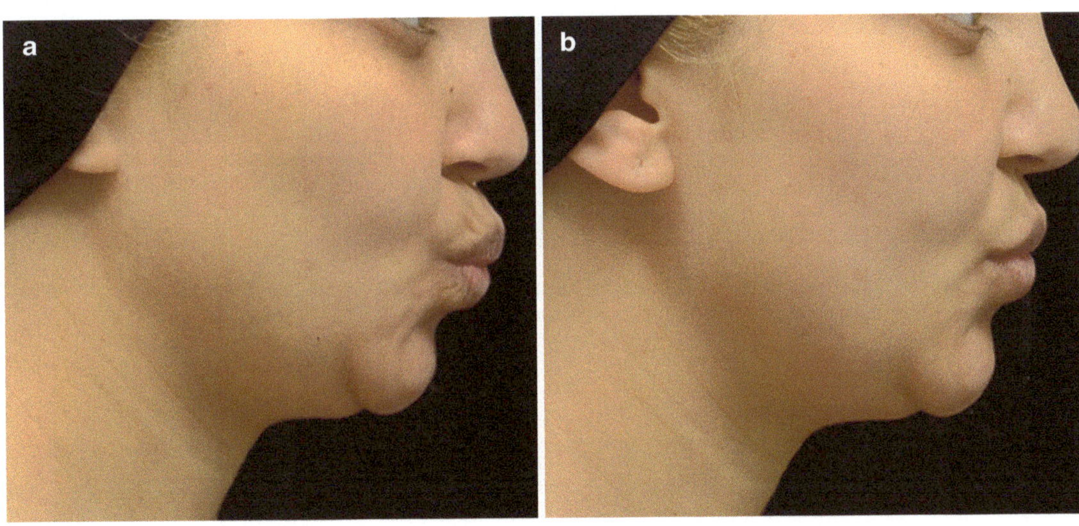

Fig. 6.76 (**a**, **b**) Profile analysis of photos before and after treatment. Note the natural aspect on animation without excessive lip projection and improvement of perioral wrinkles

Injection of BoNT-A into the levator labii superioris alaeque nasi muscle may be instead helpful in these patients. Patients must be evaluated in both static and dynamic situations. There are at least four different types of smile, and dynamic asymmetries are very common and should be demonstrated to the patient beforehand.

6.9.4 Technique

Filling the lips used to be quite painful for patients before HA products containing lidocaine came on the market. To avoid imperfect results or the necessity for frequent retouches, filling the lips should be achieved with as little pain as possible. HA products with lidocaine are

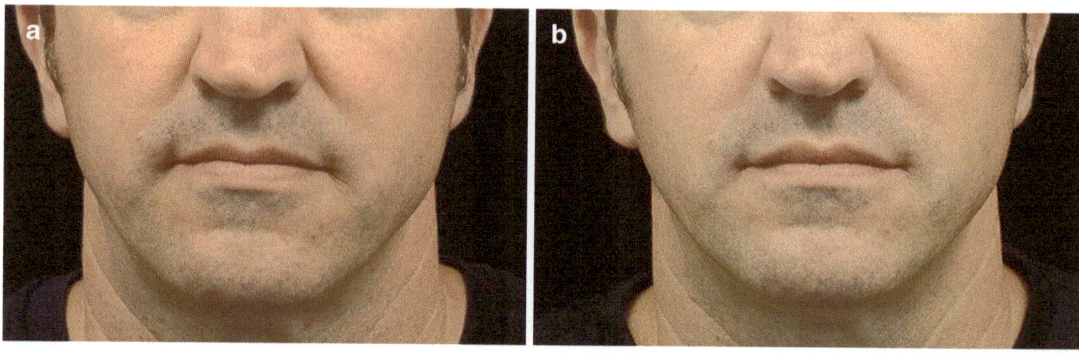

Fig. 6.77 (**a, b**) Patient with a retruded upper maxilla. Lip treatment in male patients requires a conservative approach. A total of 0.5 ml of Juvéderm Volbella has been injected into the upper lip, and 1 ml of Juvéderm Volift has been injected into the NLF per side. Note the natural result that was obtained with both procedures

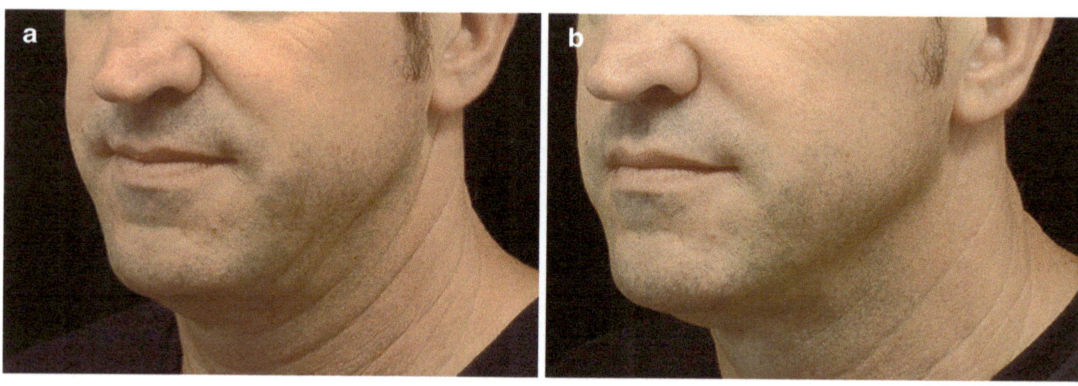

Fig. 6.78 (**a, b**) Oblique view before and after the treatment. Note the upper maxilla advancement with a slight and natural eversion of the upper lip and a more youthful appearance

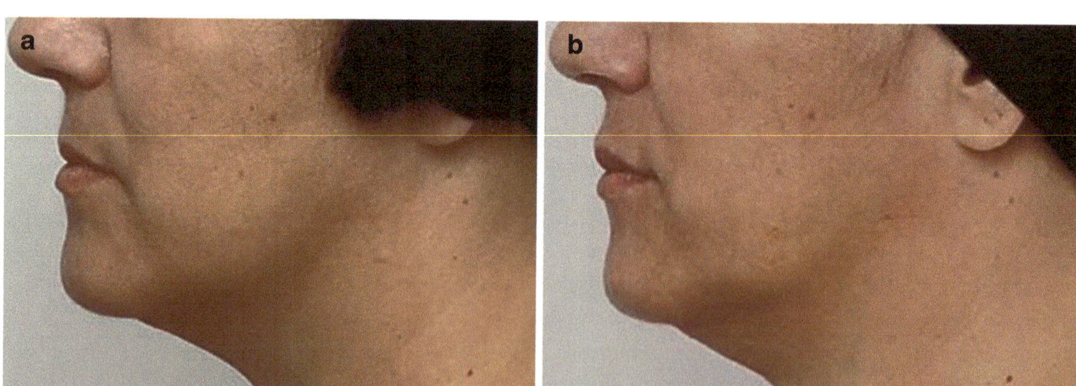

Fig. 6.79 (**a, b**) Note the retruded upper lip in comparison with the lower lip due to underbite occlusion, before treatment. Injection along the lip border and volume replacement into the medial tubercle through the mucosa lead to projection of the upper lip and more balance between the lips. Observe the nice curvature in the philtrum area. The total volume of 0.8 ml Juvéderm Ultra Plus has been injected into the upper lip and oral commissure

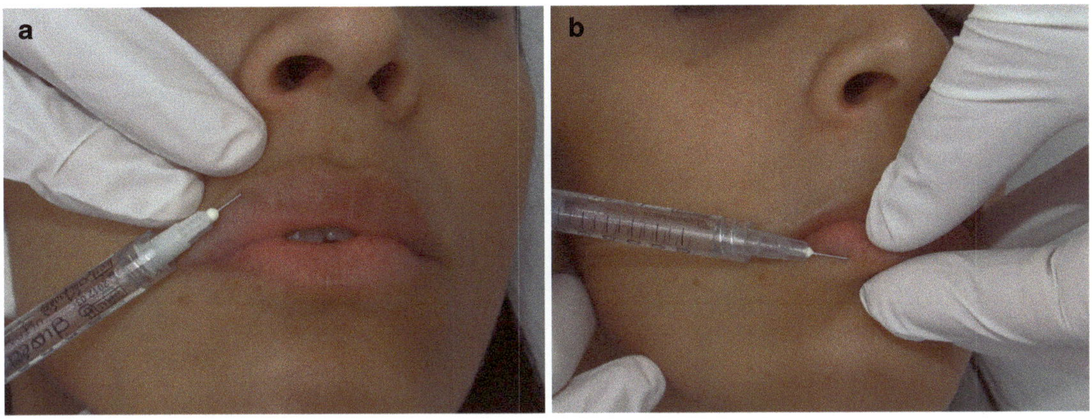

Fig. 6.80 Transition lines of both the upper (**a**) and the lower lips (**b**) are treated with an HA filler

the first choice. Prior topical anesthetics or nerve blocking might further reduce pain. For the upper lip, the infraorbital nerve may be injected followed by infiltration of lidocaine in the submucosa laterally and medially to the frenulum linguae. For the lower lip, the mentalis nerve may be blocked and infiltration into the submucosa is also beneficial. Both the intraoral and transcutaneous approach may be chosen. The intraoral approach is generally preferable as it is usually less painful (see Chap. 5). Nevertheless, in some patients topical anesthesia alone or even ice bags may be acceptable when associated with HA and lidocaine preparations.

Biodegradable products, although temporary, promote the most natural results. The lip border may be reshaped with HA to enhance lip definition (Fig. 6.80). For the vermillion, hyaluronic acid gives the volume and the mobility that only this highly hydrophilic substance may provide (Fig. 6.76). Nonbiodegradable products are less and less used for lip augmentation as the durability of HA preparations has increased.

Injections may be started from Cupid's bow or from the oral commissure. It is most important to perform it as a retrograde injection. Serial techniques increase bleeding and may lead to irregular filling. The frame of the lips (the white line) should be injected first; this will help to limit the expansion of the vermillion in both the upper and lower lips. Attention must be paid to the dental arcade at this time. If more projection is desired, the medial tubercle may be filled either from the mucosa or intraorally through the submucosa (Figs. 6.81 and 6.82). Mild perioral wrinkling may be improved only by this method. If not, direct injection into each small rhytide should be performed (Fig. 6.83). This is done best when the lip is stretched and the needle is placed directly under the rhytide.

In senile lips, a nicer look will be achieved if the entire lip structure is treated (Fig. 6.84). All perioral area should be treated in order to provide balance and natural result is mandatory (Fig. 6.85). If the lips are surrounded by elastotic skin, combinations of injectable fillers are recommended with ablative methods, such as chemical peels or laser resurfacing. The best results are obtained in those patients whose anatomic landmarks are preserved and who have soft, distensible skin.

In some cases, direct injection in the lip border may increase inversion of the lips and causing excessive protrusion if too much product is inject in trying to correct this deficiency. Preferably some senile lips and mostly young inverted lips with poor dental arcade support should be approached differently. Instead of using needles as described before, the use of a delicate cannula with submucosal injection will avoid inversion and promote lip eversion with adequate projection (Figs. 6.86 and 6.87).

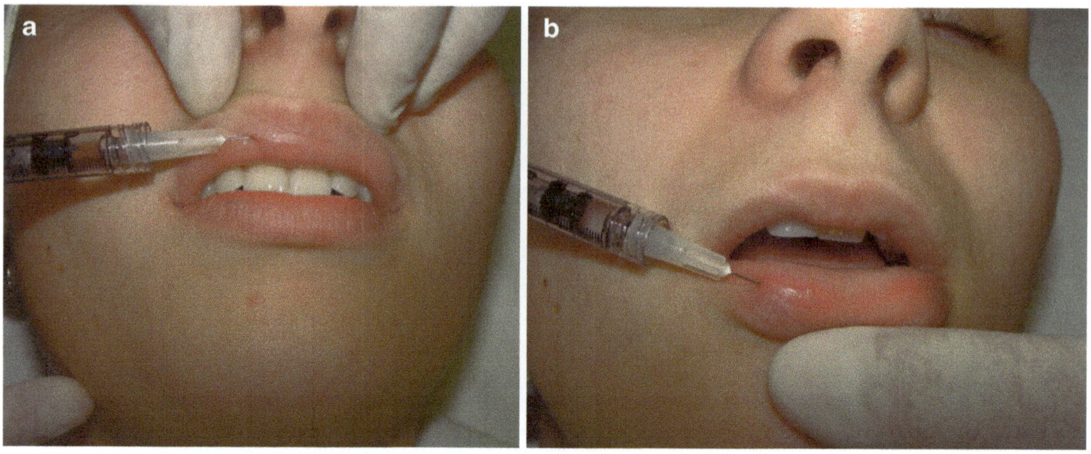

Fig. 6.81 (a, b) Augmentation of the vermillion with an HA filler

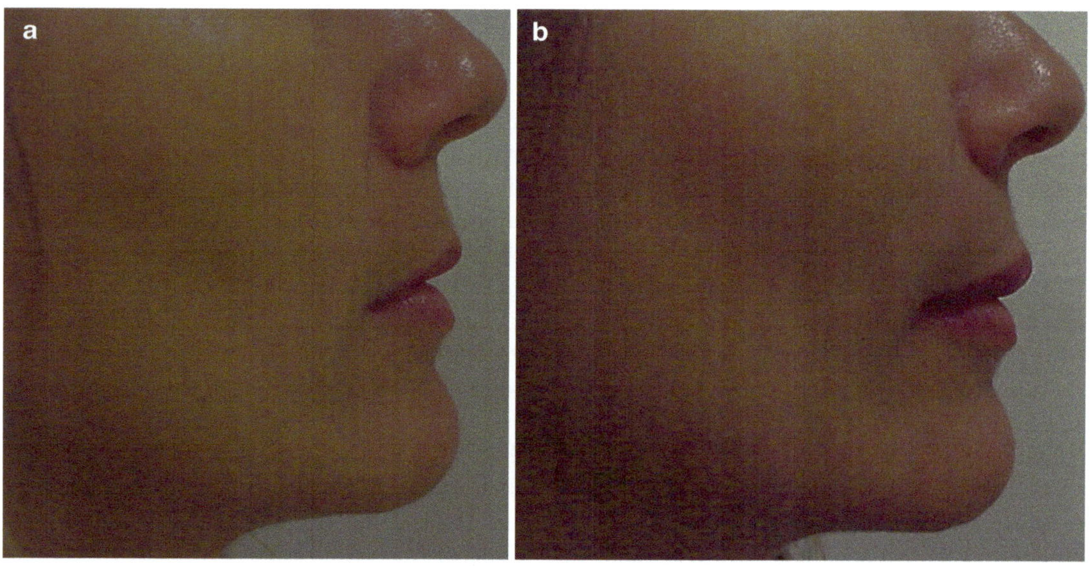

Fig. 6.82 (a, b) Filling the medial tubercle may improve the lips on profile examination

6.9.5 Complications

Lump formation and lip asymmetries are some of the complications that can result from this procedure. Swelling, ecchymosis, and redness are very common and are dependent on the type of product, quantity of material injected, and the technique used. In cases of severe swelling, a short course of oral steroids might be helpful. Nonbiodegradable products are those more often found to be associated with complications. Due to the intrinsic mobility of the lips, any capsule formation may provoke unnatural and quite obvious results.

6.9.6 Tips, Tricks and Key Points

Be careful, lips tend to look bigger when the patient is filmed or photographed. Sometimes patients ask for more material and we should show them how they would look in a photo before going any further. Avoid excessive treatment at the medial tubercle level; this may result in patients presenting a duck-like appearance in the oblique and profile analyses.

Do's
- When augmenting the lip do not only look at the patient from the front but also from both sides.
- Do educate your patient about "less is more" for lip augmentation.
- Do advice the patient that even with the newer HA products, some temporary swelling might occur.

Don'ts
- Do not forget to check the dental status of the patient. A new set of teeth or a better prosthesis might improve the lip presentation considerably.
- Do not only treat the upper lip. The lower lip needs to be in harmony with upper lip.
- Do not try to correct inverted lips with the traditional needle technique. Injecting the submucosa with cannulas might be a better option.

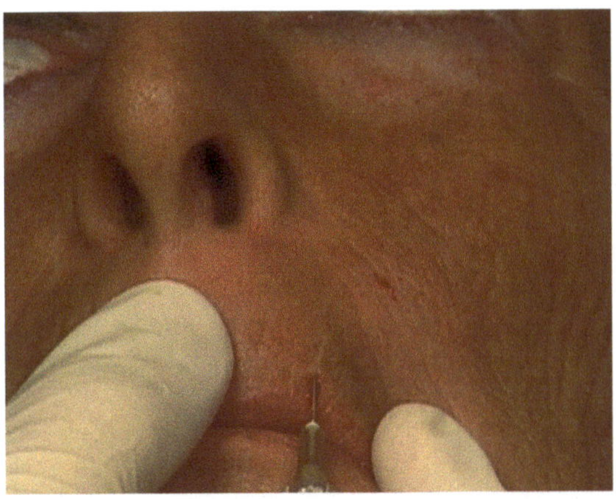

Fig. 6.83 Direct injection of a porcine collagen (Evolence Breeze) filler into the small rhytides

Key Points
- Lip reshape with HA products containing lidocaine has dramatically changed the cosmetic practice. Patient discomfort during injection was one of the main barriers for the use of injectables in the lips.
- Evaluate the lip not only statically but also during animation.
- Overtreatment should be strictly avoided.

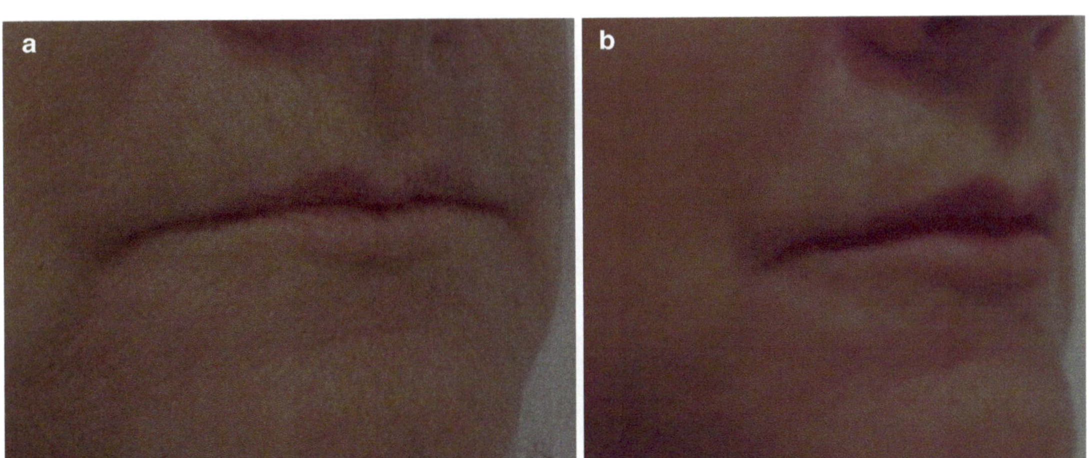

Fig. 6.84 (**a**, **b**) Filling the lips should target the restructuring of the anatomical landmarks. The philtrum has been injected as well

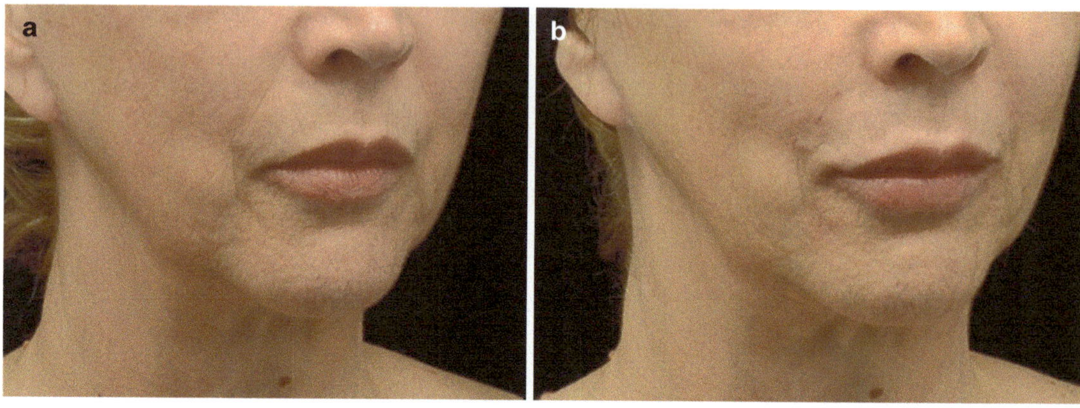

Fig. 6.85 (**a**, **b**) This 64-year-old patient presents prominent nasolabial fold (NLF) and downturn of the oral commissure with moderate degree of severity. She asked for a natural result and was in restricted budget. Result immediately after the injection of 0.4 ml of Juvéderm Volift into the NLF and 0.1 ml into the marionette lines per side. She was also submitted to lip contour with 1 ml of Juvéderm Volbella. She was very pleased with the natural result that enabled her to return to her social activities soon after treatment

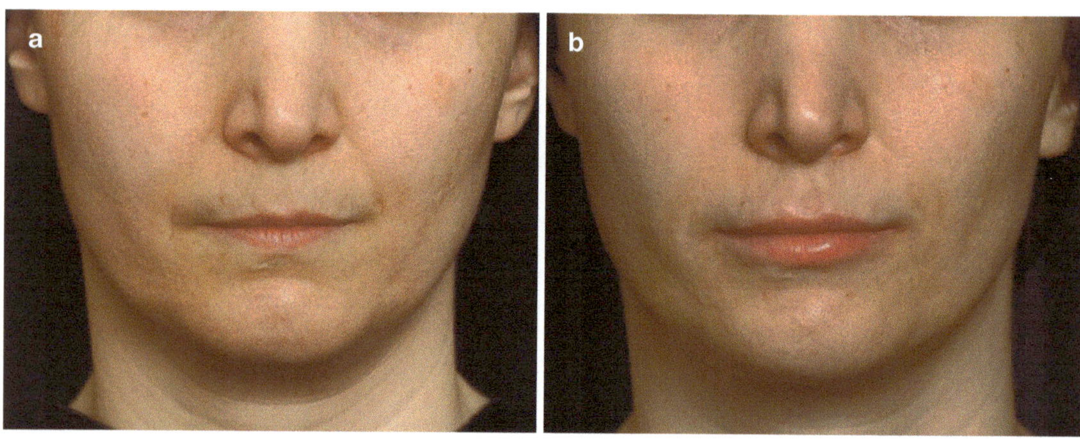

Fig. 6.86 (**a**, **b**) Inverted thin lips with flat philtrum and immediate result after the injection of both the upper and lower lips with 1.0 ml of Juvéderm Ultra Smile by a 25G blunt microcannula. After promoting deep support and eversion of the lips, lip contour and philtrum reshape were undertaken with 0.55 ml of Juvéderm Ultra Smile using a 30G needle

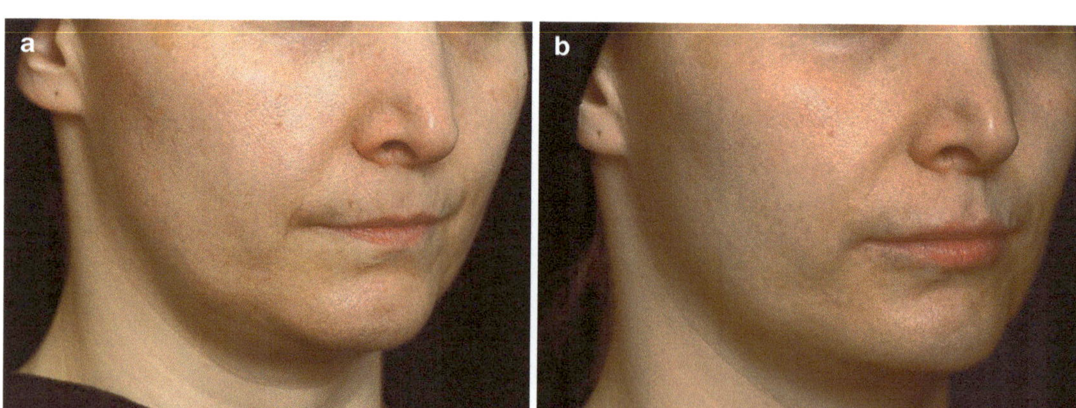

Fig. 6.87 (**a**, **b**) Oblique view: inverted thin lips with a flat philtrum before and after treatment

6.10 Marionette Lines

6.10.1 Introduction

Marionette lines are no friendly lines. They make the face appear to be sad or harder. Usually they are associated with deep nasolabial folds. In cases when just the nasolabial fold is corrected and the marionette lines disregarded (like in clinical trials on nasolabial folds), the overall picture of the treated patient might look weird.

6.10.2 Anatomy

Marionette lines might become pronounced due to muscular hyperactivity and/or elastosis. On the muscle base a hyperactivity of the depressor anguli oris and the platysma muscles might not only pull the corners of the mouth down but also contribute to these lines. However, in most of the cases, it is the increased laxity of the SMAS and the overlying elastotic skin that will provoke these lines.

6.10.3 Patient Evaluation and Selection

Patients with shallow or very deep lines are suitable for treatment (Carruthers et al. 2008, Figs. 6.88 and 6.89).

6.10.4 Technique

Pretreatment of the depressor anguli oris and the platysma muscles with BoNT-A is encouraged as it decreases the downward movements of the corner of the mouth (Fig. 6.90). Topical anesthesia is recommended. Biodegradable fillers usually give the most natural expression. The most appropriate filler must be chosen according to the depth of the lines, wrinkles, or folds. The caudal triangle at the corners of the mouth, which is formed by the margin of the lower lip and the marionette line and continues to the nasolabial fold, is injected first. Here, a triangular feathering might elevate the whole area. For deep and medium-sized lines, the retrograde tunnel technique (i.e., the filler is injected while withdrawing the needle) or the multiple injection site technique can be used. These techniques will help to blend the filler better in the surrounding area and avoid the appearance of an unnatural elevation at the area of the former fold. Deep folds usually require multilevel injections (Fig. 6.91). As for nasolabial folds, it is advisable to inject the filler medial to the fold; a more lateral injection technique would increase the visibility of the fold in patients with increased laxity of the SMAS.

6.10.5 Complications

A lateral injection will increase the visibility of the fold. In older patients with increased elastosis,

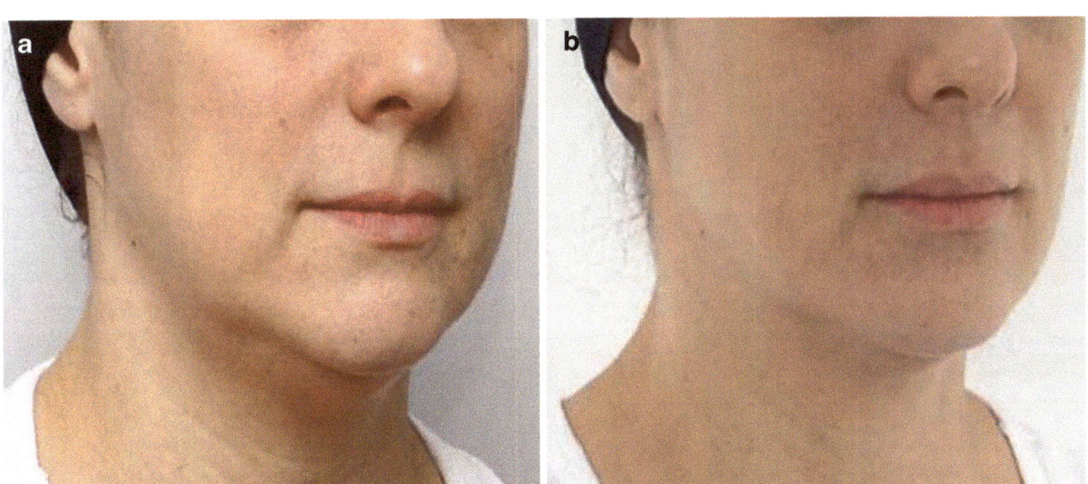

Fig. 6.88 (**a, b**) Before treatment, presence of prominent nasolabial fold, marionette lines, and prejowl sulcus. After injection of 1 ml of Juvéderm Voluma and 0.8 ml Juvéderm Ultra (Plus), all the units of the perioral area were improved. Note the improvement in the jawline as well

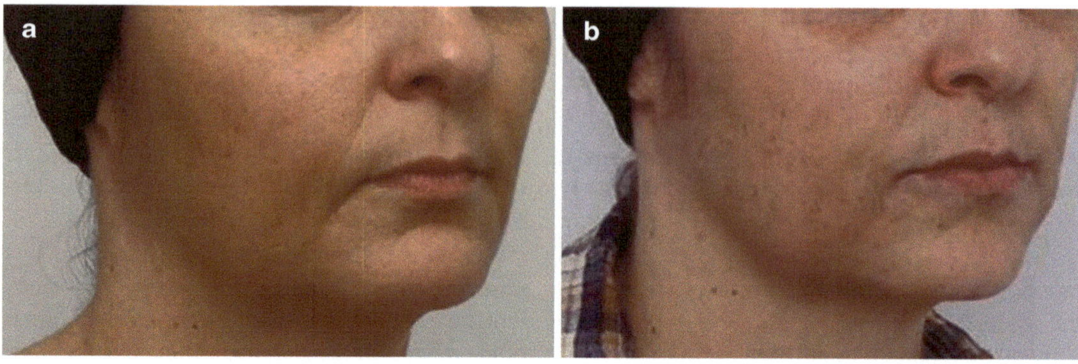

Fig. 6.89 (**a**, **b**) A difficult marionette line to treat due to the inversion of the lateral aspect of the vermillion and oral commissure. After injection of 1 ml of Juvéderm Voluma into the nasolabial fold and chin and 0.8 ml of Juvéderm Ultra Plus, eversion of the oral commissure and correction of the marionette lines were obtained

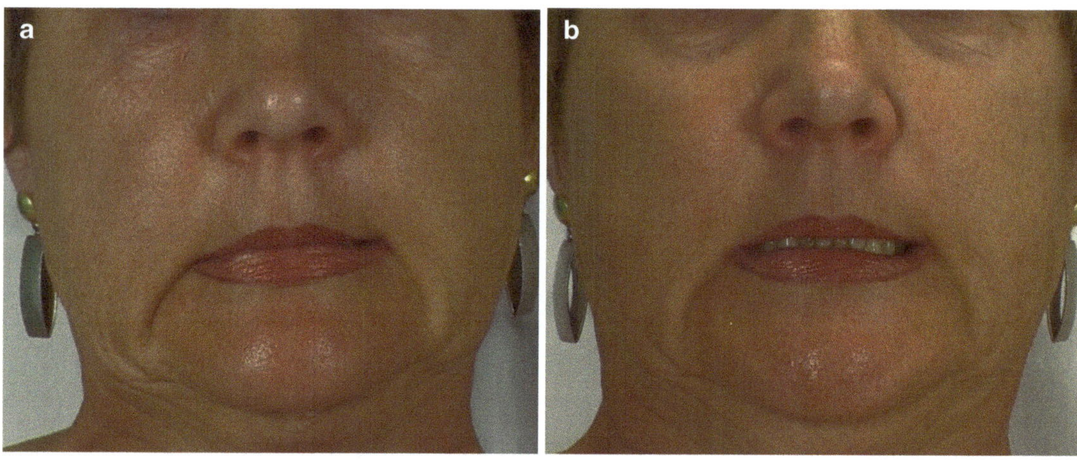

Fig. 6.90 (**a**, **b**) Marionette lines before and 1 week after treatment with BoNT-A while the patient is grimacing

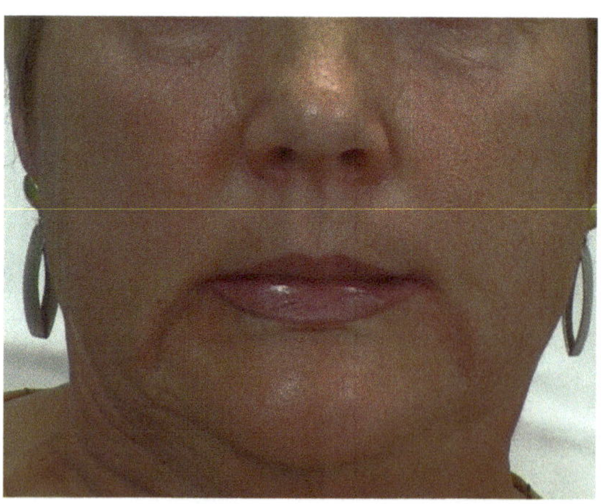

Fig. 6.91 With BoNT-A pretreated marionette lines immediately after the injection of an HA filler while the patient is grimacing

a very deep injection may have little effect other than creating an unpleasant deep lump of filler.

6.10.6 Tips, Tricks and Key Points

Do's

- Do not forget to check the dental status of the patient. With no teeth laterally or an otherwise insufficient dental correction, a treatment with an injectable filler will not be enough.
- As for nasolabial folds have the patient comfortably sit up either during the

whole procedure or at the end to make sure that you evaluate the marionette lines at maximum gravity.

- In patients with deep folds due to increased elastosis, the multilayer technique is recommended (i.e., after injecting these patients carefully with a deep filler, a filler comprising medium-sized particles should be injected more superficially to extend the dermis and thus decrease the depth of wrinkles).

Don'ts

- Do not inject too laterally in patients with saggy skin. If you inject too laterally, the fold might become more visible.
- Do not inject too much too deep. You might end up with a big lump that will stay for a long time and will remind the patient of your injection.

Key Points

- The marionette lines are an important and frequently treated indication. Overcorrection should be avoided. Repeated injections over a couple of months might yield better results.
- As for the nasolabial folds, do not undertreat this indication. Severe marionette lines might require 1 ml of a filler per side.

6.11 Jawline and Chin Reshaping

6.11.1 Introduction

The chin is a symbol of masculinity for men and sensuality for women. Any negative marks such as wrinkles, folds, or a deep oral commissure may impair the sense of beauty. Women must have a more delicate chin, with less fullness concentrated at the central part. Men, on the other hand, may have heavier features and should have a stronger chin. In all cases, a youthful and clean jawline is desired. Reshaping the mandible area promotes chin and jawline contours.

Despite the scientific studies concerning the safety of the use of silicone prostheses for chin augmentation, some patients simply refuse to be submitted to it. The use of fillers may be helpful in such cases. Patients prefer minor and minimally invasive procedures, although some doctors would indicate more complex procedures such as chin advancement. However, most patients may accept time limited results with fillers more rather than submitting to cranial surgery. The introduction of HA volumizer in the market has changed the treatment of chin and jawline reshape. High-performance, longer-lasting, and natural results are expected now.

6.11.2 Anatomy

The chin may be defined as the area between the mental foramina and the central part of the mandible. The midlateral zone can be defined as the region extending from the mental foramen posteriorly to the oblique line of the horizontal body of the mandible. The posterior lateral zone is defined as the posterior half of the horizontal body including the angle of the mandible and the first 2–4 cm of the ascending ramus. The submental area is located under the chin between the platysmal band and above the cervicomental angle.

The most suitable skin for chin and mandible reshaping is that which is soft and has mild atrophy. The fat tissue superficial to the SMAS in the mental area is densely attached to the dermis by strong fibrous septa. It makes the deep soft tissues very adherent to the skin at this level. It becomes progressively looser and more mobile lateral to the cheek and caudal to the neck.

The contraction of the mentalis muscle produces protrusion of the lower lip. This muscle arises from the mandible below the central and lateral incisors and inserts into the skin of the chin. Wrinkles can form in a cobblestone pattern where it inserts into the skin in some patients.

The chin is supplied by the mental and submental arteries: the former a branch of the inferior alveolar artery and the latter a branch of the facial artery. The venous drainage corresponds to the arterial supply. The mandible is supplied by the facial and inferior alveolar artery. The mandibular branch of the facial nerve passes just anterior to the middle portion of the mandible into the midlateral zone. The marginal branch of the facial nerve has a variable course, but its location is normally at the angle of the mandible. The greater auricular nerve is in the cervical fascia, posterior to the angle of the mandible. The mental nerve exits from the mental foramen, below the second mandibular premolar.

The aging process may be accompanied by a reduction in the size of the mandible with absorption of the alveolar processes. In older patients, there may also be soft-tissue atrophy lateral to the anterior chin, producing a deep triangle almost directly underneath the oral commissure. It is known as prejowl sulcus. With the increase of the jowl pad and soft-tissue atrophy, marionette lines and a sad mouth develop. The migration of fat down to the mandible creates the jowls that may extend below the lower mandible border. The superficial subcutaneous tissues tend to sag more than the deeper subcutaneous tissues.

6.11.3 Patient Evaluation and Selection

The ideal relationship in a patient's face is one-third upper lip and two-thirds lower lip and chin. Patients with mandibular hypoplasia appear to have a round face due to a short lower facial height. The ratio between the upper lip and lower lip and chin becomes 1:1. On the profile examination, the face presents a convex appearance, jowls, and obtuse mentocervical angle with redundant skin (Fig. 6.92).

When considering a patient for chin augmentation with fillers, evaluations of the occlusion, skeletal, and dental relationships must be performed. Patients with a normal occlusion are the best candidates for fillers. Patients with class II or III

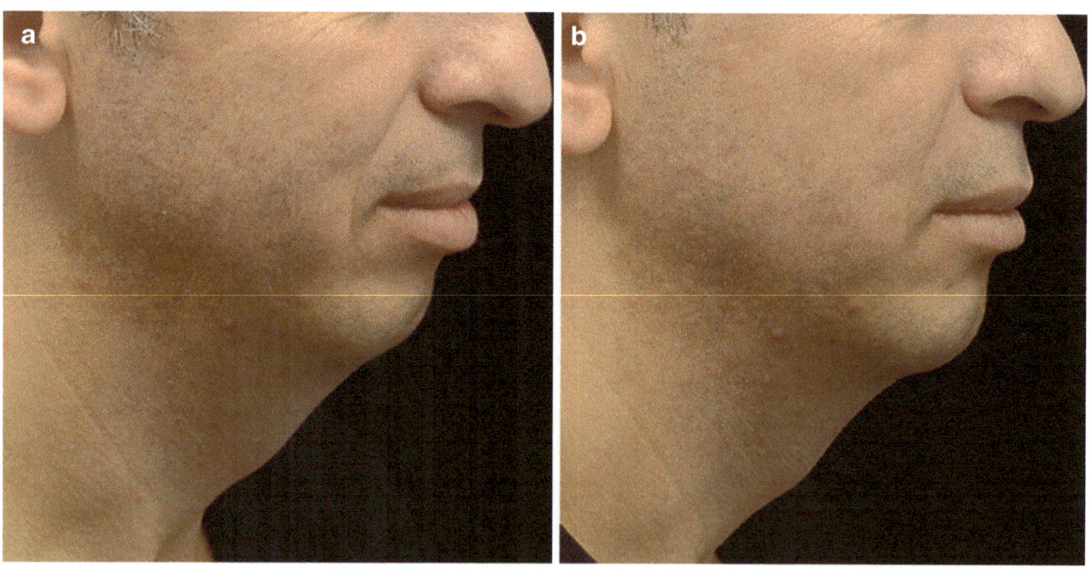

Fig. 6.92 (**a**, **b**) A male patient presenting retrusion of the upper maxilla, protrusion of the lower lip, and retruded chin. The patient was submitted to structural correction with 4 ml of Juvéderm Voluma for the chin, 1 ml of Juvéderm Volift for NLF, and 1 ml of Juvéderm Volbella for the upper lip. Note the improvement of the neck contour and the balance between the upper and the lower lip

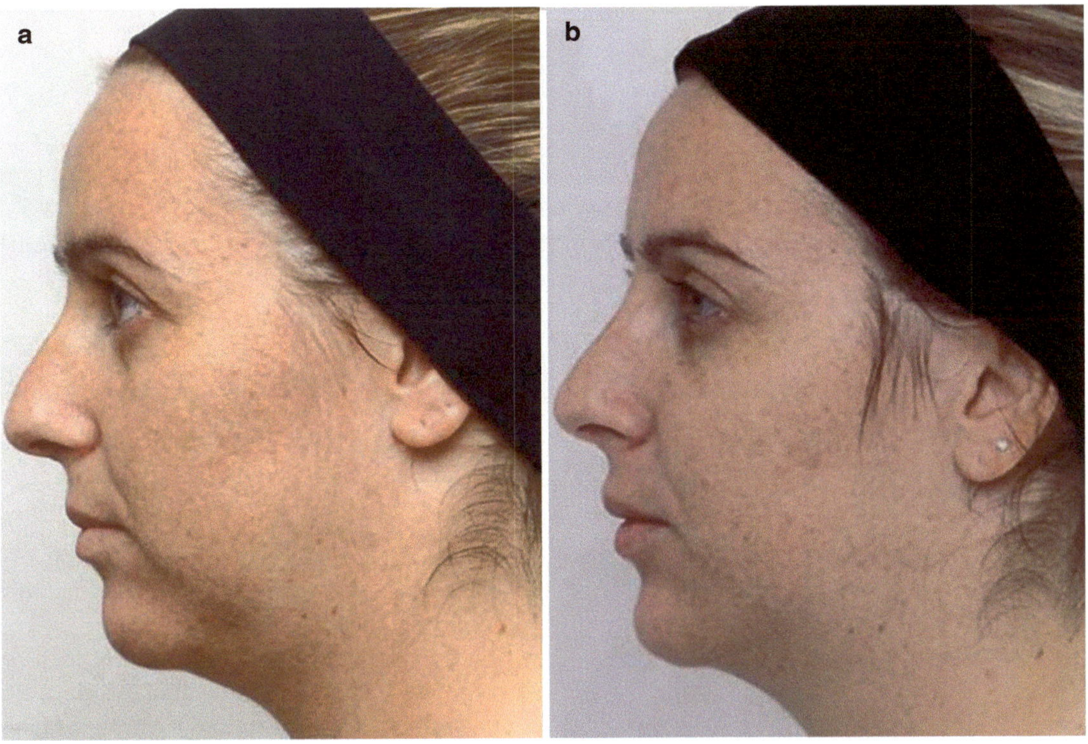

Fig. 6.93 (**a**, **b**) A female patient presenting volume loss in the mid-cheek and consequently elongated lid-cheek junction. The tip of the nose rotates downward, and an unbalance between the upper and the lower lip and the chin is seen. Volume replacement in the mid-cheek and the chin with 2 ml of Juvéderm Voluma has improved the convexity appearance of the face. Nose and lip reshape with 0.8 ml of Juvéderm Ultra Plus has also helped to improve the balance of the patient's profile

malocclusion were considered surgical candidates in the past. In some cases, avoiding extensive orthognathic surgery means giving fillers a try, while understanding their limitations and the number of sessions involved to obtain a nice result.

The classic mandibular retrognathia patient presents with a retruded mandible and convex soft-tissue profiles. Treatment involves orthodontic correction: surgical mandible advancement with osteotomy with rigid fixation.

Patients may present good chin projection and no lateral fullness. These patients are ideal candidates for fillers in these areas (Fig. 6.93). Fillers will improve chin projection and promote a jawline reshape and also improve the aspect of submental fat deposit (Fig. 6.94). Some patients may need forward and downward projection; filling into the upper and lower part of the menton may increase the distance between the mandible tip and the lip, thus balancing the face. Fillers are also suitable as a pretreatment before surgery to give an idea of the amount of projection either required or desired by the patient.

6.11.4 Technique

Fillers may be placed in the central segment alone, between the mental foramina and along the mandible body. When the central mentum and the midlateral zone are augmented, there is a resulting widening of the anterior jawline contour. Fillers in the mandibular angle will either widen or elongate the posterior mandibular angle, promoting a strong posterior jawline contour.

Before starting the injection, topical anesthesia is applied and drawings are performed to limit the area to be treated (Fig. 6.95). The filling of the mandible area associated with the nasolabial fold may promote an interesting result, especially

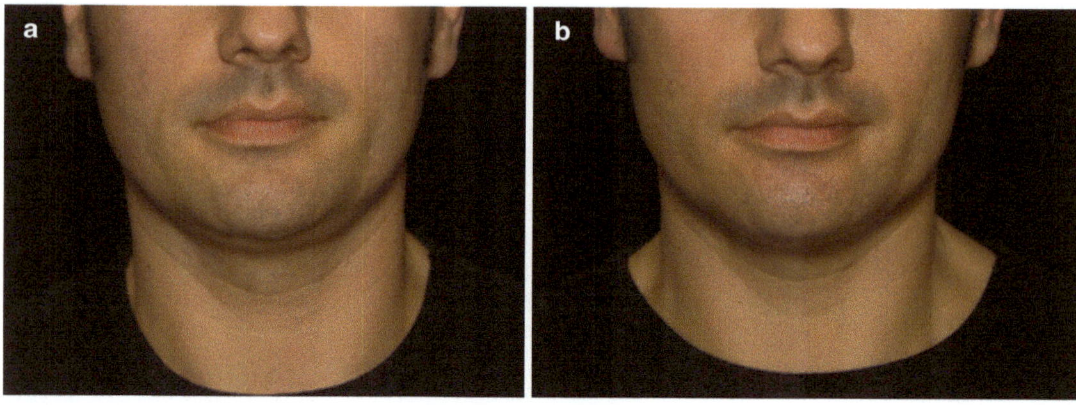

Fig. 6.94 (**a**, **b**) Due to the small size of the chin and its upward rotation, the submental fat deposit is evident. After the injection of 2 ml of Juvéderm Voluma, note the elongation of the chin and the hidden underchin fat in frontal view

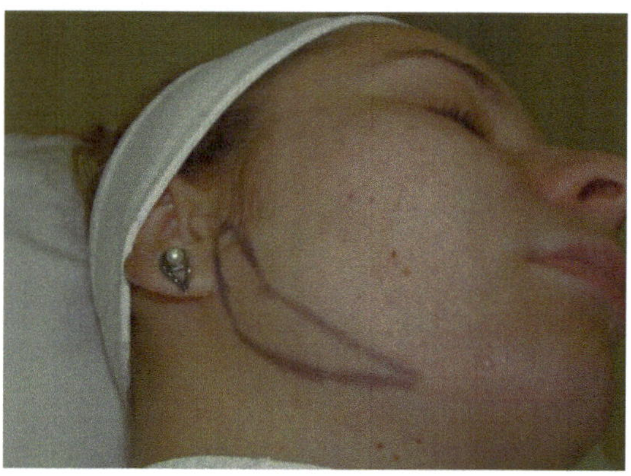

Fig. 6.95 The purpose of filling the mandibular angle is to enhance the definition of the mandibular angle. Marking the area with an eyeliner enables the physician to limit the area to be injected. The masseter and the posterior bony border of the ascending ramus are important hallmarks for mandibular angle reshaping

among patients who do not desire a surgical procedure or do not have enough time to be submitted to it (Figs. 6.96 and 6.97). A face-lift effect may be obtained (Fig. 6.98).

Depending on the physical examination, patients are only treated in the chin area for minor chin advancement and balance (Fig. 6.99). If the patient is older, the presence of jowls of mild degree can be improved with the injection of the triangle reaching from the mental foramen to the midlateral zone of the mandible. This area may not be easily expanded, and the mobility of the skin at this site must be evaluated prior to starting corrective procedures. In older patients, this triangle of soft tissue is generally atrophic, and this area may be filled because of its mobility.

Injection at the chin or jawline level may be carried out with needles or cannulas. If needles are to be used especially along the jawline, pinching the skin and keeping the needle between the fingers will protect the patient of adverse events. The facial artery is found anteriorly to the anterior margin of the masseter muscle and is deeply located. The marginal mandibular nerve is more superficial and is located at the subcutaneous level.

Retrograde injection is started by filling along the frame, followed by a soft massage to smooth the surface. Placement of the filler should be in all layers from the deep reticular dermis next to the periosteum. The multilayer technique promotes augmentation of all soft tissues within the delineated area. The use of cannula is appropriate if enhancement of vertical dimension is required. Less bruising is expected.

One of the greatest advantages of fillers is the possibility of using complementary volumes if needed. Although edema usually appears during the injection, a predictable view of the augmentation can be foreseen (Fig. 6.100).

6.11.5 Complications

In contrast to surgical procedures with implants, there is no bone resorption, no fistula, no nerve

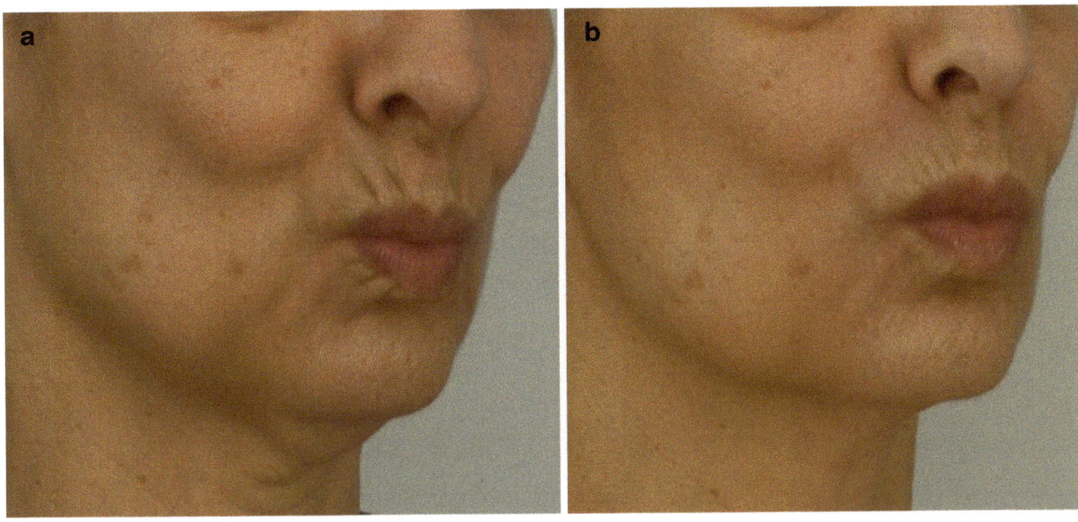

Fig. 6.96 (**a**, **b**) A female patient presenting perioral wrinkling and skin excess in the neck. This patient was submitted to lip treatment, prejowl sulcus and mandible reshape, and chin advancement with HA-based fillers. Note the improvement of the skin laxity under the chin

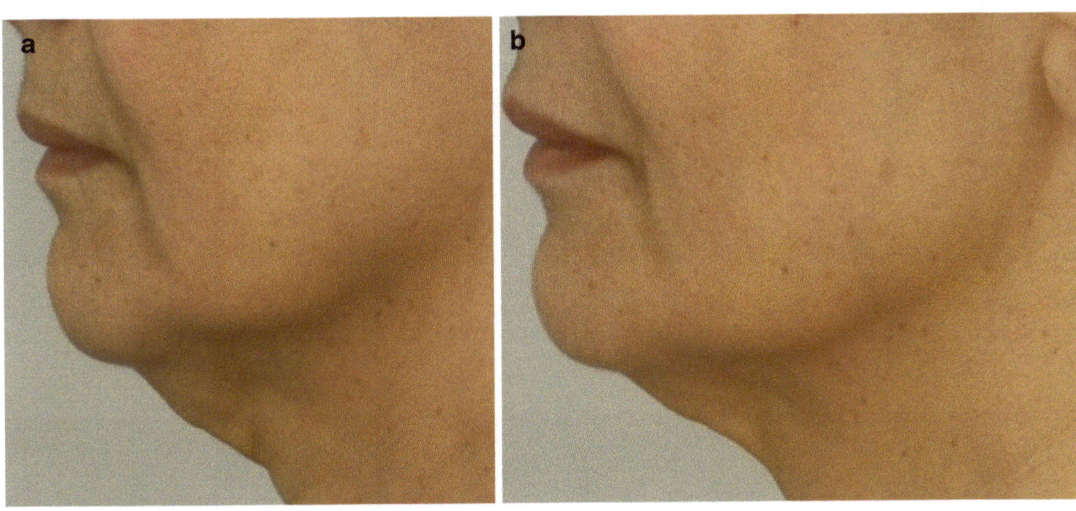

Fig. 6.97 (**a**, **b**) Profile view: before and after treatment of the lip, prejowl sulcus, and chin advancement with HA. Note that by expanding the skin with volumizers in the prejowl area and along the jawline and chin, reduction of the skin in the neck area can be obtained

damage, and rarely any extrusion or nodule formation. Chin prostheses may cause an abnormal projection, even in patients with adequate soft tissue. Mandibular and chin reshaping with fillers may only produce mild ecchymosis and edema and entails a quick recovery. Proper technique and a good choice of products may decrease these adverse events.

6.11.6 Tips, Tricks and Key Points

Do's

- Do encourage chin and jawline reshape in female patients. The loss of jawline contour leads to an older appearance.

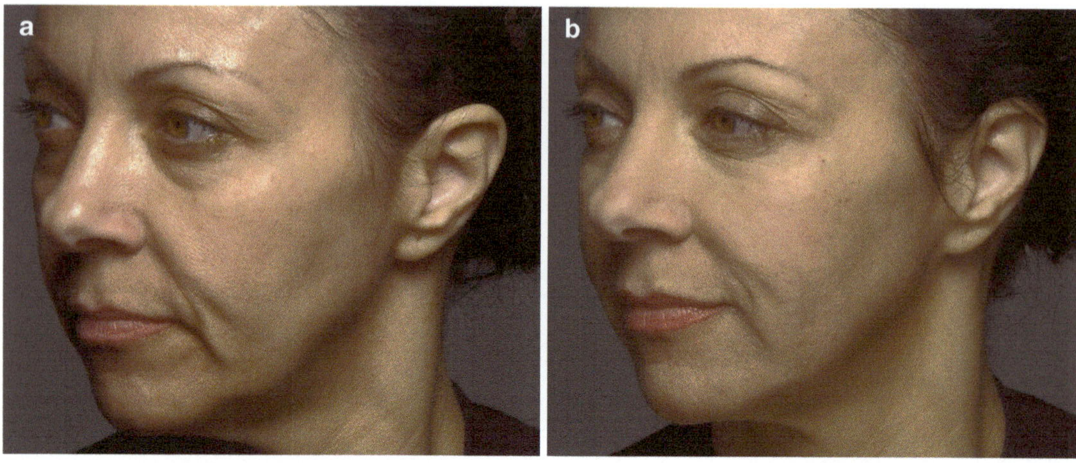

Fig. 6.98 (**a**, **b**) Mandible filling may improve the definition of the mandible and even treat mild saggy skin

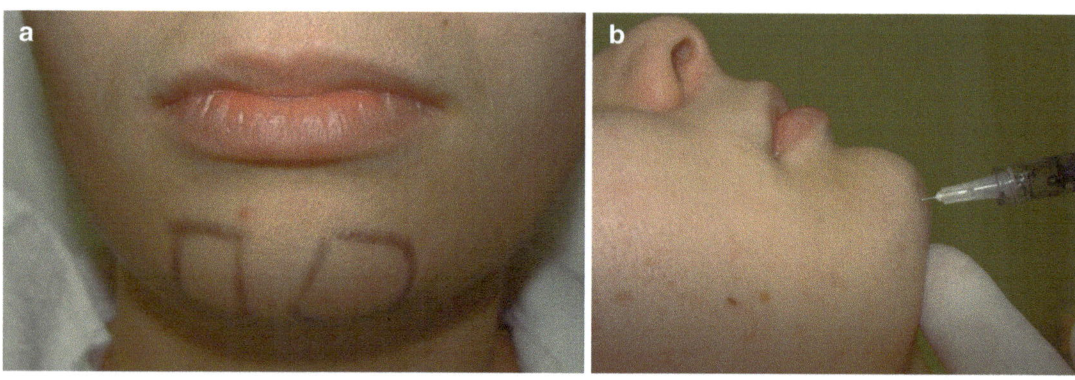

Fig. 6.99 (**a**, **b**) Either one or the other demarcation may be chosen depending on the projection desired. The *right-hand side* demarcation is for mild projection and the *left-hand side* is suitable when both mid and lateral augmentations are needed. After proper demarcation, the injection technique is started

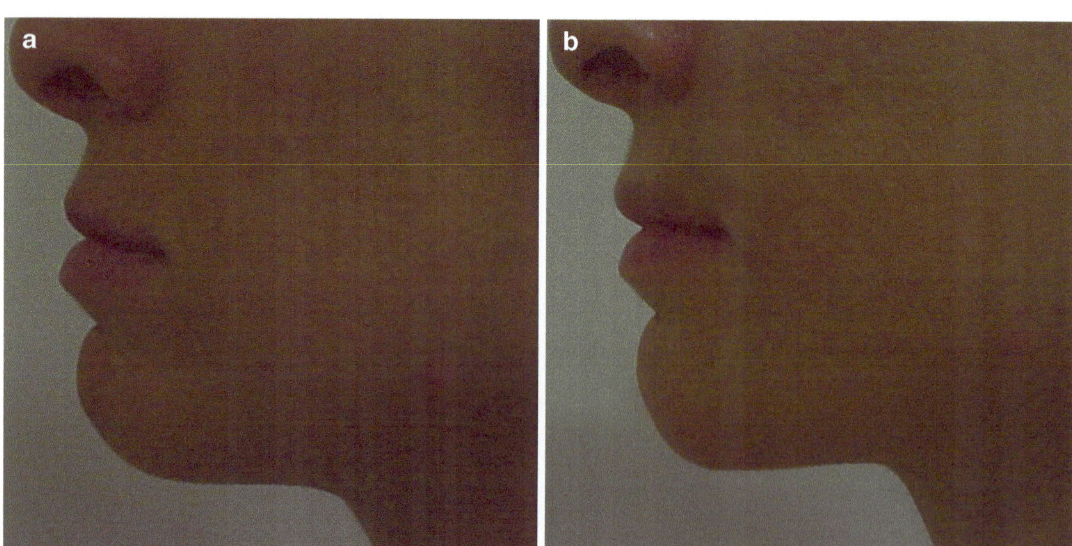

Fig. 6.100 (**a**, **b**) Chin advancement may be obtained with fillers. It is useful both as a single treatment and for surgical planning

Don'ts

- Encourage the patient to have the mentalis muscle blocked with BoNT-A before chin augmentation with volumizers. Better projection and longer-lasting results are expected.

FAQs

- Should cannulas or needles be preferred for chin and jawline injections?

  Both may be used although needles are easier to handle at these levels as long as anatomical structures are respected. Cannulas are preferable for severe cases.

6.12 Other Facial Indications for Volumizers

6.12.1 Introduction

Some patients may present with osseous malformations that usually would require surgery. Here volumizers might be an alternative.

6.12.2 Facial Advancement

Some patients may present a concave face with, e.g., class III occlusion where the LeFort I surgery would be the formal indication. Here the injection of volumizers will open new possibilities to patients reluctant to surgery (Figs. 6.101 and 6.102).

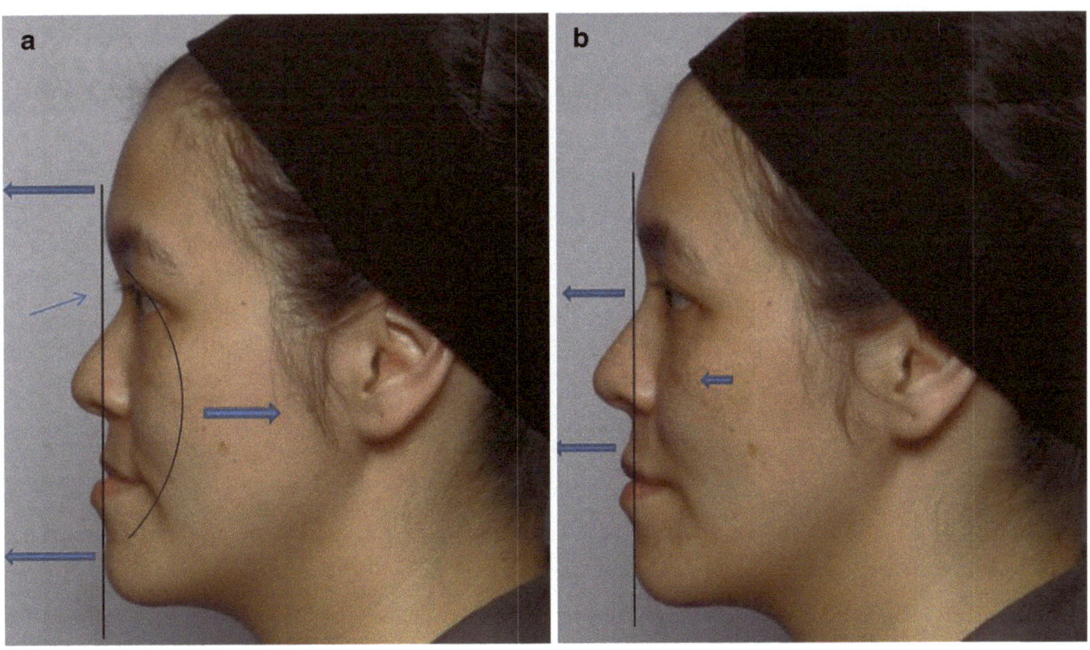

Fig. 6.101 (**a**) Patient with class III occlusion, underbite, and retruded upper maxilla. The traditional surgical indication would be LeFort I. (**b**) After midface treatment with 4 ml of Juvéderm Voluma injected into cheekbone, canine fossa, and nose and 1.2 ml of Juvéderm Ultra Plus into the lips, nonsurgical facial advancement was obtained

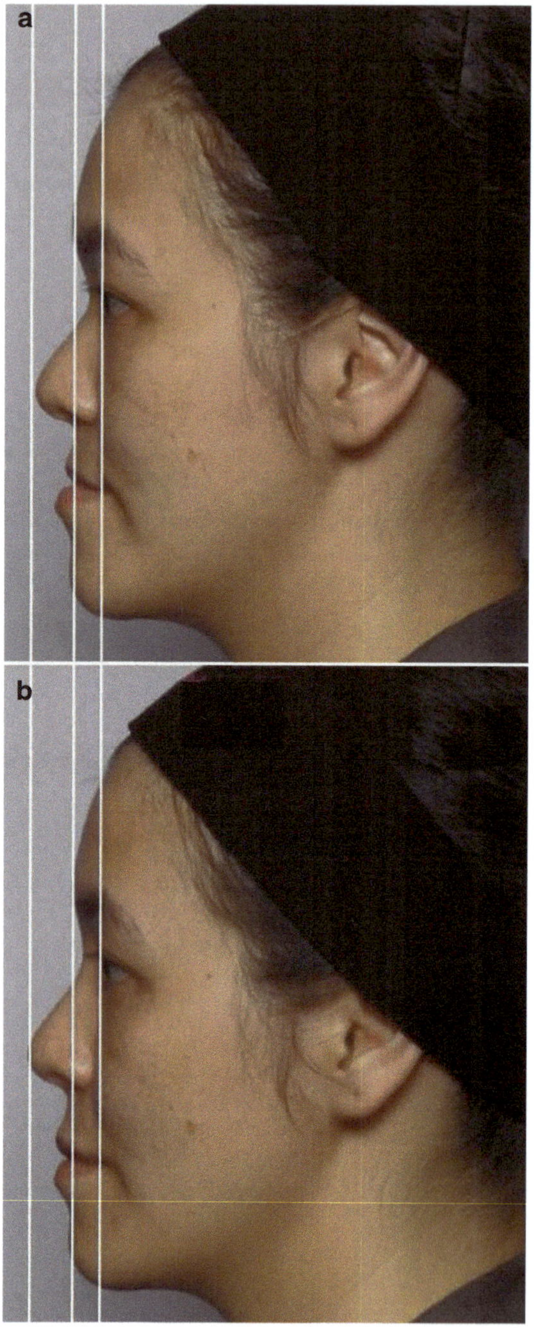

Fig. 6.102 (**a**) Concave profile before treatment. Observe the position of the nose and the upper lip. (**b**) After non-surgical advancement, a straight profile was obtained

6.12.3 Tips, Tricks and Key Points

Key Points

- Volumizers might be an alternative in patients reluctant toward surgery.

References

Bachmann F, Erdmann R, Hartmann V et al (2009) The spectrum of adverse reactions after treatment with injectable fillers in the glabellar region: results from the Injectable Filler Safety Study. Dermatol Surg 35(2):1629–1634

Carruthers A, Carruthers J, Hardas B et al (2008) A validated grading scale for marionette lines. Dermatol Surg 34(2):S167–S172

Farkas LG, Kolar JC, Munro IR (1986) Geography of the nose: a morphometric study. Aesthetic Plast Surg 10(4):191–223

Flowers RF (1993) Tear trough implants for correction of tear trough deformity. Clin Plast Surg 20:403–415

Hamra ST (1992) Composite rhytidectomy. Plast Reconstr Surg 90(1):1–13

Lambros VS (2002) The dynamics of facial aging. Paper presented at the 35th annual meeting of the American Society for Aesthetic Plastic Surgery, Las Vegas

Loeb R (1993) Naso-jugal groove leveling with fat tissue. Clin Plast Surg 20:393–401

Muzaffar AR, Mendelson BC, Adams WP Jr (2002) Surgical anatomy of the ligamentous attachments of the lower lid and lateral canthus. Plast Reconstr Surg 110(873–884):897–911

Narins RS, Dayan SH, Brandt FS et al (2008) Persistence and improvement of nasolabial fold correction with nonanimal-stabilized hyaluronic acid 100,000 gel particles/mL filler on two retreatment schedules: results up to 18 months on two retreatment schedules. Dermatol Surg 34(1):S2–S8

Pessa JE (2000) An algorithm of facial aging: verification of Lambros's theory by three-dimensional stereolithography, with reference to the pathogenesis of midfacial aging, scleral show, and the lateral suborbital trough deformity. Plast Reconstr Surg 106:479–490

Pitanguy I, Ramos AS (1966) The frontal branch of the facial nerve: the importance of its variations in face lifting. Plast Reconstr Surg 38(4):352–356

Rohrich RJ, Gunter JP, Friedman RM (1995) Nasal tip blood supply: an anatomic study validating the safety of the transcolumellar incision in rhinoplasty. Plast Reconstr Surg 95(5):795–801

Tobias GW, Binder WJ (1994) The submalar triangle: its anatomy and clinical significance. Facial Plast Surg Clin North Am 2:255

Nonfacial Indications

7

Mauricio de Maio and Berthold Rzany

Contents

7.1 **Inverted Nipple** 135
7.1.1 Introduction 135
7.1.2 Anatomy 135
7.1.3 Patient Evaluation and Selection 135
7.1.4 Techniques 136
7.1.5 Tips, Tricks and Key Points 136

7.2 **Hand Volume Replacement** 137
7.2.1 Introduction 137
7.2.2 Anatomy 138
7.2.3 Patient Evaluation and Selection 139
7.2.4 Material to Be Used 139
7.2.5 Anesthesia 139
7.2.6 Techniques 139
7.2.7 Potential Specific Adverse Events 141
7.2.8 Tips, Tricks and Key Points 142

7.3 **Penile Augmentation** 143
7.3.1 Introduction 143
7.3.2 Anatomy 143
7.3.3 Patient Evaluation and Selection 143
7.3.4 Material to Be Used 143
7.3.5 Procedure Prior to Injection 145
7.3.6 Techniques 145
7.3.7 Tips, Tricks and Key Points 147

References 147

7.1 Inverted Nipple

7.1.1 Introduction

Patients with inverted nipples are usually ashamed of their condition and may seek surgical correction, often with variable final results. Patients weary of a surgical approach might benefit from filler injections as described in this chapter.

7.1.2 Anatomy

The nipple area complex consists mostly of connective tissue and glands. Specifically, the Montgomery glands: large intermediate-stage sebaceous glands which are embryologically transitional between sweat glands and mammary glands. The Montgomery glands lead to the Morgagni tubercles, which are small (1–2-mm-diameter) raised papules on the areola. The nipple-areolar complex also contains many sensory nerve endings, smooth muscle, and an abundant lymphatic system called the subareolar or Sappey plexus (Nicholson et al. 2009).

7.1.3 Patient Evaluation and Selection

Patients that may benefit from the use of injectable fillers in the nipple area include those whose nipples are easily protruded by cold or local

M. de Maio, B. Rzany, *Injectable Fillers in Aesthetic Medicine*,
DOI 10.1007/978-3-642-45125-6_7,

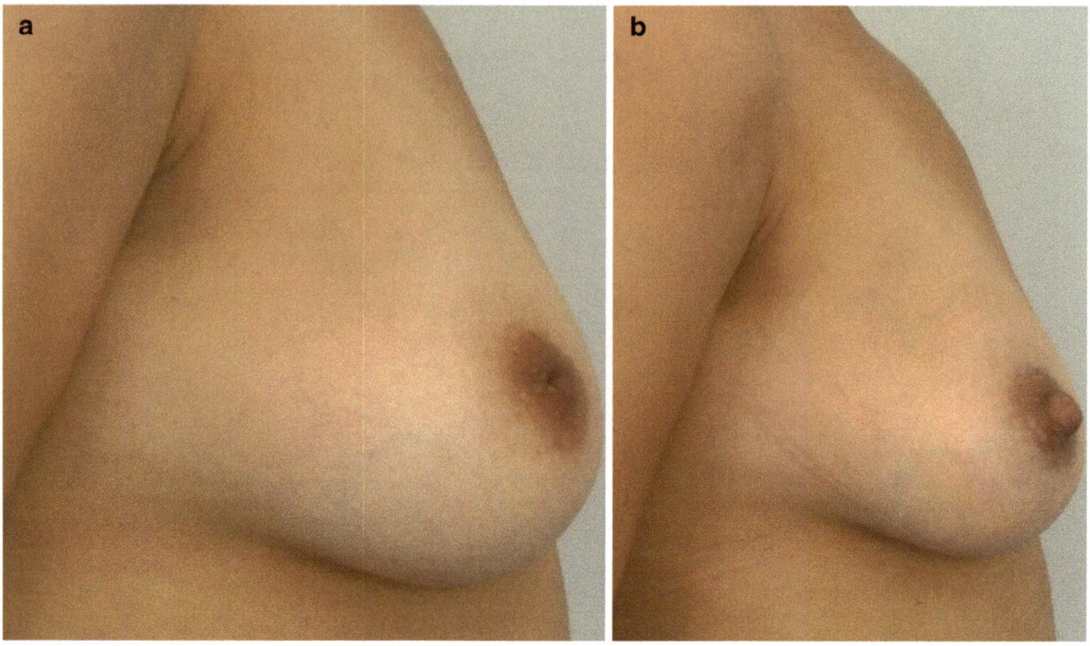

Fig. 7.1 (**a**, **b**) Inverted nipple on profile view. A total of 1.0 ml of Juvéderm Voluma was injected with a 21G blunt cannula. Full correction of the deficiency was obtained

stimulation. Patients with local retractions or previous surgery will have limited to no results. Before indicating the use of injectables for the nipple area, it is important to guarantee that patients are properly assessed and have no medical conditions in their breasts. Further, only HA products should be used.

7.1.4 Techniques

Besides providing anesthesia, the local infiltration with lidocaine of the nipple area will show the degree of correction which can be achieved. Usually a total amount of 1.0 ml is sufficient for the nipple and areola complex. It is important to inject into the nipple by bolus technique and into the areola complex by fan technique to give support at the bottom of the nipple. The use of a 21G blunt cannula is preferable since the use of needles may cause inadvertent intraductal product placement which is not desirable and may lead to cysts and injection. No antibiotics are needed. With the correct patient selection, results are expected to last up to 2 years or more (Figs. 7.1, 7.2, and 7.3).

7.1.5 Tips, Tricks and Key Points

Do's

- Inject a local anesthetic first to (1) evaluate the degree of correction that is possible and (2) provide anesthesia.
- Use medium- or high-density HAs.

Don'ts

- Do not use low-density HA products for this indication, because they are not as long-lasting and patients will be disappointed.

Key Points

- In patients with unilaterally inverted nipples, a malignancy should be ruled out beforehand. Bilaterally inverted nipples are usually benign. However again, a thorough past history and inspection should be performed before the aesthetic procedure.

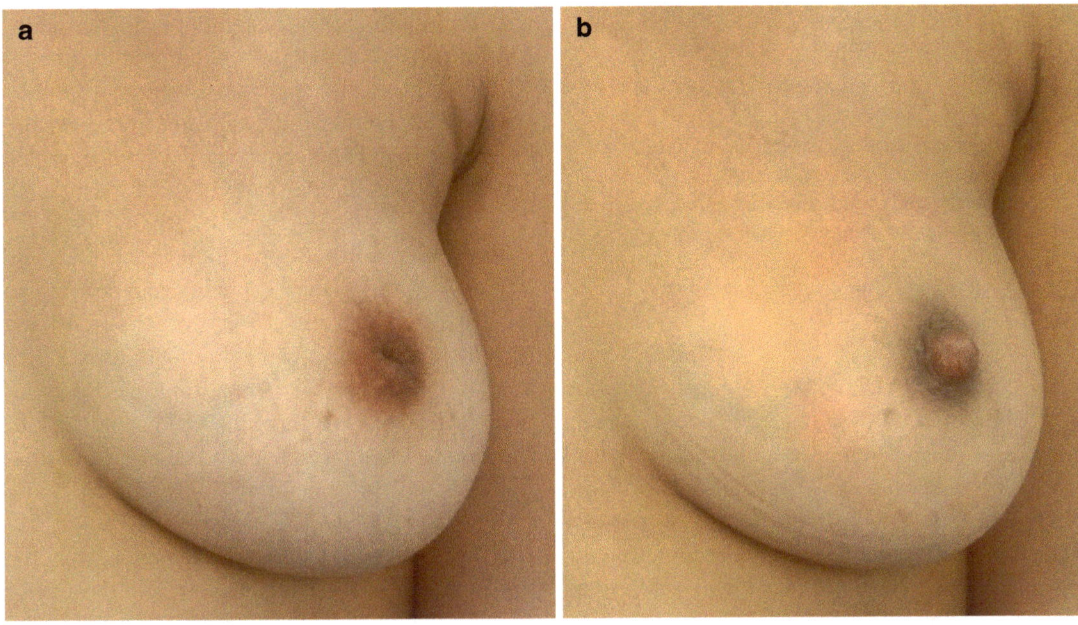

Fig. 7.2 (**a**, **b**) Frontal analysis of the correction of the inverted nipple

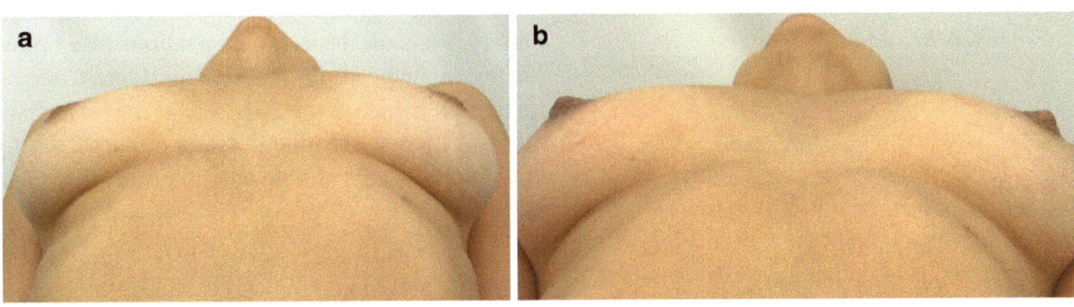

Fig. 7.3 (**a**, **b**) Bottom view: Not only the inverted nipples were corrected, but a nice projection of them was obtained

7.2 Hand Volume Replacement

Second only to the face, the dorsum of the hand is the area most visibly affected by aging. Volume loss is often accompanied here by the thinning of epidermis and dermis as well as irregular pigmentation. Therefore, injectable fillers are only one part of hand rejuvenation. To decrease pigmentation or other signs of photoaging, other tools such as lasers or chemical peels must be used to achieve overall best results.

In the past, volume replacement in hands was mainly undertaken by lipofilling. Lately, the introduction of HA volumizers and also CaHa has revolutionized this area.

7.2.1 Introduction

Volume loss of the dorsum of the hand is related to lipoatrophy. The volume loss can be graded from 0 to 4 using a recently developed clinical scale (Table 7.1) (Carruthers et al. 2008).

Lipoaugmentation (Butterwick 2002) and several fillers have been used for this indication (Abrams and Lauber 1990; Fournier 2000; Coleman 1999; Butterwick 2005; Redaelli 2006;

Table 7.1 Hand Grading Scale (Carruthers et al. 2008)

0	No loss of fatty tissue
1	Mild loss of fatty tissue and mild visibility of veins and tendons
2	Moderate loss of fatty tissue and mild visibility of veins and tendons
3	Severe loss of fatty tissue and moderate visibility of veins and tendons
4	Very severe loss of fatty tissue and marked visibility of veins and tendons

Busso and Applebaum 2007; Becker-Wegerich 2008; Man et al. 2008). The evidence, however, is quite limited. There is a small clinical trial ($n = 10$) investigating hyaluronic acid (Restylane) versus collagen (CosmoPlast). In this small study (Man et al. 2008), the HA did better than the collagen. Besides that, there is a larger case series on poly-l-lactic acid (Redaellie 2006) in which 2–4 ml of a highly diluted poly-l-lactic acid mixture was injected in 3–6 sessions as well as two case reports on hydroxylapatite (Busso and Applebaum 2007) and another on hyaluronic acid (Becker-Wegerich 2008).

7.2.2 Anatomy

The carpus is formed out of two rows – a proximal and a distal – of four carpal bones each. The metacarpus is composed of five short hollow bones. The back of the hand is covered by thin connective tissue so that the bones can be easily felt. The visible and palpable bones serve as leading structures for nerves and blood vessels from the forearm to the dorsal hand. The skin is easily movable over the superficial fascia and can be lifted in folds. Due to the loose and flexible structure of the subcutaneous connective tissue, large amounts of fluids can accumulate causing edema. The tissue flexibility offers ideal conditions for the injection and distribution of fillers. As the veins are minimally fixed by subcutaneous fat, they are to a certain extent movable, reducing the risk for puncture. Cutaneous nerves lie deeper than veins and do not follow their path. They have variable patterns of branching so that the visible veins cannot be perceived as guiding structures to protect cutaneous nerves.

Subcutaneously, the veins coming from the digiti (usually two joined by anastomoses) are continued in the dorsal metacarpal veins of which three are usually particularly well developed. The largest are the dorsal metacarpal veins at the root of the fourth digit which, after merging, become the accessory cephalic vein leading to the forearm. The dorsal metacarpal vein of the fifth digit represents the beginning of the basilica vein. A large number of anastomoses interconnect all the veins to form the venous network of the dorsal hand, which may become quite distracting with the volume loss due to aging process.

On the ulnar side, covered by veins, runs the dorsal branch of the ulnar nerve, while radially the terminal parts of the superficial branch of the radial nerve may be found. After removal of the fascia (subfascial layer), the extensor tendons and the branches of the radial artery become visible. In the region of the radial fovea, the radial artery produces the dorsal carpal branch and runs between the heads of the first dorsal interosseous into the palm of the hand. The dorsal carpal branch merges into the dorsal metacarpal arteries, which again divide into the dorsal digital arteries.

7.2.3 Patient Evaluation and Selection

Which patient is right for volume replacement of the hands? Of course, a patient that presents lipoatrophy of the dorsum of the hand. Some patients may complain of mild to moderate prominence of the vein or tendon, while others are only bothered by a severe skeletonized appearance of the hands. Depending on the grade of lipoatrophy, the choice of filler may vary. Please find below the different stages of volume loss with patients of various ages (Fig. 7.4).

There are other hand positions that are useful for evaluating volume loss and prominence of the tendons (Fig. 7.5) and veins (Fig. 7.6) as follows:

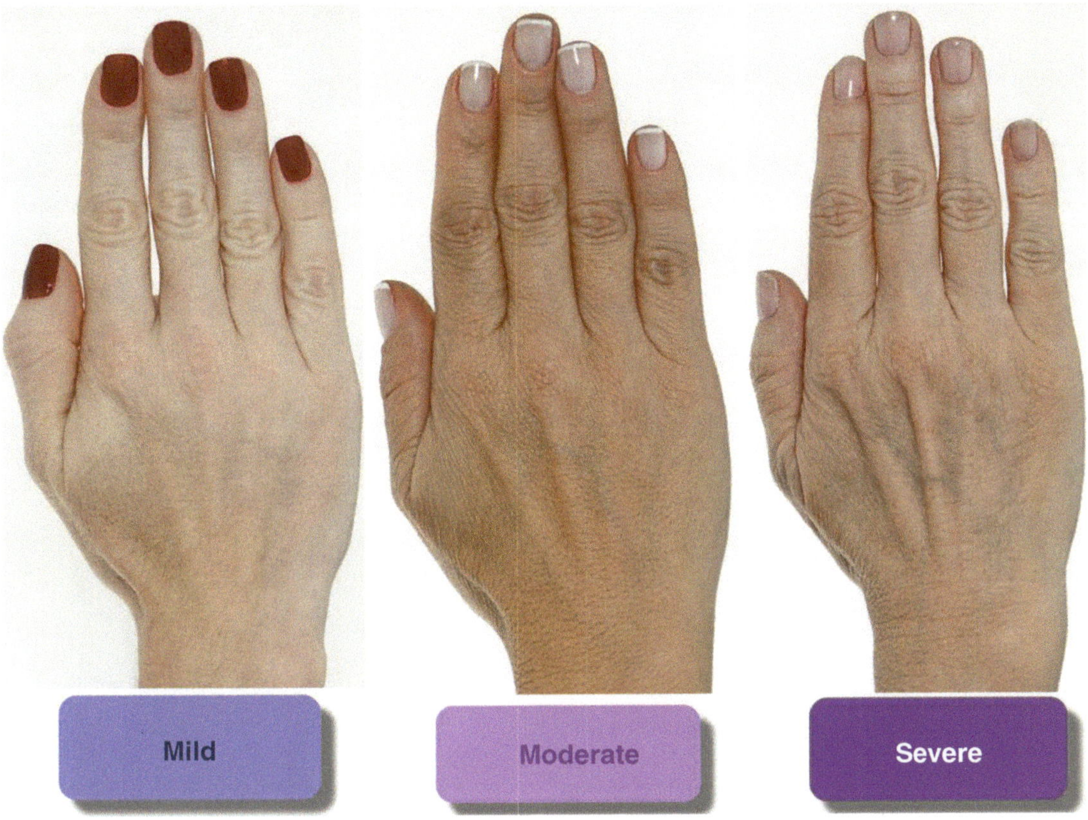

Fig. 7.4 Different stages of volume loss of the dorsum of the hands. These are best candidates for volume replacement

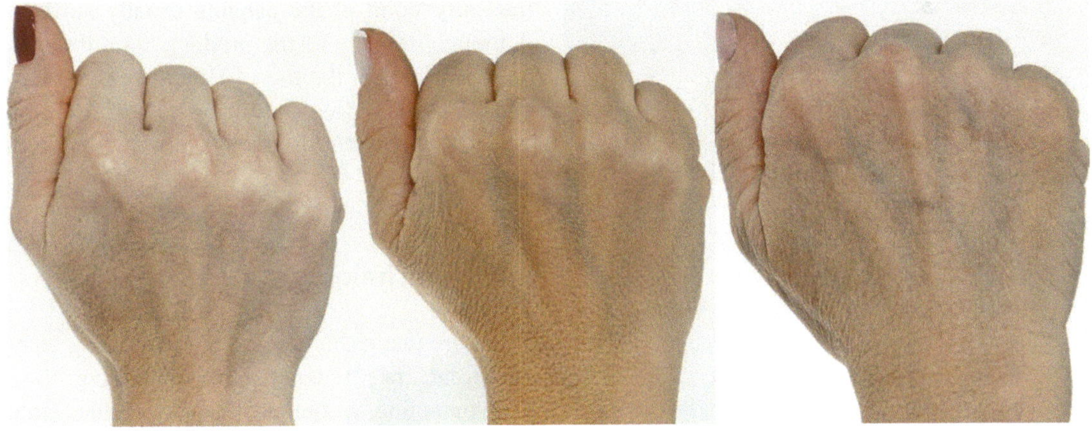

Fig. 7.5 Forming a fist to show the tendons

7.2.4 Material to Be Used

Several fillers have been used for hand augmentation. Which one should be chosen? This depends on the indication. For patients with severe elastosis, at first, a superficial filler should be used to strengthen the dermis. In the second step, the volume loss can be addressed with fillers intended

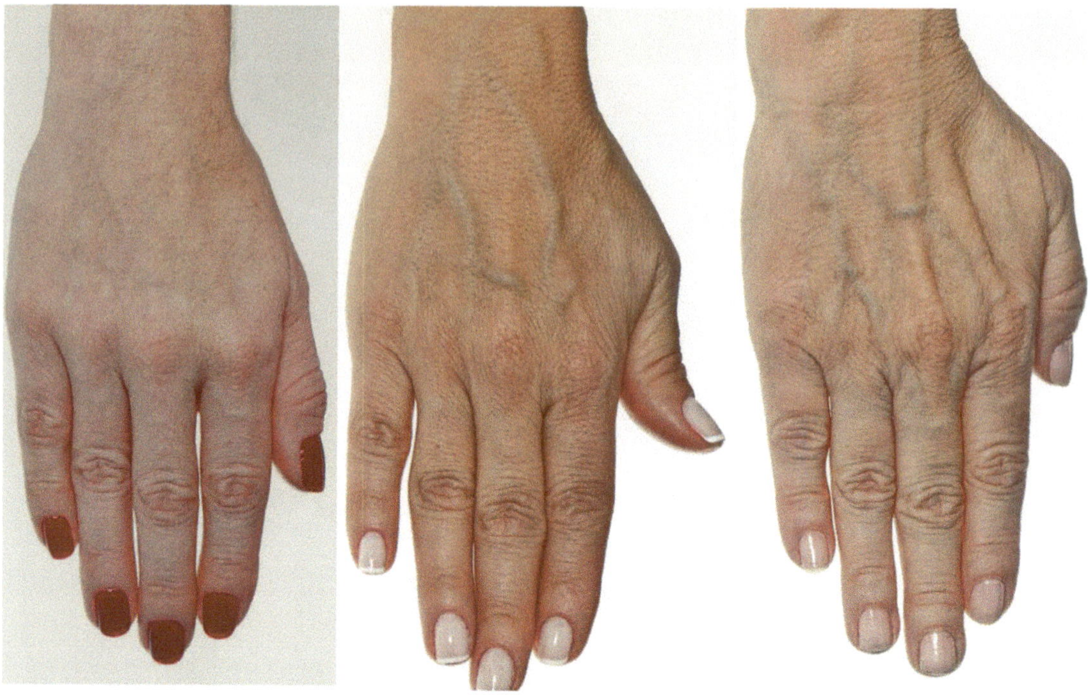

Fig. 7.6 Increased venous congestions with hands down

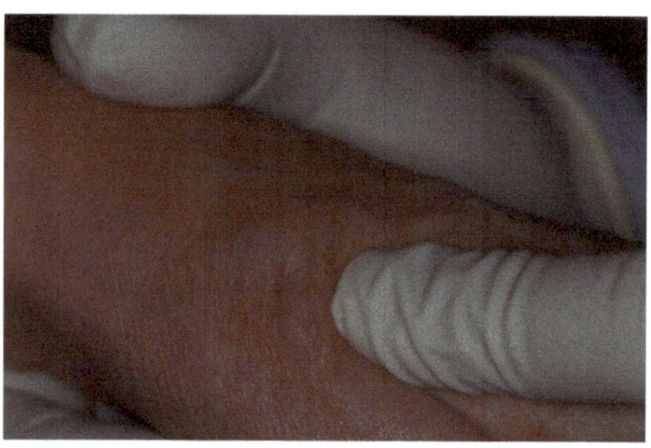

Fig. 7.7 Encapsulated bluish lumps of HA (Macrolane VRF20) which is still visible after 3 months in a patient with very thin skin. The patient did not complain. Otherwise, an injection of hyaluronidase would have removed the HA lump

for deeper injections, e.g., Juvéderm Voluma or Macrolane (although with Macrolane encapsulation has been seen (Fig. 7.7)) or CaHA.

7.2.5 Anesthesia

The dorsum of the hand is not a very painful area. Usually a topical anesthetic should suffice. When using hydroxylapatite, mixing with a local anesthetic (lidocaine) is recommended. Edelson (2009) mixes 1.3 ml of CaHA combined with 0.5 ml lidocaine. When working with blunt cannulas, local infiltration of 0.1 ml of lidocaine into the entry point of the cannula usually suffices. Although delivery of the products with the cannula is tolerable, the use of HA-containing lidocaine has further lessened the discomfort during the anterograde/retrograde movement with cannulas.

7.2.6 Techniques

There are two techniques: (1) the tunneling technique and the (2) tenting technique (Fig. 7.8). The tunneling technique can be divided into superficial tunneling (intradermal injections) and subdermal injections.

7.2.6.1 Superficial Tunneling Technique

This technique is best used when the dorsum of the hand is stretched. For this purpose, the patient must form a fist and then, for example, a

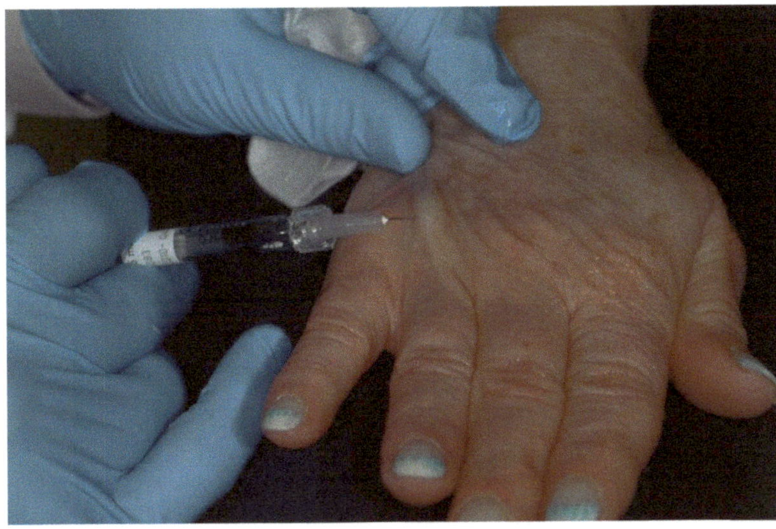

Fig. 7.8 Injection of HA in tenting technique

hyaluronic acid preparation can be injected with a 30 gauge needle (Man et al. 2008; Redaelli 2006).

7.2.6.2 Deep Tunneling Technique

For this technique, a blunt cannula is used. Different cannula gauges can be used at this level including 18, 21, or 25. As the blunt cannula does not allow the penetration of the dermis, a small incision with needles must be made at the dorsum of the hand. The cannula is inserted into this incision, and then the material (usually hyaluronic acid) is distributed subcutaneously by anterograde and retrograde technique. For experienced hands, this is a very fast technique (Hartmann et al. 2010). Regardless of the injection's volume, slight massaging should be performed to produce an aesthetic and uniform result. Please find below the result of the hand volume replacement both with hands shut (Fig. 7.9), hands up (Fig. 7.10), and hands down (Fig. 7.11).

7.2.6.3 Tenting Technique

The tenting technique is straightforward. 0.2 ml or more is injected forming a small nodule. This nodule will then be massaged into the dorsum of the hand (Becker-Wegerich 2008; Busso and Applebaum 2007; Hartmann et al. 2010).

7.2.7 Potential Specific Adverse Events

Besides the typical adverse events as hematoma and swelling, some specific adverse events or unwanted results may occur which will be discussed briefly.

7.2.7.1 The Pin Cushion Hand

If a high volume is used and the epidermis/dermis is very thin, the whole dorsum of the hand may take on the appearance of a pin cushion. This is not the usual desirable effect.

In this case, it is recommended to strengthen the dermis by a superficial HA injection before applying a large volume subcutaneously. Here, a low-density HA filler is recommended.

7.2.7.2 Visible Depots

In patients with extensive elastosis, depots of the filler may be visible as lumps. To avoid this, the first step is to use a suitable filler as an HA indicated for superficial injections to strengthen the dermis. In the second step, the deep filler should be used.

7.2.7.3 Paraesthesias

In some patients, paraesthesias have been reported after deep injections with large cannulas. These paraesthesias usually disappear after a couple of weeks and are hardly bothersome to most patients.

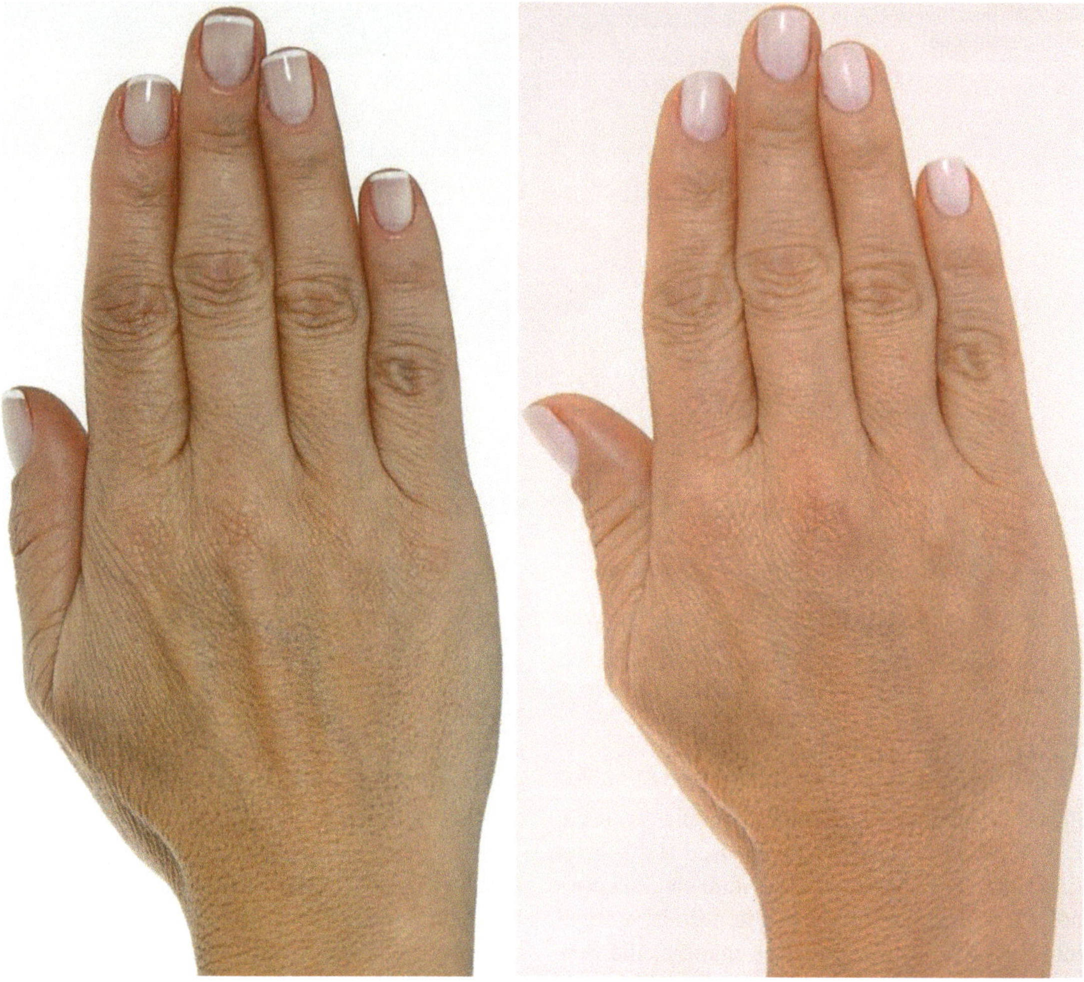

Fig. 7.9 Before and after augmentation by a 21G cannula and a total of 1.6 ml of Juvéderm 4

7.2.8 Tips, Tricks and Key Points

Do's

- In a moderate up to very severe lipoatrophy status, use a sufficient amount of material. In severe lipoatrophy, 5 ml of a hyaluronic acid preparation per hand is recommended.

Don'ts

- Do not apply great bulks of material (between 5 and 10 ml) to patients with very thin skin of the dorsum of the hands. The substance could be visible and/or the whole hand could look like a pin cushion, especially while using large volumes.

Key Points

- Several materials have been used for hand augmentation. As for other indications, each filler must be injected according to its specifities.
- Superficial injections must be done in tunnel technique.
- Deeper injections can be done by either tenting technique or tunneling technique.

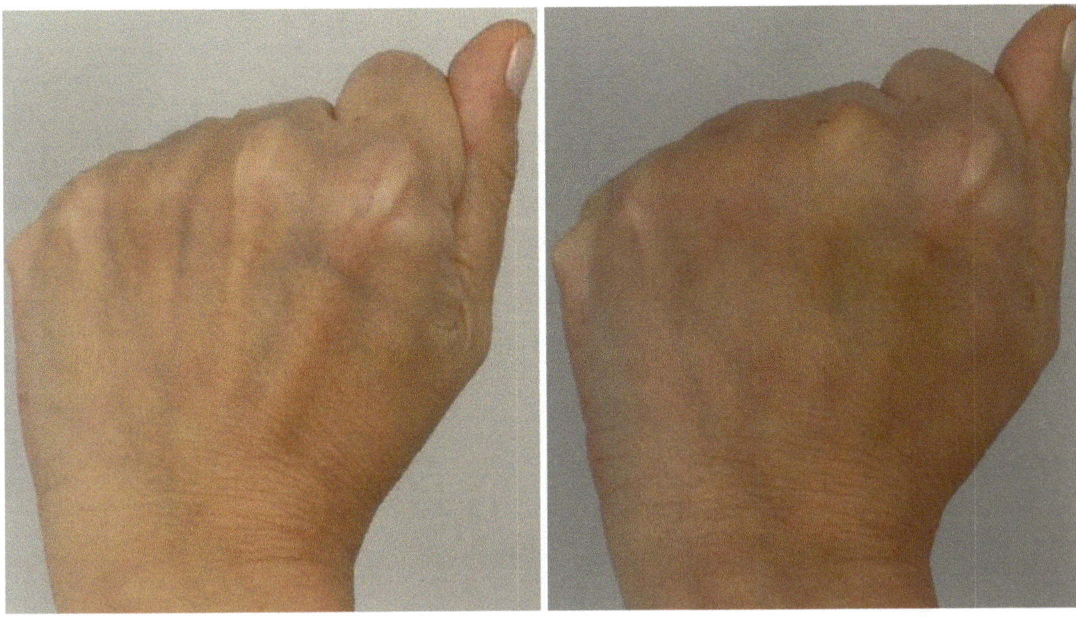

Fig. 7.10 Before and after augmentation with an 18G cannula and with 1 ml of Juvéderm Voluma

7.3 Penile Augmentation

7.3.1 Introduction

Penile size – flaccid and/or erected – varies considerably. Size – with the exception of the micropenis – does not reflect functionality. However, size matters, at least in the eye of the beholder.

7.3.2 Anatomy

The penis basically consists of the two corpora cavernosa and the corpus spongiosum which contains the urethra. The two corpora cavernosa, which are essential for the erection, are bound together by the tunica albuginea. Several layers of tunicas enclose the penis. The superficial penile veins lead between these layers. Above the tunicas is the skin which ends up in the prepuce of the penis. The prepuce can be divided into the outer and the inner layer.

7.3.3 Patient Evaluation and Selection

Most patients are quite shy about this indication. Therefore, it is advisable to establish a trustful atmosphere between patient and physician before clinical examination. As with every other indication in aesthetic medicine, it is a must to rule out dysmorphobia. Psychologically stable men with realistic expectations are the best type of patients.

The inspection should include a thorough examination of the penis. How long is the penis at inspection? How long can it be extended if the glans penis is taken and stretched? Is the patient circumcised or not?

7.3.4 Material to Be Used

Most evidence for shaft augmentation can be found for lipofilling (Abecassis et al. 2010; Panfilov 2006). Literature for fillers is scarce. There is a quite enthusiastic paper about the use of silicon (polydimethylsiloxane oil) for shaft augmentation (Yacobi et al. 2007). This paper reports on the results for over 300 men. The mean measured penile circumference is 9.5 cm (7.5–11.5 cm) pretreatment and increases up to 12.1 cm (10.3–15.3 cm) posttreatment (mean increase of 27 % in circumference and 0.84 cm in diameter). The silicon was injected in a tenting technique using an 18 gauge needle. The mean follow-up was after 20 months with a range of

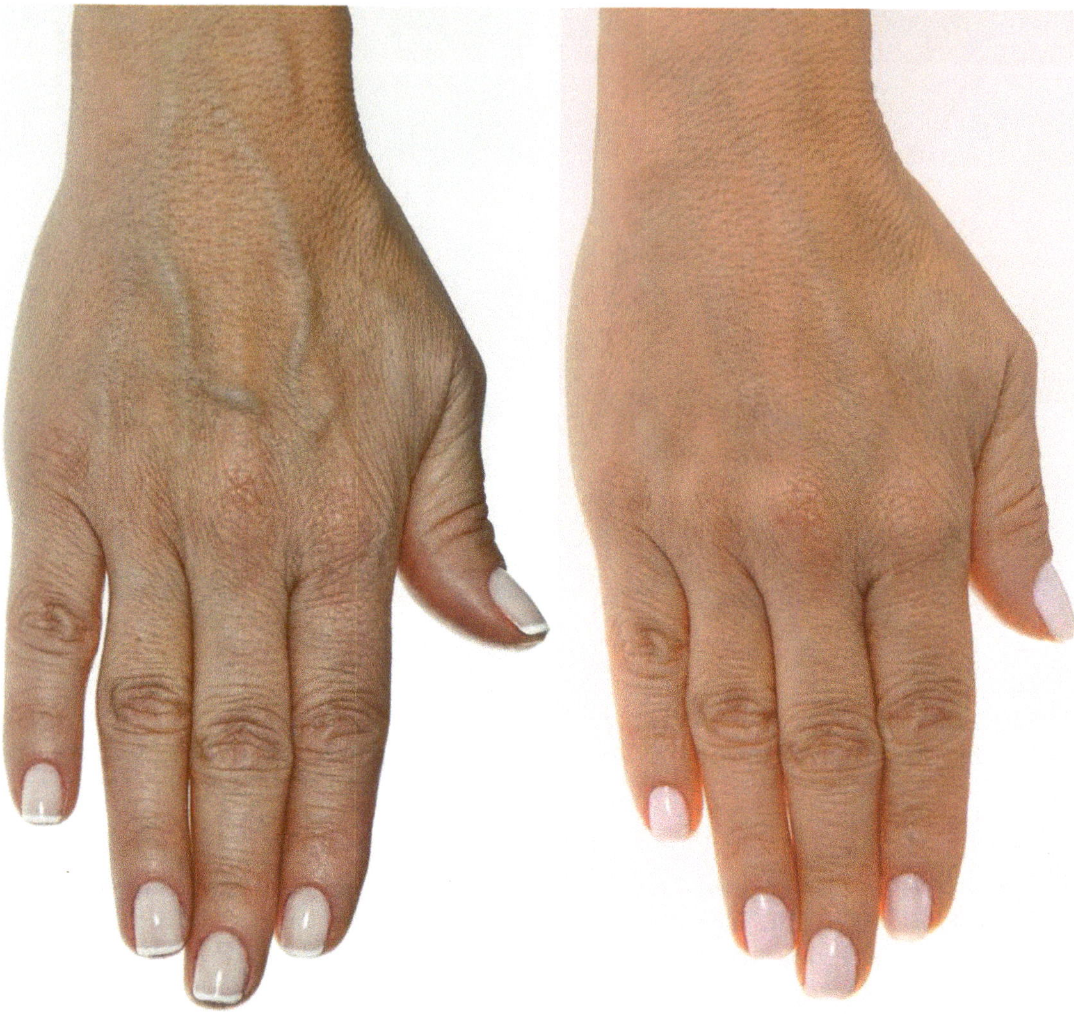

Fig. 7.11 Same hand positioned down. The degree of venous congestions is significantly decreased

1–36 months. No complications were reported. Sexual intercourse could be resumed after 8 h. However, two things must be considered: (1) silicon has been associated with partly horrendous adverse effects (García Díez et al. 2005; Vardia et al. 2008), and (2) the study size and the follow-up period do not allow to detect rare and/or delayed adverse events.

For the augmentation of the glans penis, evidence can also be found. Kim et al. (2003) report in a large case series: 100 patients with a subjective small penis (Group I) and 87 patients with a small glans after dermofat graft (Group II) were treated with HA. In all patients, 2 ml of the HA was injected subcutaneously into the glans penis. One year after the injection, the glandular circumference had significantly increased in maximum compared to basal circumference of 9.13 ± 0.64 cm in Group I ($p = 0.01$) and 9.49 ± 1.05 cm in Group II ($p = 0.01$). Net increase of glandular circumference in maximum after glans augmentation was 14.93 ± 0.80 mm in Group I and 14.78 ± 0.89 mm in Group II. No abnormal reaction in area feeling, texture, or color was described. In most cases, initial discoloration by glandular swelling recovered to a normal state within 2 weeks.

Concerning the limited evidence, which one should be chosen? In the interest of the patient's well-being and the doctor's safe sleep, it is recommendable to use HAs for this indication as unwanted results or adverse reactions might be more easily corrected.

7.3.5 Procedure Prior to Injection

Prior to injection, a local anesthesia is inevitable. A penile block anesthesia with a standard local anesthetic (no epinephrine!) is sufficient. Kim et al. (2003) report glandular enhancement after EMLA application only. A concomitant antibiotic therapy, e.g., with clindamycin or ciprofloxacin, is recommendable.

7.3.6 Techniques

Several techniques are known for elongation and augmentation. Elongation is discussed only briefly as it is a surgical procedure.

7.3.6.1 The Elongation of the Penis

A real elongation of the penis requires a surgical intervention, for example, the dissection of the suspensory ligament (Abecassis 2010; Vardia et al. 2008). This procedure combined with fat augmentation might increase the penis length by about 2.5 cm (Abecassis et al. 2010). However, even with a mere filling of the shaft, a slight elongation of the penis will be achievable as the weight of the injected HA will lengthen the penis somewhat.

7.3.6.2 The Augmentation of the Penis Shaft

The augmentation of the penis shaft leads to a visibly bigger penis. According to Abecassis (2010), the increase using lipofilling is about 2.6 cm in circumference. To achieve this dimension, the injectable filler must be placed between the tunicas. Usually a bilateral injection technique between the tunicas is used. The injection can be done either top down by placing the injections at the beginning of the penis shaft or bottom up (pre-coronally). In that case, the material is injected from the prepuce area upward (Abecassis 2010).

Using blunt cannulas associated with proper antisepsis, technique and HA products will guarantee a safe treatment. The nerve block anesthesia at the dorsal penile base is required. Please find below before and after photos for penile treatment (Figs. 7.12, 7.13, and 7.14).

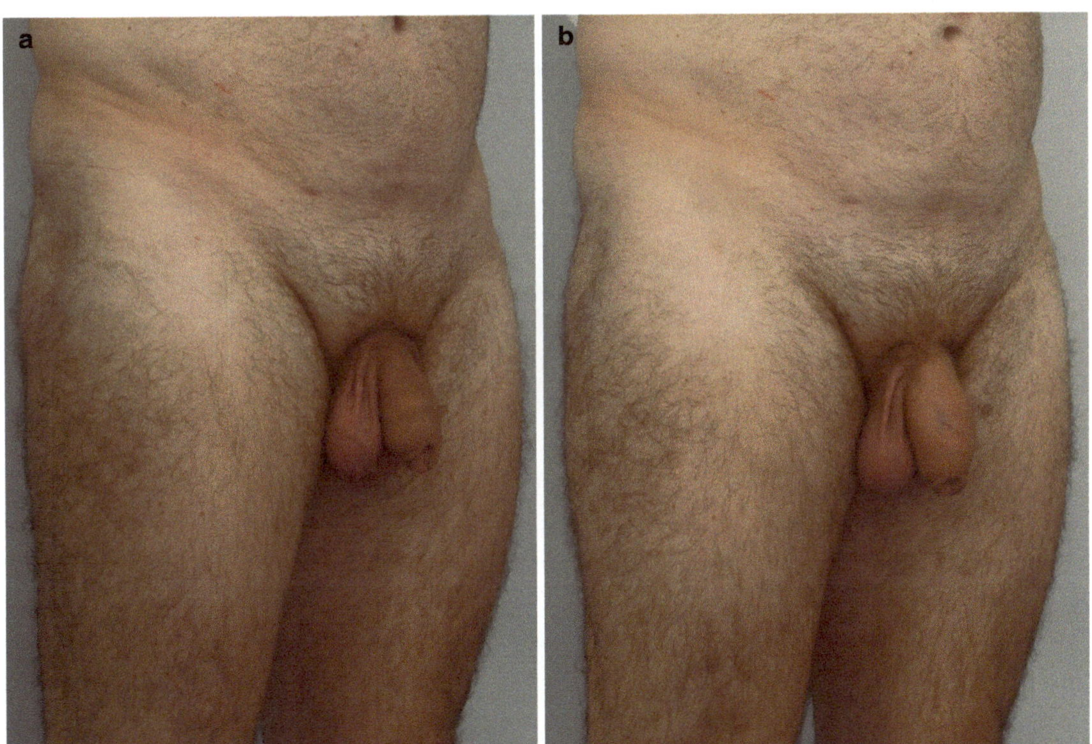

Fig. 7.12 (**a**, **b**) Increase of the length and diameter of the penis after the injection of 10 ml of Macrolane VRF20. A blunt 21G cannula was inserted at the foreskin as the entry point

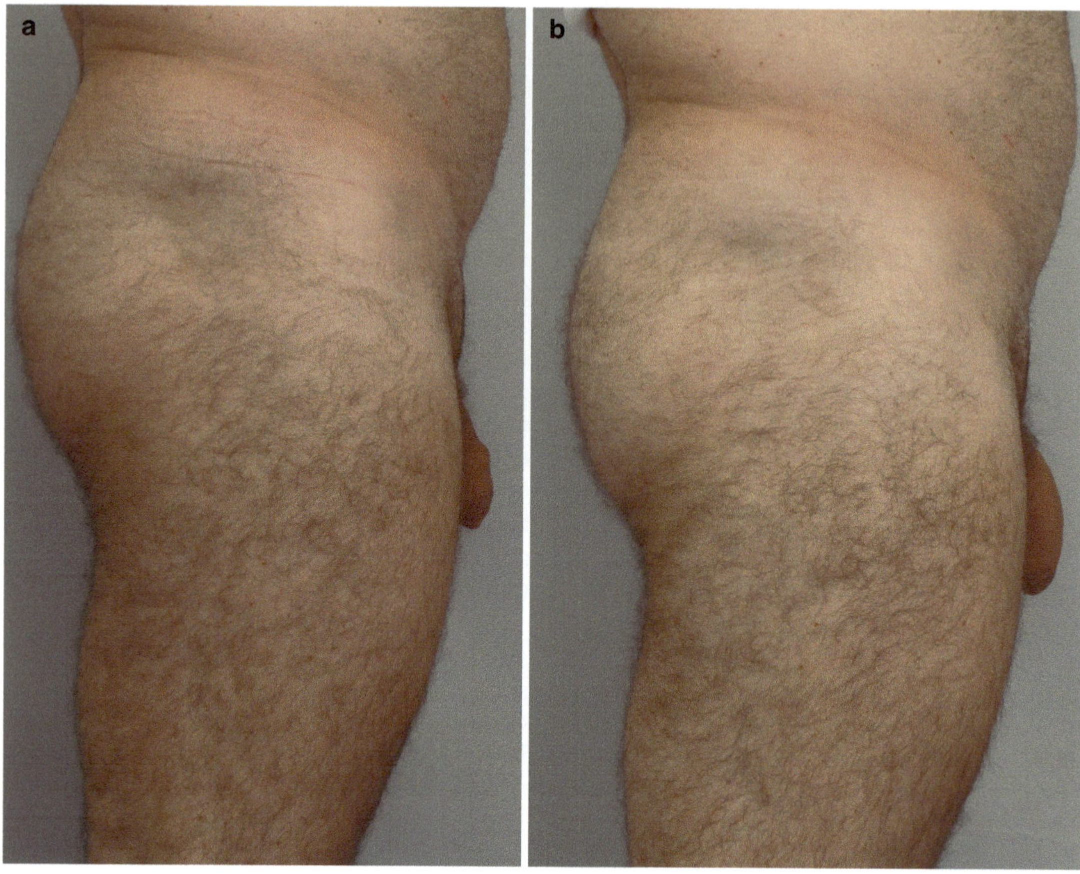

Fig. 7.13 (**a**, **b**) Profile view after penile elongation with 10 ml of Macrolane VRF20

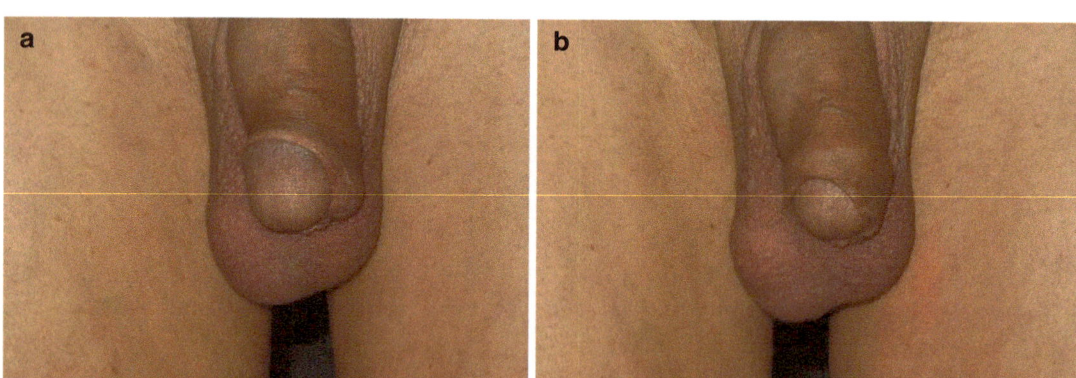

Fig. 7.14 (**a**, **b**) Before and 14 days after erasing a large HA nodule after Macrolane VRF20 injection in the left foreskin area with hyaluronidase (Hylase Dessau, 1:150). Please not another lump of the material on the right side of the shaft

7.3.6.3 The Augmentation of the Glans Penis

The augmentation of the glans penis is done either after or without shaft augmentation. The HA is injected in the glans. Kim et al. (2003) describe the injection based on a fanning technique using Restylane Perlane.

7.3.7 Tips, Tricks and Key Points

Do's

- Take the time for a thorough anamnesis of the patient. This is an area of the body where dysmorphia is a known challenge. Patients with diagnosed dysmorphia should not be treated.
- Always take photographs beforehand. Besides the frontal view, a lateral view should be done. If possible, the penis should be photographed in flaccid as well as in erected state. Patient can do this easily enough themselves or under standardized conditions in the doctor's office using an automatic release.
- Inject enough material. 20 ml of an HA is usually not sufficient.
- After creating a larger shaft with HAs, having a closer look at the glans penis is recommended. If the glans penis is small compared to the shaft, an additional augmentation of the glans penis should be considered as well.

Don'ts

- Do not inject too superficially. If you inject superficially in uncircumcised penises from top down, the material may end up in the prepuce making it look like a big tear.

Key Points

- Penile augmentation may lead to a longer penis in flaccid state. It will not change the length of the penis in erected state.
- Do not try to treat a patient based on the instructions in this book. Find a colleague who can teach you this procedure. Basically, it is an easy treatment. However, some avoidable errors might occur.
- If you overcorrect with an HA, hyaluronidase can be used to obtain a better result. Dosing is mandatory (e.g., the volume of hyaluronidase should match the amount of HA that needs to be dissolved (Fig. 7.13)).

References

Inverted Nipple

McCarthy CM, VanLaeken N, Lennox P et al (2010) The efficacy of Artecoll injections for the augmentation of nipple projection in breast reconstruction. Eplasty 10:e7

Nicholson BT, Harvey JA, Cohen MA (2009) Nipple-areolar complex: normal anatomy and benign and malignant processes. Radiographics 29(2):509–523

Hand Volume Replacement

Abrams HL, Lauber JS (1990) Hand rejuvenation. The state of the art. Dermatol Clin 8(3):553–561

Becker-Wegerich P (2008) New indications for hyaluronic acid of the NASHA-gel-generation–highlights from aesthetical dermatology in clinical daily routine. J Dtsch Dermatol Ges 6(3):S3–S20

Busso M, Applebaum D (2007) Hand augmentation with Radiesse® (Calcium hydroxylapatite). Dermatol Ther 20:385–387

Butterwick KJ (2002) Lipoaugmentation for aging hands: a comparison of the longevity and aesthetic results of centrifuged versus noncentrifuged fat. Dermatol Surg 28:987–991

Butterwick KJ (2005) Rejuvenation of the aging hand. Dermatol Clin 23:515–527

Carruthers A, Carey W, De Lorenzi C et al (2005) Randomized, doubleblind comparison of the efficacy of two hyaluronic acid derivatives, restylane perlane and hylaform, in the treatment of nasolabial folds. Dermatol Surg 31:1591–1598

Carruthers A, Carruthers J, Hardas B et al (2008) A validated hand grading scale. Dermatol Surg 34(2): S179–S183

Coleman WP III (1999) Fat transplantation. Dermatol Clin 17(4):891–898

Edelson KL (2009) Hand recontouring with calcium hydroxylapatite (Radiesse). J Cosmet Dermatol 8(1): 44–51

Fournier P (2000) Fat grafting: my technique. Dermatol Surg 26:1117–1128

Hartmann V, Bachmann F, Plaschke M et al (2010) Hand augmentation with stabilized hyaluronic acid (Macrolane VRF20 and Restylane Vital, Restylane Vital Light). J Dtsch Dermatol Ges 8(1):41–44

Lindqvist C, Tveten S, Bondevik BE et al (2005) A randomized, evaluator-blind, multicenter comparison of the efficacy and tolerability of Perlane versus Zyplast in the correction of nasolabial folds. Plast Reconstr Surg 115(1):282–289

Man J, Rao J, Goldman M (2008) A double-blind, comparative study of nonanimalstabilized hyaluronic acid versus human collagen for tissue augmentation of the dorsal hands. Dermatol Surg 34:1026–1031

Narins RS, Brandt F, Leyden J et al (2003) A randomized, double-blind, multicenter comparison of the efficacy and tolerability of Restylane versus Zyplast for the correction of nasolabial folds. Dermatol Surg 29(6): 588–595

Redaelli A (2006) Cosmetic use of polylactic acid for hand rejuvenation: report on 27 patients. J Cosmet Dermatol 5:233–238

Penile Augmentation

Abecassis M, Berreby S, Boccara D (2010) Penile enhancement surgery: widening and lengthening lipopenisculpture. Ann Chir Plast Esthet 55(2):135–142

García Díez F, Izquierdo García FM, Benéitez Alvarez ME et al (2005) Penile silicone granuloma. Arch Esp Urol 58(5):457–460

Kim JJ, Kwak TI, Jeon BG et al (2003) Human glans penis augmentation using injectable hyaluronic acid gel. Int J Impot Res 15:439–443

Panfilov DE (2006) Augmentative phalloplasty. Aesthetic Plast Surg 30:183–197

Vardia Y, Harshaib Y, Gilb T, Gruenwald A (2008) Critical analysis of penile enhancement procedures for patients with normal penile size: surgical techniques, success, and complications. Eur Urol 54(5):1042–1050

Yacobi Y, Tsivian A, Grinberg R et al (2007) Short-term results of incremental penile girth enhancement using liquid injectable silicone: words of praise for a change. Asian J Androl 9:408–413

Safety: Assessment and Treatment of Adverse Reactions

8

Berthold Rzany

Contents

8.1 **Introduction** ... 149
8.2 **Epidemiology** ... 150
8.3 **Identification of the Responsible Filler** ... 150
8.4 **Potential Risk Factors** ... 150
8.4.1 The Doctor as a Risk Factor ... 151
8.4.2 The Product as a Risk Factor ... 151
8.4.3 The Patient as a Risk Factor ... 151
8.4.4 The Biofilm Theory ... 152
8.5 **Treatment of Adverse Reactions** ... 152
8.5.1 Bluish Discoloration ... 152
8.5.2 Hypersensitivity Reaction ... 153
8.5.3 Acute Vascular Reaction ... 153
8.5.4 Nodule Formation ... 154
8.5.5 Abscess Formation ... 156
8.6 **Guiding the Patient** ... 157
References ... 157

8.1 Introduction

A multitude of adverse reactions can occur after the injection of fillers. It is important to understand that there is NO risk-free filler. Even when using biodegradable fillers with a good scientific background, adverse reactions may occur. Fortunately, severe adverse reactions as nodule formation or even ulcerations are rare for most fillers.

In general, adverse reactions can be grouped depending on time after onset into acute, subacute, and delayed reactions (Table 8.1). "Subacute" is somewhat vaguely defined; it basically means something that happens in the weeks after injection.

Table 8.1 Possible adverse reactions to fillers

Immediate reactions (within 72 h after injection) (more common)	Transient erythema Transient edema Transient induration Transient pruritus Transient ecchymosis
Subacute reactions (rare)	Abscess formation Discoloration (i.e., bluish) Persistent local symptoms (hypersensitivity reactions): erythema, edema, induration, pruritus, hyperpigmentation Local necrosis Reactivation of herpes
Delayed reactions (rare)	Nodule formation Abscess formation Ulcerations

M. de Maio, B. Rzany, *Injectable Fillers in Aesthetic Medicine*,
DOI 10.1007/978-3-642-45125-6_8,

Key Points

- Every injectable filler can elicit an adverse reaction.
- Adverse reactions can be grouped according to their occurrence after the initial injection.
- Basically we can distinguish between acute, subacute, and delayed reactions.

8.2 Epidemiology

Adverse reactions may be also grouped into frequent and rare ones. The frequent reactions are easy to detect, especially if they are acute, e.g., if you see an immediate swelling during lip augmentation. If the event is rare and delayed, it is much more difficult to detect.

Having good safety data from a clinical trial does not necessarily mean that you have a safe filler in your hands. Clinical trials usually cover a time period ranging 6–12 months. Anything beyond that would require separate reporting (Strom 1994).

So how do we get information about these reactions? There are three basic sources: (1) the companies, (2) the agencies (e.g., the BfArM, the FDA), and (3) specialized adverse reaction registries as the Berlin registry (Zielke et al. 2008). However, one must be aware that these sources only collect the data. We, the treating physicians, must actually report the data.

Do's

- Communicate and/or report adverse reactions and their therapy.

Key Points

- Frequent and acute adverse reactions are easy to detect.
- Rare and delayed reactions require much more effort.
- Only if we report the adverse reactions we do see these reactions will become known.

8.3 Identification of the Responsible Filler

In an ideal world, the patients know with which filler they were injected. In reality, this is often not the case. Patients rarely remember the name or might confuse the filler with a popular brand name, e.g., sometimes Restylane is used synonymously with filler.

How can this issue be solved? A thorough past history analysis, which might include going back to the treating physician, might be the first step. If this is not helpful, the next step is a biopsy. The biopsy may allow identification of the group of fillers, e.g., biodegradable versus permanent as well as specific fillers as PLLA. However, not every pathologist is familiar with this task. A diagnosis of "foreign body reaction" is only partially helpful. If the pathologist seems to be insecure, the paper from Dadzie et al. (2008) might be helpful.

Key Points

- Identification of the causal filler is very important.
- In case of uncertainty (e.g., nodules are suspicious of an adverse reaction to Dermalive but only biodegradable filler injections have been reported), a biopsy is recommended.
- Be aware the biopsy might distinguish between groups of fillers but not between fillers of one group (e.g., the different HA fillers).

8.4 Potential Risk Factors

What are the risk factors for these reactions? We would be pleased to know them because no decent physician would like to have one of his patients develop one of these reactions. However, most of the risk factors have remained unknown thus far. The main reason is that they are difficult to study, as most of the reactions are rare and delayed. Therefore, investigating them would require the efforts of multicenter case-control studies with a duration of at least a couple of years.

In summary, present knowledge is based on case reports and case series and therefore needs to be viewed cautiously.

Roughly three groups of risk factors can be distinguished:

1. The doctor
2. The product
3. The patient

8.4.1 The Doctor as a Risk Factor

When do we as doctors become a risk factor? (1) When we use products of questionable origin, (2) when we inject the wrong product for the wrong area or when we inject too aggressively (there is some evidence that arterial embolization might be caused by high-pressure injections), (3) when we insufficiently dilute the product (see PLLA), and (4) when we do not do the local disinfection properly prior to the injection – especially when we are using cannulas. Furthermore, this has been reported before – when we share syringes between different patients. This might sound economical, but might be associated with an increased risk of infections.

8.4.2 The Product as a Risk Factor

Substances with a rough irregular surface seem to have a higher risk for adverse reactions. There are basically three examples for that: (1) PLLA, which has a strong tissue-stimulating ability especially when not correctly diluted upon injection (Rossner et al. 2009b); (2) hydroxyethylmethacrylate in a fixed combination with hyaluronic acid (Dermalive) (Rossner et al. 2009a), which to our best knowledge is currently for the sake of everybody no longer being produced; and (3) polymethylmethacrylate and collagen, when modifying the surface structure of the rate of adverse reactions could be reduced. There are also some suggestions that some HAs might have an increased risk of adverse reactions. Be specifically suspicious of HAs where no good clinical trial data exists (e.g., this is true for the majority CE-marked HA products in Europe).

8.4.3 The Patient as a Risk Factor

When is the patient a risk factor? As said before, we do not know a lot about the origin of these adverse reactions. However, there is some evidence that active autoimmune diseases, such as rheumatoid arthritis, or a treatment with interferon might increase the risk of adverse reactions specifically when using a tissue stimulation filler such as PLLA.

Do's

- Take a thorough past history in your aesthetic patients.
- If a patient reappears in your office for a reinjection, take a few minutes and ask him/her if a new medical condition did arise.

Don'ts

- Do not do routine laboratory screening tests in your patients. There is no evidence that they are helpful.
- Do not do skin testing (except for bovine collagen) as skin testing would only make sense in patients with a delayed-type allergy.

Key Points

- There is no sense of an undirected laboratory screening for autoimmune diseases prior to an injection.
- However, it is highly advisable to ask prior to the injection the patient if he/she is aware of any current medical conditions.

8.4.4 The Biofilm Theory

The biofilm theory is momentarily quite en vogue. The theory comes from a group of Danish physicians working on adverse reactions to polyacrylamide and who discovered bacterial proteins next to polyacrylamide depots. It basically states that bacteria, either from the injection or from an infection close to the area of the injection, and the filler form matrix-enclosed aggregates, termed biofilm. The biofilm will then trigger a foreign body reaction that is difficult to treat. The administration of steroids is considered contraindicated as it might lead to abscesses (Bjarnsholt et al. 2009). The Bjarnsholt et al. (2009) publication is a small publication covering eight patients with complications to polyacrylamide. The theory is based on the detection of bacterial material close to the injected filler. This was done/discovered by FISH (fluorescence in situ hybridization) technique. The patients, however, were not only treated with antibiotics but also with immunosuppressive therapy including steroids and surgery. In contrast to Bjarnsholt et al. who focused on polyacrylamide (Aquamid), L. Wiest et al. (2009) were not able to detect any bacterial residues when examining nodules after hydroxyethylmethacrylate and hyaluronic acid (Dermalive) injections.

Currently, the theory seems to be too lightly appraised by physicians and applied to any adverse reaction against any filler - even an HA filler (Marusza et al. 2012).

Don'ts

- Do not believe in any therapeutic recommendation before there is some clinical proof that a therapy suggestion based on a theoretical concept really works.

Key Points

- The biofilm theory is quite popular at the moment although only limited evidence backs it up. Recommendations based on this theory must be carefully reviewed. For instance, nothing speaks against thorough disinfection before injection. However, steroids have proven to be very helpful, especially in patients with nodule formation, and should not be disregarded.

8.5 Treatment of Adverse Reactions

As said before, adverse reactions to fillers are not common and so our knowledge of how to treat them is limited to expert opinions and the reporting of case series. Therefore, even these recommendations have to be critically reviewed.

8.5.1 Bluish Discoloration

Bluish discolorations that arise after injections of hyaluronic acid may be treated with hyaluronidase (Fig. 8.1). The volume of the injected hyaluronidase should reflect the volume of the injected HA that causes the bluish discoloration.

Key Points

- Use hyaluronidase to dissolve the HA which causes the bluish discoloration. Inject tiny little papules along the line.

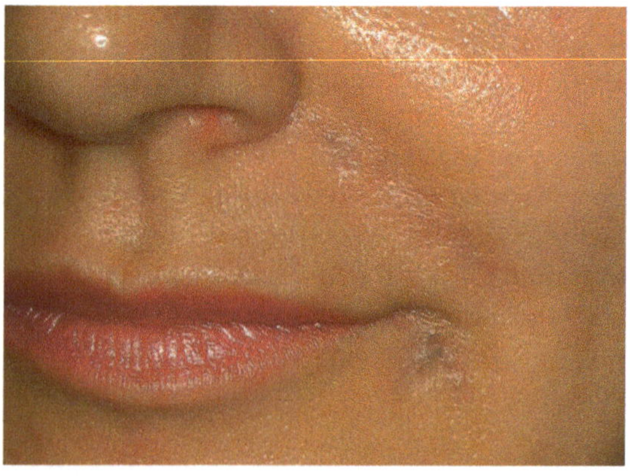

Fig. 8.1 Bluish discoloration after injection of an HA (Restylane)

8.5.2 Hypersensitivity Reaction

Bovine collagen was the only preparation with a significant risk of hypersensitivity reactions (Fig. 8.2). Treatment of contact dermatitis after collagen injection is usually straightforward and involves topical and oral glucocorticosteroids (oral pulse; see below).

Key Points

- The treatment of hypersensitivity reactions after bovine collagen was straightforward and involved topical and oral glucocorticosteroids.

8.5.3 Acute Vascular Reaction

If the injected filler occludes an artery, patients will report immediate pain and the injector might even see a whitish vascular reaction. Usually these reactions can be seen when injecting the glabella/forehead area or the nasolabial folds. It is assumed that high-pressure injections increase the risk of embolization. Besides cutaneous reactions (e.g., necrosis of the glabella/forehead area or the alae nasi), there are recent reports of blindness after filler injections (Lazzeri et al. 2012 and 2013; Kim and Choi 2013; Park et al. 2012).

In case an HA was injected, hyaluronidase should immediately be used. 1 to 3 ml of hyaluronidase should be injected around the HA depot following the flow of the artery to make sure that all the HA that was injected dissolves (Rzany et al. 2009). The additional use of topicals that enhance the blood flow in this area might be helpful. Both measures, however, only make sense in the immediate hours after the injection. From animal studies, we know that an occlusion was reversible in a 4-h period (Kim et al. 2011). After 24 h, when there are already erythematous and pustular changes (Fig. 8.3), the damage is too far progressed and the injection of hyaluronidase will not be helpful anymore.

Do's

- In case of a likely vascular occlusion, immediately stop the injection.
- In case of an (extremely rare) event of visual disturbances, have the patient immediately transferred to an ophthalmologist.
- In case hyaluronic acid was used, hyaluronidase should be injected in the area where the filler was injected and in the area of the supposed arterial distribution as soon as possible (see below).

Don'ts

- Do not inject the hyaluronidase too late. From animal studies (rabbit ears), we do know that hyaluronidase should be injected at least 4 h after the occlusion.

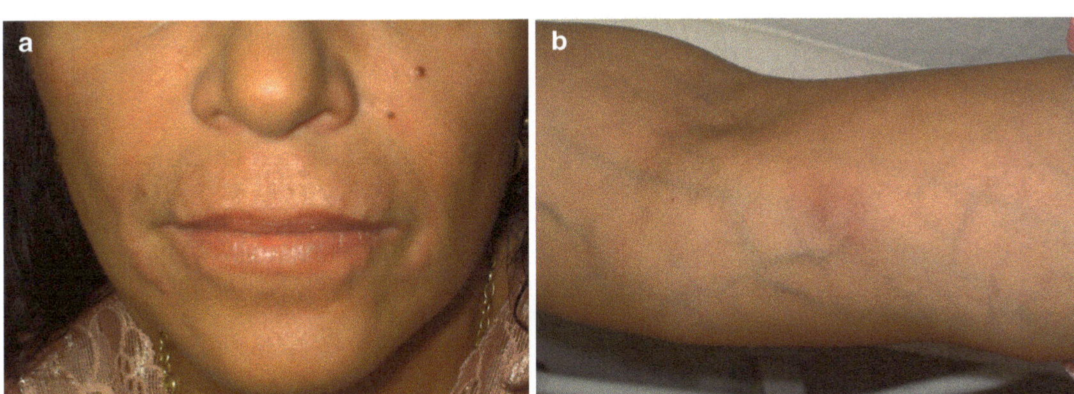

Fig. 8.2 (**a, b**) Acute inflammation of injection and testing sites 2 weeks after injection of bovine collagen and 4 weeks after the second skin test (Zyderm I and II)

Key Points

- Act immediately if there is the possibility of a vascular occlusion.
- Stop the injection.
- If an HA was used, inject hyaluronidase.
- Do not forget that hyaluronidase of animal origin (this is the hyaluronidase available in Europe) might elicit allergic reactions.

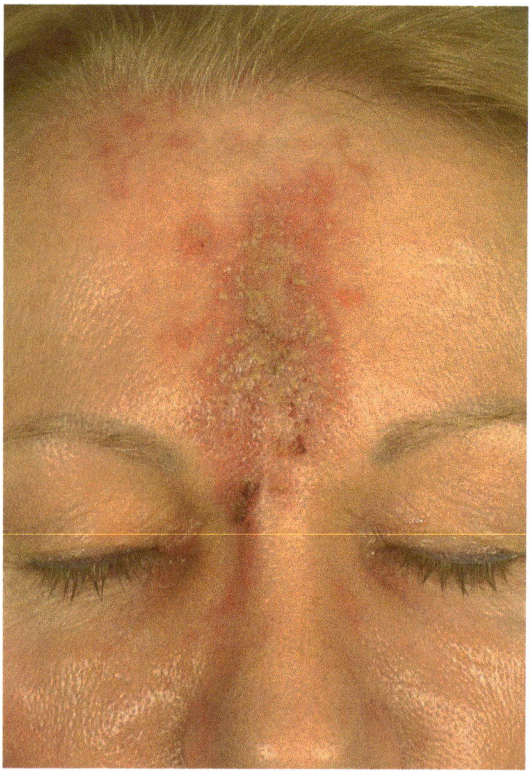

Fig. 8.3 Forehead showing a patchy macular erythema and pustule formation a couple of days after an injection of an HA filler in the glabellar region. This represents a typical clinical finding for an arterial occlusion after a filler injection

8.5.4 Nodule Formation

Nodule formation is usually the clinical sign of a foreign body reaction around the injected filler (Fig. 8.4). There is no filler that cannot elicit such a reaction. There are several possibilities to treat these reactions (Table 8.2). The evidence for the treatment of these reactions, however, is based on case reports and case series - if any; hence, the level of evidence is not as high as it should be.

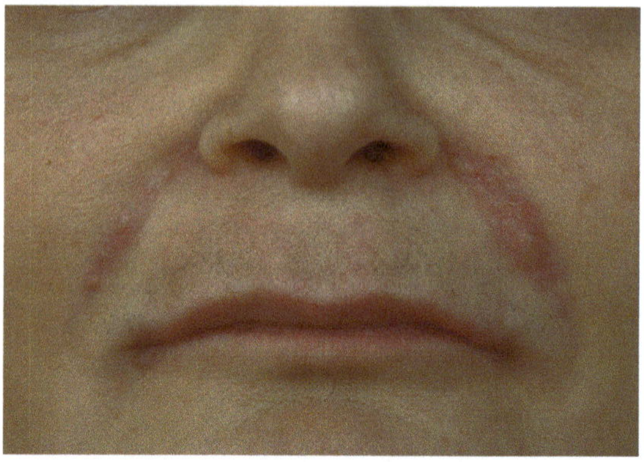

Fig. 8.4 Nodule formation approximately 5 months after injection of a combination of hydroxyethylmethacrylate and hyaluronic acid (Dermalive)

Table 8.2 Therapy for nodules (foreign body reactions)

Step 1	If the nodule formation is traceable to an HA filler, hyaluronidase should be injected first
Step 2a	Steroid injections therapy Injection of triamcinolonacetonide 10 or 40 mg if possible directly into or beneath the granuloma. Injections at weekly intervals until an improvement can be seen. Then the intervals can be extended. 5-Fluorouracil can be also added to triamcinolonacetonide 10 or 40 mg. The procedure is basically the same
Step 2b	Oral pulse steroid therapy with, e.g., methylprednisolone tablets of 40 mg. Day 1 and 2: 1 ½ tablets (e.g., 60 mg) Day 3 and 4: 1 tablet (40 mg) Day 5 and 6: ½ tablet (20 mg) Then no tablets will be given for approximately 1 week. Afterward the therapy is resumed. Now after treatment, the period without treatment will be extended to 2 weeks, then to 3 weeks, etc. (see text)
Step 3	If there is no improvement, a laser (Cassuto et al. 2009) or a surgical intervention may be considered. Please note that laser or surgery might also be a first step, e.g., on solitary lip nodule

8.5.4.1 Intralesional Injections

Steroids

Injecting steroids into the nodules will decrease the foreign body reactions and subsequently lead to a decrease of the nodules. Patients are treated with triamcinolonacetonide, either 10 mg in 1 ml or 40 mg in 1 ml. A local anesthetic may be added in a 1:1 ratio. Please note that triamcinolonacetonide 40 mg may induce severe atrophy in areas with underlying fatty tissue. The steroid should be injected directly into or beneath the granuloma. If this is not possible (granulomas due to HEMA are particularly difficult to penetrate), the steroid should be injected around the granulomatous tissue. Per granuloma the injected volume should not exceed 0.05–0.1 ml per injection point. Initially the injections should be performed weekly. If the granulomatous tissue reduces, subsequent injections can be carried out every 2 weeks. The duration of therapy varies among patients. The aim of the treatment should be to make the granulomatous reaction less visible.

5-FU

Besides steroids 5-fluorouracil (5-FU) might be injected (50 mg/ml). As with all therapeutic approaches, evidence is very limited. Following the treatment recommendations for keloids, a dose of 50 mg/ml might be used (Fitzpatrick 1999; Nast et al. 2012). Wiest et al. (2009) report a mixture of triamcinolonacetonide 10 mg/ml, 1 ml lidocaine, and 5-fluorouracil (250 mg/ml). As with steroids, the injections should not exceed an injected volume of 0.05–0.1 ml per injection point.

When injecting steroids, atrophy of the fatty tissue might occur, as in the forehead region (Fig. 8.5) or the lip region. This can be corrected with a biodegradable filler (e.g., hyaluronic acid, if the source of the initial reaction is not hyaluronic acid but another filler).

8.5.4.2 Oral Pulse Steroid Therapy

When treating patients with foreign body reactions with an oral pulse steroid therapy, we are basically treating these patients like patients with

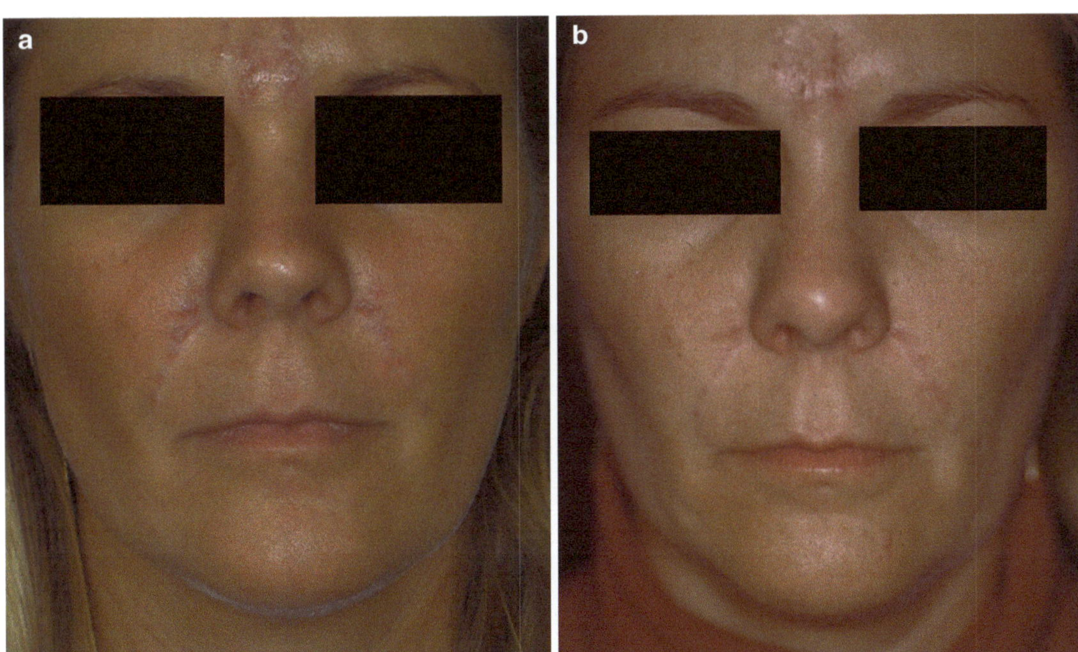

Fig. 8.5 (**a, b**) Nodular reaction 2 years after injection of a combination of hydroxyethylmethacrylate and hyaluronic acid (Dermalive). Five months before and after repeated injections of triamcinolonacetonide 40 mg (11 treatments)

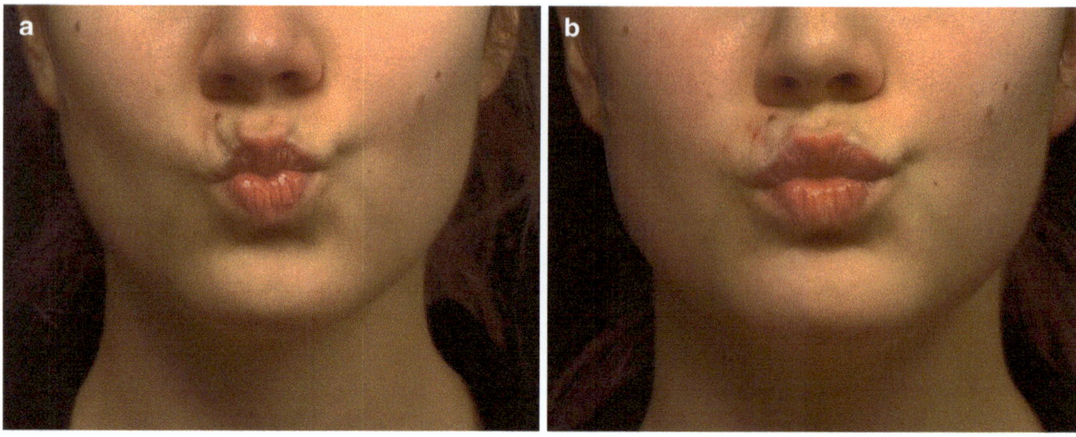

Fig. 8.6 (**a**) Focal lipoatrophy after steroid injections in the upper lip to decrease nodule formation after PLLA. (**b**) The same patient after correction of the focal lipoatrophy with an HA

autoimmune reactions. In contrast to autoimmune diseases, the recommended dosages are lower. When prescribing methylprednisolone tablets of 40 mg, the patient will take 1 ½ tablets (e.g., 60 mg) in the first 2 days followed by 2 days of 1 tablet (40 mg) followed by an additional 2 days of ½ tablet (20 mg). Then, no tablets will be given for approximately 1 week. Then the therapy is resumed. The period without treatment will be extended to 2 weeks and then to 3 weeks. The intervals may be further extended or decreased depending on the treatment response. Usually the treatment is continued for 6–12 months (Fig. 8.6). The pulse therapy can be resumed when the nodules became visible or painful again.

Usually no serious adverse events occur in these patients. Patients with steroid-sensitive diseases as diabetes mellitus should be monitored carefully. As some patients might have the tendency to switch to a continuous oral steroid intake, the tablets should only be prescribed in small quantities.

8.5.4.3 Other Medical Options

A further case report suggests that oral 200–600 mg allopurinol per day given over 16 weeks is helpful. However, this particular patient was also treated with topical steroids and the results have never been confirmed by another paper (Reisberger et al. 2003). In a couple of patients, oral fumaric acid (used for the treatment of psoriasis) has also been tried. Last not least: antibiotics that have some immunomodulatory potential. In some cases of inflammed nodules the use of low dose doxycyclin for at least 4-6 weeks might be another approach to try. Again, there is not enough evidence to recommend either of these treatment approaches.

8.5.4.4 Laser Therapy

Daniel Cassuto et al. (2009) report 21 patients where they drilled small holes with a lithium triborate laser at 532 nm into the nodules and then squeezed out the granulomatous material and the filler material.

8.5.4.5 Surgery for Granulomatous Reactions

Plastic surgery might be helpful for those patients where granulomatous reactions are limited to defined areas. Patients should be aware that all surgical interventions lead to some kind of scarring.

8.5.5 Abscess Formation

Abscess formation is another common adverse reaction pattern (Fig. 8.7) must be drained. Smaller abscesses may simply be drained with a large needle (e.g., 19 gauge). Larger abscesses will require an incision by a scalpel.

If the abscess is of possible bacterial origin, an adequate antibiotic response is required. An antibiotic that focuses on infections of the skin is

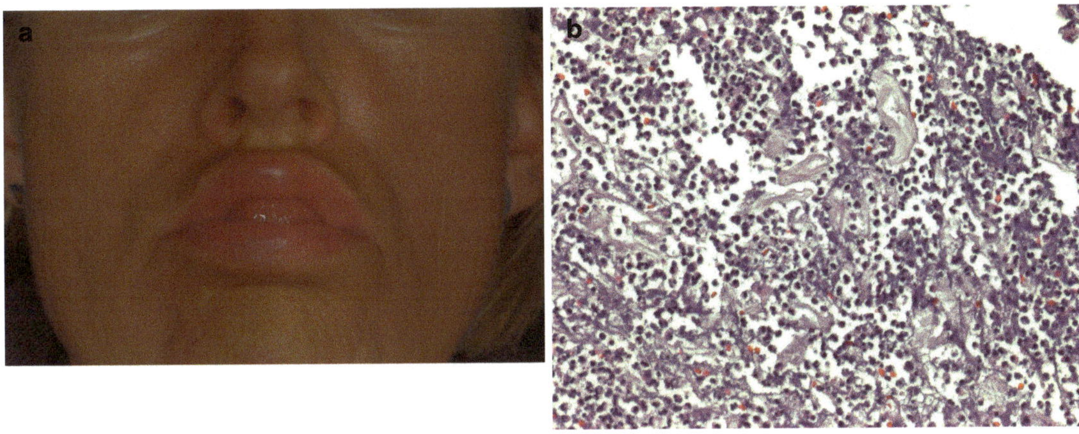

Fig. 8.7 (**a**) Abscess formation several months after injection of a porcine collagen (EVOLENCE BREEZE). (**b**) The histopathology shows a huge amount of neutrophil granulocytes around the injected collagen

recommended. Prior to the treatment a bacterial culture to identify the pathogen is encouraged.

Key Points
- Drain the abscesses in the first step.
- In case of an assumed bacterial infection, an appropriate antibiotic treatment must be initiated.
- If an adverse reaction occurs, the first goal is to find out about the filler or the fillers that have been injected.
- In unclear cases a biopsy is highly encouraged.
- The treatment should be based on the clinic of the adverse reaction.
- Every step should be openly communicated with the patient.

8.6 Guiding the Patient

Patients with adverse reactions usually feel very insecure. Patients need to be guided. The goal should always be to reduce the visible impact of the adverse reaction, not to remove all injected filler material, which, in some cases of nonbiodegradable injectables, is not possible. The patient should understand this aim and not focus on something that might not be achievable.

Key Points
- There is no filler with nil risk.
- Therefore all patients need to be informed about the potential of an – even delayed – adverse reaction.

References

Bjarnsholt T, Tolker-Nielsen T, Givskov M et al (2009) Detection of bacteria by fluorescence in situ hybridization in culture-negative soft tissue filler lesions. Dermatol Surg 35(2):1620–1624

Cassuto D, Marangoni O, De Santis G et al (2009) Advanced laser techniques for filler-induced complications. Dermatol Surg 35(2):1689–1695

Dadzie OE, Mahalingam M, Parada M et al (2008) Adverse cutaneous reactions to soft tissue fillers–a review of the histological features. J Cutan Pathol 35:536–548

Fitzpatrick RE (1999) Treatment of inflamed hypertrophic scars using intralesional 5-FU. Dermatol Surg 25(3):224–232

Kim YJ, Choi KS (2013) Bilateral blindness after filler injection. Plast Reconstr Surg 131(2):298e–299e

Kim DW, Yoon ES, Ji YH et al (2011) Vascular complications of hyaluronic acid fillers and the role of hyaluronidase in management. J Plast Reconstr Aesthet Surg 64(12):1590–1595

Lazzeri D, Agostini T, Figus M et al (2012) Blindness following cosmetic injections of the face. Plast Reconstr Surg 129(4):995–1012

Lazzeri S, Figus M, Nardi M et al (2013) Iatrogenic retinal artery occlusion caused by cosmetic facial filler injections. Am J Ophthalmol 155(2):407–408

Marusza W, Mlynarczyk G, Olszanski R et al (2012) Probable biofilm formation in the cheek as a complication of soft tissue filler resulting from improper endodontic treatment of tooth 16. Int J Nanomedicine 7:1441–1447

Nast A, Eming S, Fluhr J et al (2012) German S2k guidelines for the therapy of pathological scars (hypertrophic scars and keloids). J Dtsch Dermatol Ges 10(10):747–760

Park SW, Woo SJ, Park KH et al (2012) Iatrogenic retinal artery occlusion caused by cosmetic facial filler injections. Am J Ophthalmol 154(4):653–662

Reisberger EM, Landthaler M, Wiest L (2003) Foreign body granulomas caused by polymethylmethacrylate microspheres: successful treatment with allopurinol. Arch Dermatol 139(1):17–20

Rossner M, Rossner F, Bachmann F et al (2009a) Risk of severe adverse reactions to an injectable filler based on a fix composed of hydroxyethylmethacrylate and ethylmethacrylate with hyaluronic acid. Dermatol Surg 35(1):367–374

Rossner F, Rossner M, Hartmann V et al (2009b) Decrease of reported adverse events to injectable polylactic acid after recommending an increased dilution: 8-year results from the Injectable Filler Safety-Study. J Cosmet Dermatol 8(1):14–18

Rzany B, Becker-Wegerich P, Bachmann F et al (2009) Hyaluronidase in the correction of hyaluronic acid-based fillers: a review and a recommendation for use. J Cosmet Dermatol 8(4):317–323

Strom BL (1994) What is pharmacoepidemiology? In: Strom BL (ed) Pharmacoepidemiology, 2nd edn. Wiley, New York

Wiest LG, Stolz W, Schroeder JA (2009) Electron microscopic documentation of late changes in permanent fillers and clinical management of granulomas in affected patients. Dermatol Surg 35(2):1681–1688

Zielke H, Wölber L, Wiest L et al (2008) Risk profiles of different injectable fillers: results from the Injectable Filler Safety Study (IFS Study). Dermatol Surg 34(3):326–335

Combination Therapy

9

Contents

9.1 **Introduction** 159

9.2 **Lasers and Fillers** 159

9.3 **Chemical Peels and Fillers** 161

9.4 **Botulinum Toxin and Fillers** 162

9.5 **Facial Plastic Surgery and Fillers** 166

9.6 **Topical Drugs in Combination with Fillers** 167

9.7 **Eye Rejuvenation as an Example for Combination Therapy** 167

9.7.1 Step 1: Improvement of Eyelashes 167

9.7.2 Step 2: Restoration of Volume Loss 167

9.7.3 Step 3: Decreasing Muscular Activity by BoNT-A 169

9.7.4 Step 4: Develop a Plan for Maintenance Therapy 170

References 171

9.1 Introduction

Aging is a complex process. Single therapies, for example, botulinum toxin and injectable fillers, might be insufficient in dealing with all the signs that appear with time. Instead of using one method exclusively, the tendency in aesthetic medicine nowadays is toward combined therapies. When analyzing the aging face, it becomes clear that aging signs such as saggy skin, static and dynamic wrinkles, deep folds, and hyperpigmented spots may result from various etiologies. Therefore, it is comprehensible for physicians that multiple therapies should be suggested to the patients, though for patients such an approach might not appear as obvious at the first time. Patients should be educated that the most natural appearance can be attained in using multiple treatments.

The introduction of HAs with higher viscosity (volumizers) has changed the way HA injectable fillers were combined with lasers. Specifically when using the fractional lasers in contrast to traditional Er:YAG and CO_2 ablative lasers, both procedures can be combined in one session.

9.2 Lasers and Fillers

Both interventions can be used effectively for the treatment of static wrinkles. The depth of the wrinkles, skin type, and recovery time after the procedure may influence the choice of either method. Usually, patients with a fair complexion benefit from laser resurfacing. Patients with a dark

M. de Maio, B. Rzany, *Injectable Fillers in Aesthetic Medicine*,
DOI 10.1007/978-3-642-45125-6_9, © Springer-Verlag Berlin Heidelberg 2014

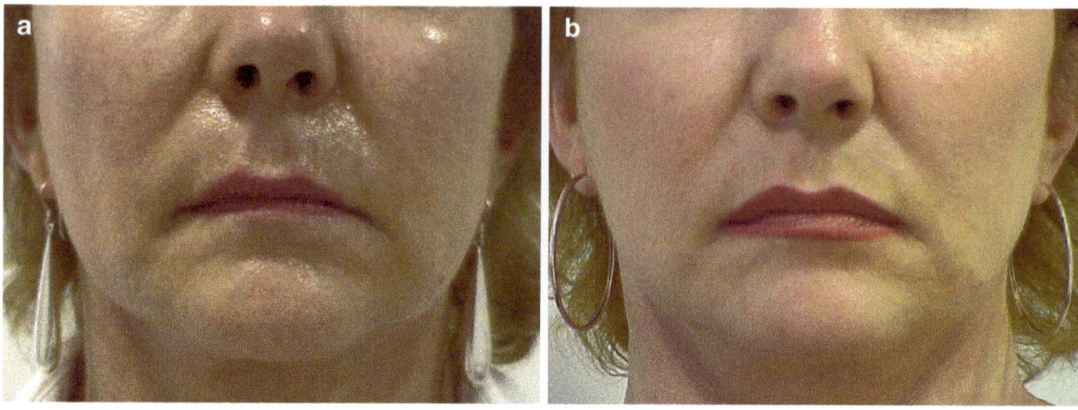

Fig. 9.1 (**a**) Patient before treatment to improve the lips and balance the asymmetries. (**b**) Same patient. Submitted to laser resurfacing. Fillers were injected 6 months later

complexion specifically in the hands of a less experienced physician may present hyper- and/or hypopigmentation after laser resurfacing. In patients with fair and sun-damaged skin showing a full-face fine wrinkling, laser skin resurfacing may be the treatment of choice to decrease the number of rhytides by increasing the dermal strength. Awaiting the inflammatory phase to subside, in a next step, biodegradable fillers may be injected into deeper wrinkles. The degree of collagen remodeling that occurs following laser treatment varies, depending on laser aggressiveness and levels of enzymes, such as collagenases, which must have stabilized before any biodegradable products are injected. The appropriate time for beginning filler treatment is at the subsiding erythema.

Some patients cannot schedule the required recovery time for a laser resurfacing. Those may prefer fillers to improve the appearance of wrinkles and scars until the time is appropriate for laser resurfacing. The advent of fractional lasers which are characterized by a much faster recovery time allows to use both tools in one session. Therefore, combining both of the methods may be more feasible.

Patients with darker skin are not suitable for aggressive laser resurfacing. For these patients, the combination of a mild exfoliative method or even a fractional laser device and fillers is appropriate. Skin resurfacing should improve skin quality, and fillers should be used to treat deeper defects. Mid-exfoliative methods as well as fractional lasers can be combined with fillers in the same session.

Fillers must be seen as the primary therapy for volume loss of the deep dermis or subcutaneous fat. In contrast, laser resurfacing is the first method to be used for superficial rhytides and elastotic and pigmented skin due to sun damage. For complex scars, both methods should be used. If any resurfacing method reaches the deep dermis or in case of bacterial or viral infections, scar tissue may result. This complication has also been dramatically reduced by the use of fractional lasers. Fillers injected too superficially into rhytides may result in nodule or "sausage" formations and cause irregularities in the skin – specifically when not appropriate fillers are used. When full-face resurfacing is performed, laser resurfacing as well as a deep peel may in some cases decrease the depth of the nasolabial fold, especially a superficial crease, as it tightens the skin from both of the cheeks and upper lips. An aggressive therapy, however, may result in scar tissue formations. Patients with deep nasolabial folds may benefit from a combined therapy with fillers and laser. As a rule, the injection of fillers into the dermis should not be carried out until laser-induced collagen remodeling has ceased. If injection of nonbiodegradable fillers or fat transfer is to be carried out in the subdermal layers (fat or muscle), it may be possible to combine them in the same session. Fillers should be injected immediately before laser resurfacing has begun. Vertical lines of the upper and lower lip benefit from laser resurfacing. Results can be quite impressive. If partial improvement is obtained, fillers can be used to achieve better results after laser resurfacing (Fig. 9.1).

Other lasers may be helpful as well. Vascular lasers such as the KTP laser will reduce telangiectasias and facial erythema. Pigment lasers such as the Rubin laser will decrease lentigines – not only in the face but also in all sun-exposed areas such as the décolleté and the hands.

Key Points

- A combination of fillers and lasers is possible in the same session depending on the layer in which the tools are used.

FAQs

- Which one is better: dermal fillers or laser resurfacing?

  For extensive superficial facial wrinkling, laser resurfacing, even fractionated laser resurfacing, is still superior to dermal fillers.
- When should fractional lasers and injectable fillers be combined?

  For patients with fair skin, multiple superficial wrinkles, folds, and creases, both methods produce synergistic results.
- What is the right order of procedures?

  If a full-face resurfacing is planned, the resurfacing should lead, and the filler should follow after the inflammation has subsided. If a fractionated mode is used, the order is not as important. The same applies for vascular and pigmented lesion lasers.

9.3 Chemical Peels and Fillers

Chemical peels are also important tools for the removal of superficial wrinkles. Although patients may find the word laser more appealing, depending on the skin type and the time required from recovery, superficial or medium-depth peels are better suited for some patients – and of course more economical. The rules are the same as for laser resurfacing: there are advantages and disadvantages with lasers, chemical peels, and dermabrasion (with the latter being mostly used for acne scar treatment). Combining any of these resurfacing methods may amplify the advantages of each and reduce the disadvantages.

Superficial peels must be used over a course of several sessions to produce a visible result. Since they only exert effects in the epidermis, the recovery time is quite quick, and skin conditioning can be obtained. There is no problem with performing superficial chemical peels and dermal or subdermal fillers in the same session. Fillers must be injected first and the superficial peel applied soon after. Patients must be warned that skin redness may be more prominent at the points of injection. It may be the perfect method for a "lunch-time" visit. Patients can return to their social or professional activities immediately after.

On the contrary, medium-depth peels, such as trichloroacetic acid peels, require at least 1 week away from work and social activities. When the effect of the chemical peel extends down to the dermis, dermal fillers should not be injected in the same session. Injections should only be made when the collagen remodeling has ceased and skin redness fades. In general, dermal filler injection can take place sooner after chemical peels than after deep laser resurfacing.

Key Points

- Superficial chemical peels are beneficial for skin conditioning, and the association with fillers is very favorable because it tends to enhance overall skin appearance.
- Deep peels should not be combined with fillers in the same session. Here, the peel should precede the filler.

9.4 Botulinum Toxin and Fillers

The use of BoNT-A has changed the way cosmetic procedures are handled. Nonsurgical treatment of wrinkles used to consist of filling (with collagen) or peels, both of which were focused on static rhytides. At the time, dynamic wrinkles could only be treated by a surgical approach and only in a few areas, such as the forehead and glabella. Muscle action may affect the duration of biodegradable fillers. Therefore, the inhibition of muscular activity with BoNT-A might have a beneficial effect on the durability of a filler, especially in the upper third of the face. Furthermore, as the study of the Carruthers et al. (2010) clearly shows the combination of BoNT-A and filler in the same area has a clear advantage over the only BoNT-A therapy of the lower third of the face as with the combination, adverse effects of BoNT-A become less recognizable.

The aging process triggers a change in muscular behavior. Continuous contraction of specific muscles may lead to static rhytides. For such wrinkles, BoNT-A alone might even be the only method required. In severe cases, however, the dermis is so affected by both muscular hyperactivity and sun damage that fillers and even other interventions need to be used. Although the onset of the BoNT-A effect starts after 24–72 h, a period of 15 days is advisable before treatment with fillers in the same area in order to avoid over- or undercorrection. Experienced practitioners, however, may inject both BoNT-A and fillers in one session.

Glabellar lines result from the action of the corrugator and procerus muscles. Surgical section of both muscles often produces imperfect results and may cause a distorted frown line. BoNT-A is the optimal solution to treat this area, and fillers may be used as complementary treatment (see Fig. 6.2). This is the case when the wrinkle is very deep; some wrinkles are so deep that they seem to be like scars and are therefore uncorrectable even by the combination of BoNT-A with fillers. In these cases, subcision or direct excision may be considered. Horizontal lines on the forehead are caused by excessive movement of the frontalis muscle. BoNT-A is usually the single method needed in this area. However, specifically in patients with severe elastosis, BoNT-A is often associated with unwanted brow ptosis. Depending on the skin's thickness and wrinkle depth, fillers may be very helpful as the only or adjunctive treatment here. After the effects of BoNT-A are at their maximum, fillers can be injected into the remaining wrinkles. The use of combination treatment with BoNT-A and fillers is also interesting in the oral commissure (Carruthers and Carruthers 2004, de Maio 2003). BoNT-A inhibits the hyperactivity of the depressor anguli oris muscle, and fillers promote structural support (Fig. 9.2; see Figs. 6.90 and 6.91).

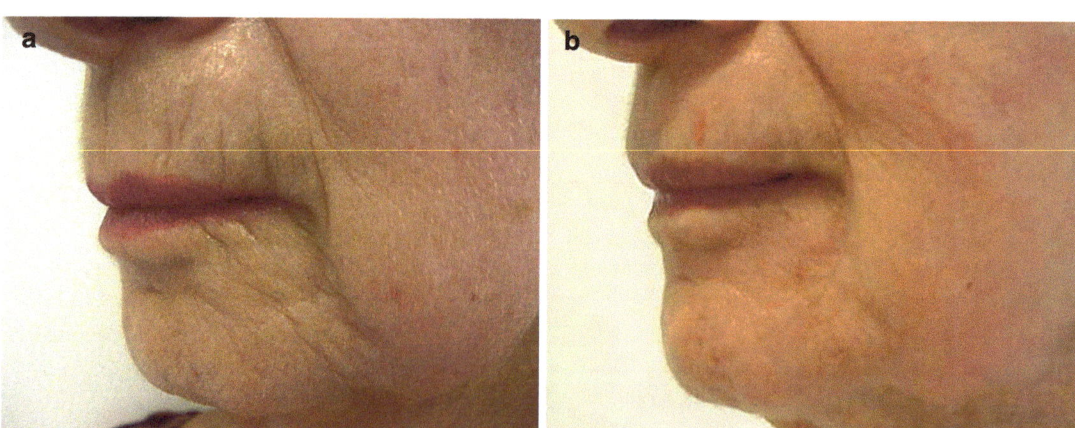

Fig. 9.2 (a) Patient before treatment to improve perioral wrinkles. (b) Dermal fillers were injected into the perioral wrinkles and into the oral commissure. BoNT-A was injected to block both the overcontraction of the orbicularis oris in the upper and lower lip and into the depressor anguli oris

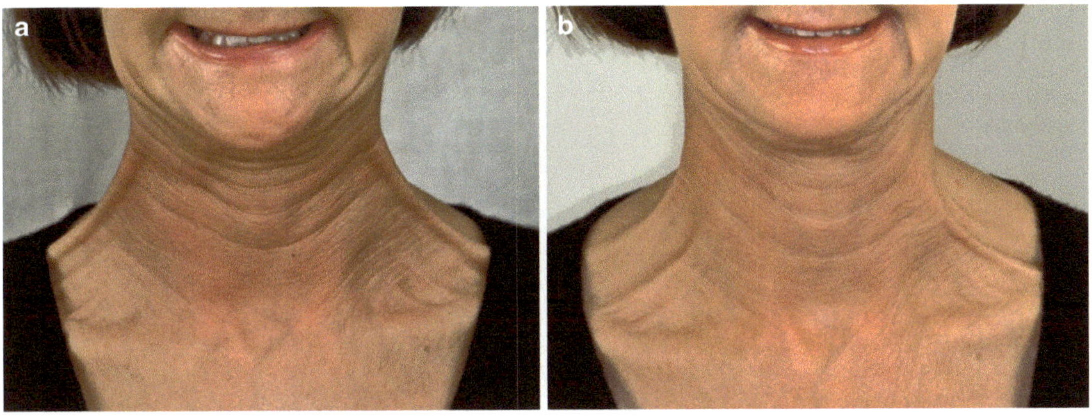

Fig. 9.3 (**a**) On animation, excessive action of the DAO and platysma bands is observed. (**b**) After the combined treatment, the reduction of DAO, platysma, and mentalis action is clearly visible. Juvéderm Ultra 3 was injected into the lips and oral commissure. Juvéderm Voluma was injected into the chin

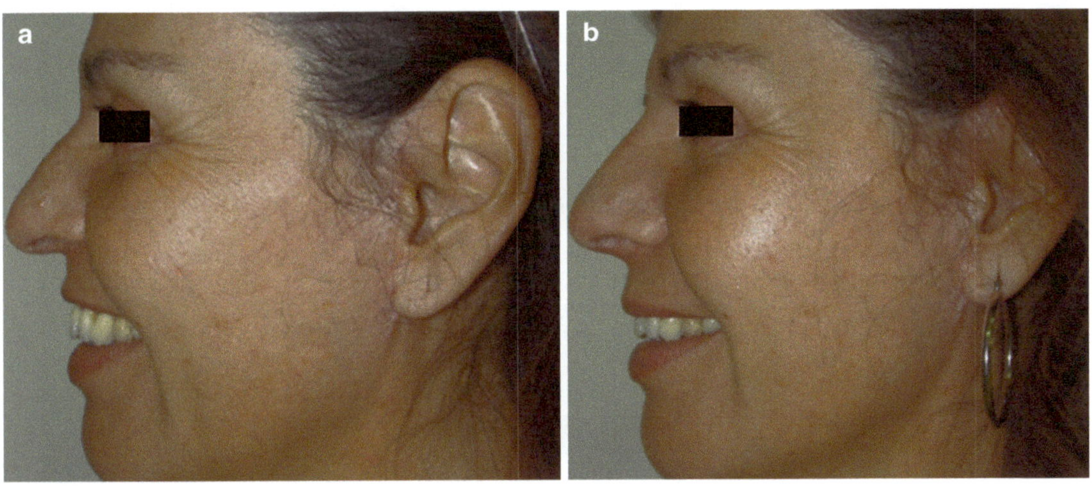

Fig. 9.4 (**a**) Patient before treatment to reshape the nose. (**b**) This patient submitted to nasal reshaping with fillers and botulinum toxin to block the depressor muscle of the septum. There is a change in the laugh line and an elevation of the tip of the nose

Platysmal bands reduce or disappear with BoNT-A. However, some of the horizontal lines on the neck require complementary treatment with fillers. Fillers may be injected in one session or after the BoNT-A effect has appeared (Fig. 9.3).

Other areas in which both methods can be combined are in the nose and nasolabial folds. As mentioned earlier (Chap. 6), nose reshaping may be conducted with fillers. Here, fillers can be effectively combined with BoNT-A, which will block the action of the depressor muscle of the septum and thus lift the tip of the nose (Figs. 9.4 and 9.5).

Treating the nasolabial fold is feasible with BoNT-A, but it must be conducted only in very few cases where muscular action plays an important role. In this situation, the opposite happens: fillers should be injected first into the nasolabial fold, and BoNT-A may be injected subsequently to decrease the muscular puffiness next to the nasal flare. Symmetry can also be achieved in selected cases (Fig. 9.6). Care should be taken because asymmetry is not an

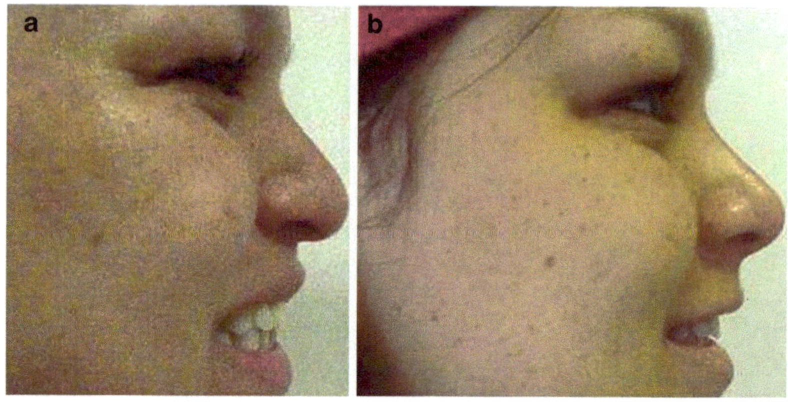

Fig. 9.5 (a) On animation, there is excessive downturn of the tip of the nose. It is a typical case where combination therapy of fillers and BoNT-A works. (b) After the treatment, observe the change of nasal tip position and laugh line resulting in a softer look

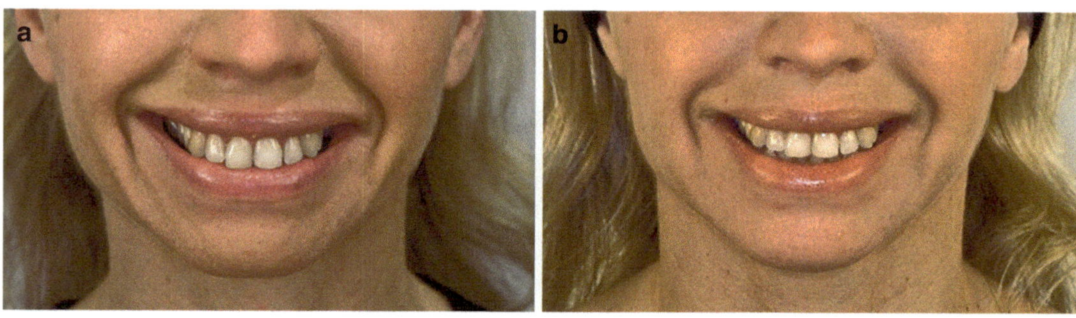

Fig. 9.6 (a) On animation, observe overactivity of the M. zygomaticus major on the right and the DAO on the left. Observe also the widening of the nasal flare due to action of M. alaeque nasi labii superioris levator. (b) After the combined treatment of BoNT-A into the muscles previously mentioned and Juvéderm 3 into the nasolabial fold, balanced symmetry was achieved

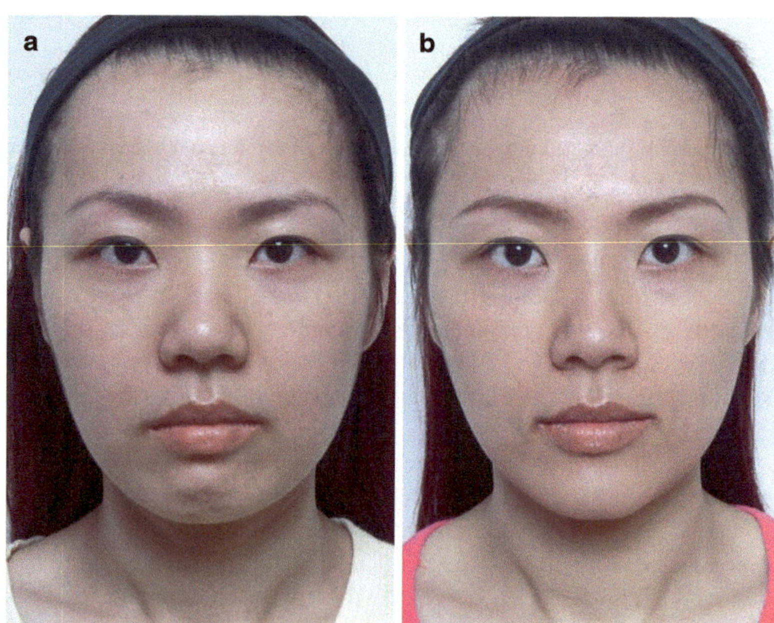

Fig 9.7 (a) Young patient before full-face beauty makeover. (b) BoNT-A was injected into the glabella, crow's feet, chin, and masseter. Observe the slimming of the face and better aspect of the chin. Juvéderm Voluma was injected into the cheekbones in order to reduce infraorbital volume loss and into the nose and chin to improve projection. Juvéderm Ultra Plus was injected into lip and oral commissure

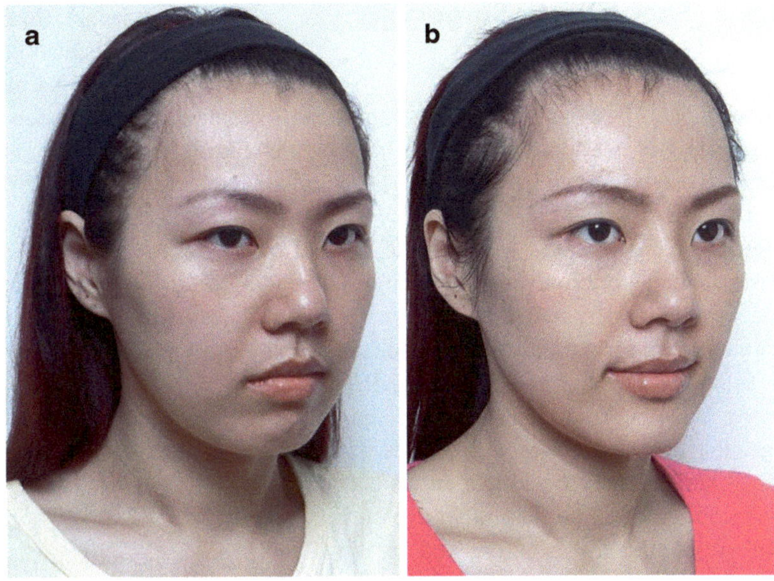

Fig. 9.8 (**a**, **b**) Same patient in oblique view. Observe softer and more attractive appearance. After the treatment, she has a happier look and balanced proportion (and could not quit smiling for the photo)

uncommon occurrence. BoNT-A should be injected to flatten this area. The "gummy smile" may also be treated with fillers and BoNT-A. The former is used to make the lips thicker and the latter to inhibit hyperactivity of the alaeque nasi labii superioris levator and the labii superioris muscles.

One of the most striking uses of combination of fillers with BoNT-A is the possibility of beautifying a young patient, leading to a higher standard in beauty perception – full-face makeover (Figs. 9.7 and 9.8).

Key Points

- The combination therapy of botulinum toxin and fillers has changed cosmetic practice. With only these two tools, the number of surgical procedures has decreased over the years.
- The global approach of the face with injectable fillers and BoNT-A has given outstanding results, sometimes superior to surgery.

FAQs

- Where do both procedures deliver their best outcome?

  BoNT-A is the best tool for the upper third of the face, while injectable fillers are unbeatable for the mid- and lower thirds. Neck treatments have been showing stimulating results with BoNT-A.
- Which treatment should be performed first if the same area is treated?

  Usually the treatment with BoNT-A should precede, and then after the BoNT-A effect is present, the filler should be administered in a second step. However, experienced user professionals might inject BoNT-A and filler at the same time.
- What is the advantage of combining BoNT-A and fillers in the lower face?

  With the combination therapy, adverse events of BoNT-A in this tricky area become less recognizable (Carruthers et al. 2010).

9.5 Facial Plastic Surgery and Fillers

Such as BoNT-A has changed the approach to remodeling of the upper face, fillers have revolutionized the surgical approach to the face. Minimal facial surgery with a quicker recovery time combined with fillers is the treatment of choice for cosmetic facial improvement. In addition to treating wrinkles, fillers may be used to promote the volumetric augmentation that was unachievable in facial surgery (de Maio 2004) (Fig. 9.9).

As facial subcutaneous tissue decreases with age, the flattened appearance of the face after facial surgery may no longer be considered an issue. Fillers may be helpful in eye surgery for both reshaping the eyebrow and treating tear-trough deformities and even to improve the appearance of sunken eyes after excessive eye-bag removal. When saddle deformity results from rhinoplasty, fillers are perfect allies, because they can promptly correct the deformity without the need for a second surgical review (see Fig. 6.47). Fillers can be used to lift the tip of the nose in situations where surgery is either unsuccessful or inadvisable. Malar and chin augmentation with fillers is also very helpful during facial surgery, promoting a more harmonious result. If the mandible angle becomes too flat after skin traction, fillers may also be used to diminish this effect with volumetric augmentation.

In conclusion, the combination of fillers with other methods in aesthetic medicine is quite rewarding when they are viewed as more than just dermal fillers but also as tools to enhance the volume of fat and muscle.

Key Points

- The need of an extensive full-face lift has decreased over the years. BoNT-A can effectively tackle the aging process in the upper third of the face. Volumizers and dermal fillers have reduced the aging signs from the mid- and lower thirds. Important: skin laxity still needs a surgical approach. However, the necessity of extensive undermining and skin resection has decreased drastically.

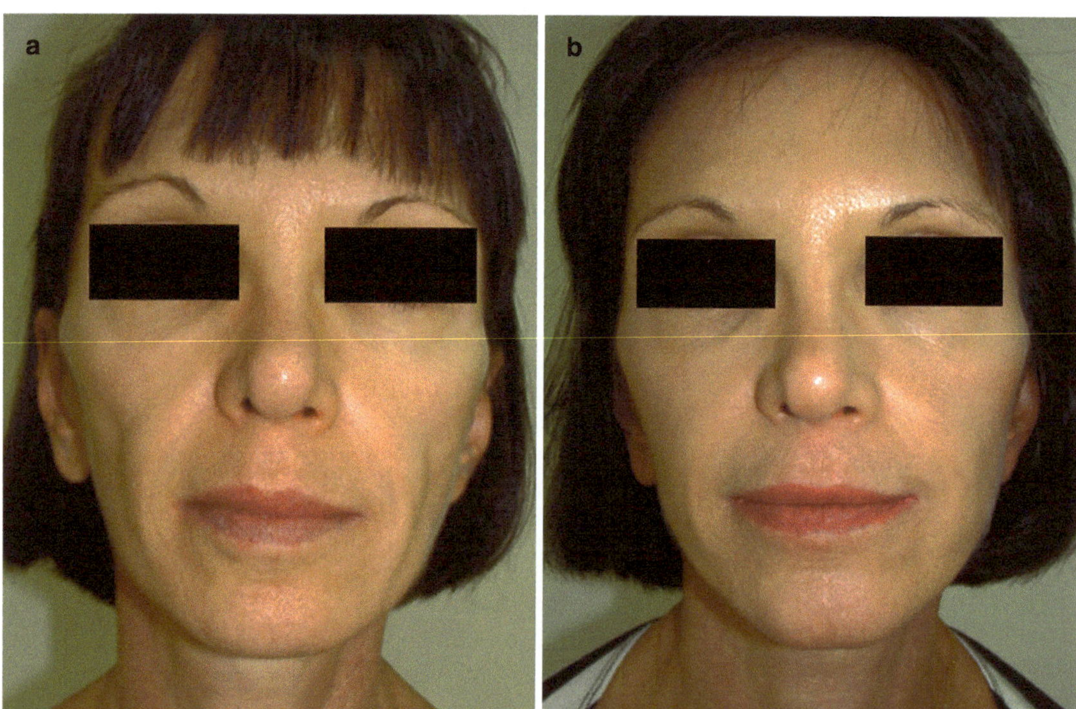

Fig. 9.9 (**a**) Patient before treatment. (**b**) Same patient. Submitted to minimum invasive surgery and full-face filling for volumetric improvement

9.6 Topical Drugs in Combination with Fillers

Besides topical vitamin A preparations as tretinoin and topical estrogens, the evidence for the clinical efficacy of topical drugs is very limited. Topical drugs can be combined with filler treatments. In case of multiple punctures after a filler treatment, it might be wise to wait 24 h before restarting the topical treatment.

Key Points

- Topical drug therapy can be combined with filler treatment.
- Specifically in patients with severe elastosis, the combination of a PLLA therapy with external tretinoin application has been recommended (Schierle and Casas 2011).

9.7 Eye Rejuvenation as an Example for Combination Therapy

The natural youthful and attractive frame of the eye is represented by fullness, lack of prominent transitions, and wrinkles with beautiful contours of the eyelids. In contrast, the aging eye is typically hollowed out and dominated by the shadows of the lid sulcus, skin excess, eyebrow droop, skeletonized orbital rim, and deflated cheek. Furthermore, eyelashes are often shorter and rarified. In addition to botulinum toxin and injectable fillers, nonsurgical "eye rejuvenation" might also include a topical drug, bimatoprost 0.03 % (Latisse), which is known to increase length, thickness, and darkness of eyelashes (please note that Latisse is not available in all countries).

9.7.1 Step 1: Improvement of Eyelashes

In eye rejuvenation, this is step 1 (hook) in making the patient aware of the importance of this area, especially when they are resistant to alternatives such as injectables or surgery. The effect of bimatoprost 0.03 %, prostaglandin eye drops, on eyelashes was first seen in a clinical trial on glaucoma, where some patients were forced to trim their eyelashes periodically to prevent them from hitting their eyeglasses. This leads to further studies and in 2008 to the FDA approval of Latisse (Allergan) for eyelash hypotrichosis. Here the bimatoprost solution was not used as an eye drop but as a topical product which was applied to the upper eyelashes using an applicator. The bimatoprost ophthalmic solution 0.03 % must be applied daily to the skin of the upper eyelid margin at the base of the eyelashes using the accompanying applicators. Excessive application around the eye must be avoided since resulting from the drop-skin contact, pigmentary changes were reported.

The ritualistic daily application on the upper eyelid margin helps patients focus on the eye area. The improvement seen in the eyelashes includes length, thickness, and darkness (Fig. 9.10). This product produces effective results on a home care basis with minimal adverse events giving the patient a very positive experience. It may also help strengthen the patient/physician relationship.

9.7.2 Step 2: Restoration of Volume Loss

In the lower eyelid, the loss of orbital volume may cause the infraorbital hollow and create a sharp distinction line or shadow separating the lower eyelid from the cheek. This same loss of orbital volume may reveal the underlying orbital fat provoking the eye bags. At the cheek level, the anterior view determines the volume loss creating the midface depression. Cheek ptosis with a depression parallel to the nasolabial fold and the presence of the malar mound are important aging signs that are seen midface (Fig. 9.11).

Step 2 focuses on the volume loss. The restoration of volume loss in the cheekbones and midcheek will lead to shortening of the lid-cheek junction. Correcting the infraorbital hollow and the malar depression will decrease the sharp transition between these two segments (Fig. 9.12).

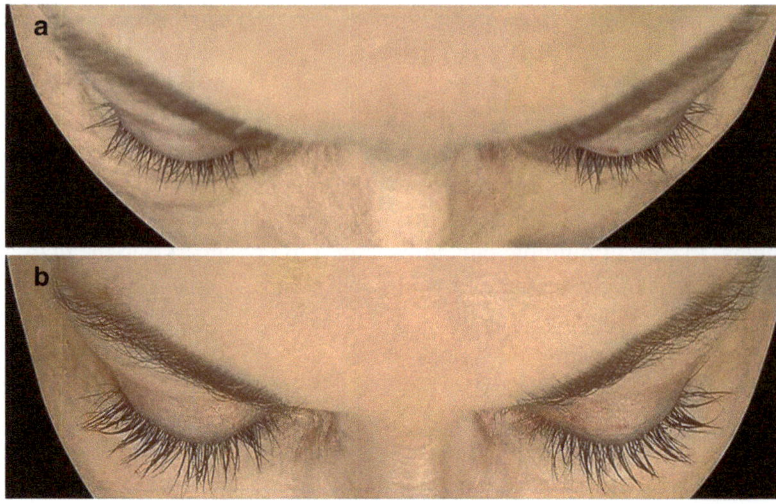

Fig. 9.10 (**a**, **b**) Step 1 – patient before and after 4 months of daily use of bimatoprost 0.03 %. The improvement of the eyelashes is easily identified by the patient and may bring awareness to the eye area. The communication with the patient about further treatments may be facilitated after seeing the improvement in the eyelashes

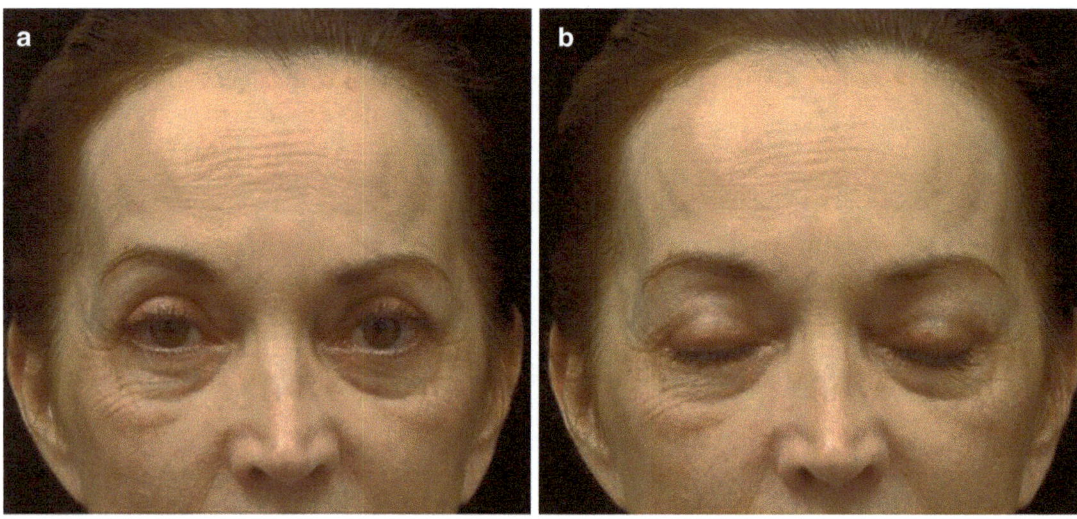

Fig. 9.11 (**a**, **b**) Same patient before treatment with eyes opened and closed: the presence of volume loss in the periorbital area is evident. Further aging signs include elongated lid-cheek junction, skin excess in the lower eyelid, eye bags, malar mound, and static periorbital wrinkles

Treatment in the infraorbital area starts with the marking. The patient should be in an upward position and lean its head forward, chin facing down and eyes looking up. This position enables more accurate distinction of the elongated lid-cheek junction and accentuates the volume loss along the infraorbital and cheekbones and mid-cheek areas. In general, volume replacement in the infraorbital and cheekbone areas should come first and may completely or partially solve problems at the lid-cheek junction when it is not a real tear-trough deformity. If direct injection into the tear trough is needed, the volume requirement will be lower and so will the risk of adverse events. Care should be taken when the malar mound is present. Aggressive attempts to overfill a malar mound can increase the deformity provoking prolonged and greater swelling. It is most recommendable to volumize the surroundings and leave the malar mound untouched (Fig. 9.13) (see also Sect. 6.5).

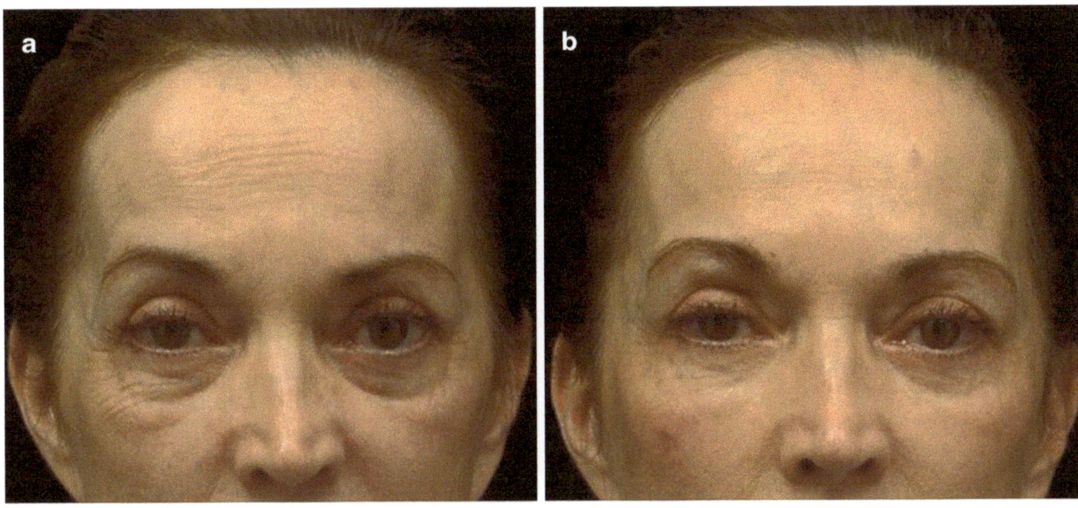

Fig. 9.12 (**a, b**) Step 2 – observe the shortening of the lid-cheek junction and the improvement of the tired look and skin excess in the lower eyelid after the treatment of the cheekbones and mid-cheek with 1 ml Juvéderm Voluma per side. The infraorbital volume loss was treated with Juvéderm Refine (0.3 ml per side). The upper part of the nasolabial fold also improved without direct injection

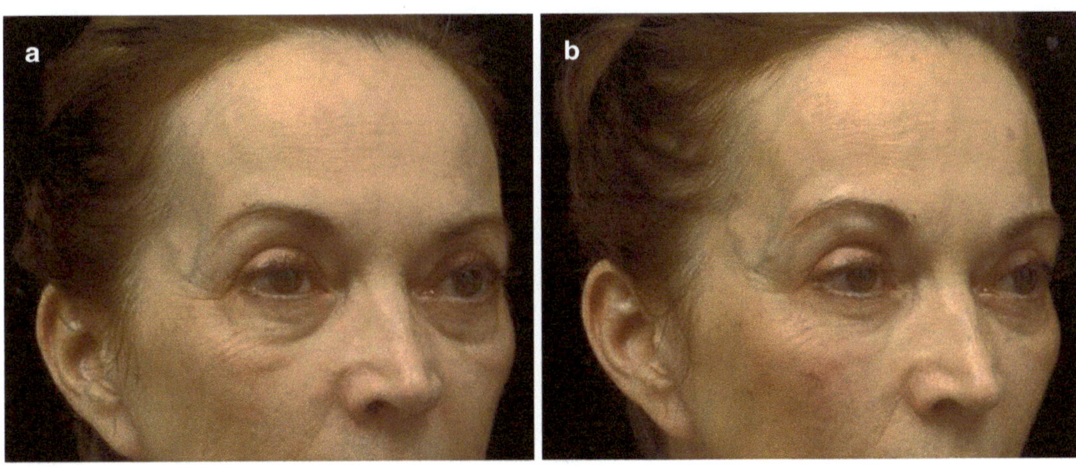

Fig. 9.13 (**a, b**) The malar mound must be handled with caution. Direct injection into the zygomatic retaining ligament without providing support to the malar fat pad may lead to prolonged edema and should be avoided at this level. Lifting the upper and lower cheek will smooth this area. The posttreatment picture shows correction of the volume loss in the cheekbones and infraorbital hollow and improvement of the malar mound

9.7.3 Step 3: Decreasing Muscular Activity by BoNT-A

BoNT-A has revolutionized the treatment for eye rejuvenation. With precise injection sites in the corrugators and procerus muscles, elevation of the eyebrows and reduction of glabella lines are obtained. A weakening of the brow depressors allows the frontalis muscle to act unopposed, resulting in brow elevation. Step 3 may comprise the treatment of the glabella area. The dynamic component of wrinkles for the eye rejuvenation may be carried out 15 days before the filling process. Other alternatives are also possible including both treatments in one session or even after the filler component is completed as seen below (Figs. 9.14 and 9.15).

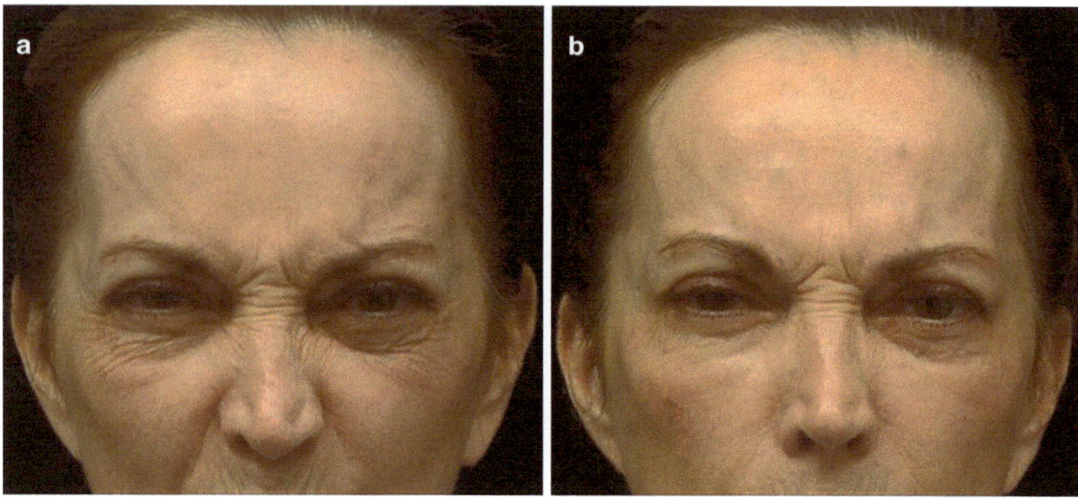

Fig. 9.14 (**a**, **b**) Again same patient before and after the treatment with HA-based products only as described above. Note the visible glabella lines and crow's feet when the patient is frowning in the picture before treatment. The picture after treatment shows the improvement of the dynamic periorbital wrinkles after the injection of HA

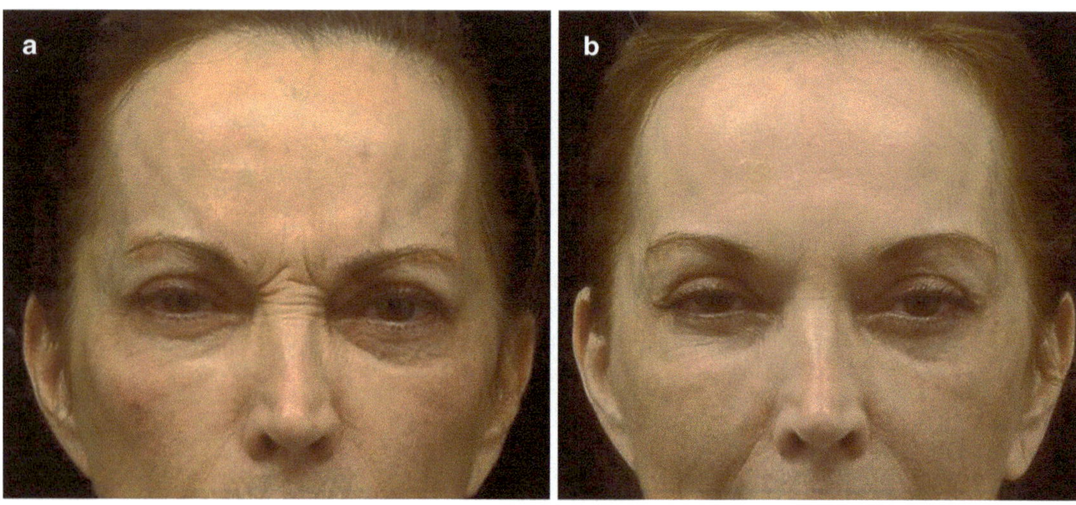

Fig 9.15 (**a**, **b**) The patient has been treated with a total of 20 U of BOTOX® injected into the corrugator and procerus. Note the improvement of the glabella area and the lifting of the eyebrows. The beauty of the curved and longer eyelashes can be more appreciated now

9.7.4 Step 4: Develop a Plan for Maintenance Therapy

Step 4 is of utmost importance as we are working with temporary products. It is important to remember: "We do not go to sleep looking young and wake up the following morning looking old." Aging is a continuous process that starts with mild aging signs, to moderate, that become severe and lead to very severe aesthetic problems. With that understanding in mind, we need to communicate with our patients and make them aware that the aging process can be effectively slowed down. If we do not have a follow-up plan, we will always be starting from nothing. Book 2 or 3 visits per year for your patients for touch-ups and/or reevaluation. Patients need and appreciate your attention.

Table 9.1 The 4-step approach to periocular rejuvenation

Step	Action
1	Build up confidence and trust with patients with bimatoprost[a]
2	Treat the first priority, the most important component in aging sign that may lead to the most dramatic impact for the patient such as volume loss in the mid-cheek, glabella line, eyebrow lift, or skin resurfacing
3	Treat all other components to promote the global approach for eye rejuvenation
4	Create a follow-up plan that will maintain the results and effectively slow down the aging process

[a]Please note that this product is not available in all countries

As a conclusion, with the introduction of new techniques and HA products of longer durability, we can now say that it is possible to deliver effective results with injectables previously only obtainable by surgical procedures. Some patients may be reluctant to any minimal invasive procedures and be skeptical toward the benefits of injectables for eye rejuvenation. The 4-step plan may be helpful in those cases but will also prove helpful for any other patients presented with periocular aging (Table 9.1).

Key Points

- Combination therapy might be specifically rewarding in eye rejuvenation. The step 4 plan might help colleagues to achieve the uttermost benefit.
- Other step $4 \pm x$ plans for other indications might follow a similar approach.

References

Carruthers J, Carruthers A (2004) Aesthetic botulinum A toxin in the mid and lower face and neck. Dermatol Surg 29(5):468–476

Carruthers A, Carruthers J, Monheit GD, Davis PG, Tardie G (2010) Multicenter, randomized, parallel-group study of the safety and effectiveness of onabotulinumtoxinA and hyaluronic acid dermal fillers (24-mg/ml smooth, cohesive gel) alone and in combination for lower facial rejuvenation. Dermatol Surg 36(Suppl 4):2121–2134

de Maio M (2003) Botulinum toxin in association with other rejuvenation methods. J Cosmet Laser Ther 5(3–4):210–212

de Maio M (2004) The minimal approach: an innovation in facial cosmetic procedures. Aesthetic Plast Surg 28(5):295–300

Schierle CF, Casas LA (2011) Nonsurgical rejuvenation of the aging face with injectable poly-L-lactic acid for restoration of soft tissue volume. Aesthet Surg J 31(1):95–109

Index

A

Abscess, 3, 6, 7, 9, 13, 15, 149, 152, 156–157
Acute vascular reaction, 153–154
Adverse reactions, 3, 4, 7–15, 36, 144, 149–157
Alginates, 2, 8
Anesthesia, 34, 37, 61–68, 71, 97, 113, 136, 140, 145
Asian patients, 23, 73, 80–83, 93, 94, 102
Asians, 23

B

Biodegradable fillers, 1–11, 13–16
Biofilm, 12, 152
"Blind spot" of self-perception, 23
Bluish discoloration, 7, 149, 152
Botulinum toxin A (BoNT-A), 22, 25, 27, 35, 45, 57, 70–74, 76, 77, 79, 99, 108, 114, 117, 123, 124, 131, 162–166, 169–170

C

Calcium hydroxylapatite (CaHa), 2, 5, 10–11
Cheek, 3, 7, 9, 28, 37, 49, 50, 53–55, 64, 70, 74, 95–97, 106, 107, 110, 111, 125, 127, 160, 167–169, 171
Cheekbones, 23, 38, 42, 51, 53–55, 81, 90, 95–97, 108, 109, 131, 164, 167–169
Chemical peels, 119, 137, 161
CIA. *See* Cosmetic investment advisor (CIA)
Combination of nonbiodegradable and biodegradable fillers, 13–15
Combination therapy, 15, 74, 159–171
Cosmetic investment advisor (CIA), 45, 46, 58–59

D

Dextranes, 2, 7, 8
Documentation, 12, 14, 31–34, 49, 77, 78
Dysmorphia, 36, 147
The dysmorphic patient, 28, 37

E

Earlobe, 112–114
Epicanthal fold, 80–82
Eyebrow, 23, 49, 64, 70, 71, 73–80, 84, 166, 167, 169–171

F

Facial plastic surgery, 166
Facial thirds system, 25
First consultation, 22, 24, 27, 32
Forehead and glabella, 70–74, 77, 153, 162

H

Hand volume replacement, 137–143
Hyaluronic acid, 2, 3, 5–7, 10, 14, 15, 67, 72, 85, 105, 111, 119, 138, 141, 142, 151–155
Hyaluronidase, 5, 35, 83, 105, 111, 140, 146, 147, 152–154
Hydroxyethylmethacrylate (HEMA), 14, 15, 151, 152, 154, 155

I

Ideal patient, 25, 43
Intralesional injections steroids, 155
Inverted nipple, 135–137

L

Lips, 3, 6, 9, 10, 13, 16, 23, 28, 32, 34–36, 38, 42, 44, 62, 64, 65, 67, 68, 84, 85, 93, 95, 96, 99, 100, 102, 108, 114–123, 125–127, 129, 131, 132, 150, 154–156, 160, 162–165

M

Marionette lines, 53–55, 107, 111, 122–126
MdM 8-point lift, 52–56
Merz aesthetics scales, 32

N

Nasolabial folds, 5, 9, 10, 12, 22, 23, 42, 43, 45, 49, 53, 54, 64, 67, 83, 84, 90, 91, 93, 97, 106–111, 118, 122–125, 127, 153, 160, 163, 164, 167, 169
Nerve block, 37, 61, 63–68, 78, 90, 101, 119, 145
New products, 4, 6, 16, 43
Nodule, 7–10, 12, 14, 15, 38, 96, 129, 141, 146, 149, 150, 152, 154–157, 160

M. de Maio, B. Rzany, *Injectable Fillers in Aesthetic Medicine*,
DOI 10.1007/978-3-642-45125-6, © Springer-Verlag Berlin Heidelberg 2014

NO GO area, 53, 54, 92, 94
Nonbiodegradable fillers, 11–13, 36, 38, 160
Nose, 23, 49–51, 64, 68, 80–82, 84, 85, 97–106, 114, 127, 131, 163, 164, 166

O

Oral pulse steroid therapy, 154–156

P

Penile augmentation, 143–147
Photographs, 23–25, 32–35, 77, 90, 120, 147
PLLA. *See* Poly-l-lactic acid (PLLA)
Polyacrylamide, 11–13, 42, 152
Polyalkylimide, 11, 13
Poly-l-lactic acid (PLLA), 2, 8, 9, 15, 42, 68, 95–97, 110, 111, 138, 150, 151, 156, 167
Polymethylmethacrylate (PMMA) and collagen, 14, 151

S

Scales, 5, 9, 12, 23, 32, 49, 137, 138
Silicone, 11–12, 41, 42, 125
Sunken upper eyelid, 80–83

T

Tear trough and infraorbital area, 70, 85–89
Temples, 9, 21, 45, 74–76
Topical anesthesia, 33, 37, 62–63, 87, 90, 92, 101, 119, 123, 127
Treatment plan(ing), 21, 23–25, 32, 33, 41–58, 75, 77

FSC
www.fsc.org
MIX
Papier | Fördert
gute Waldnutzung
FSC® C083411

Kolibri 360 GmbH
Ferdinand-Jühlke-Straße 7
99095 Erfurt, Deutschland
produktsicherheit@kolibri360.de